Contact Lenses A–Z

To Suzanne, Zoe and Bruce

Publisher: Caroline Makepeace
Development editor: Robert Edwards
Production Controller: Chris Jarvis
Desk editor: Claire Hutchins
Cover designer: Alan Studholme
Grading scale artwork: Terry R. Tarrant
Schematic artwork: Kathy Underwood and Lisa Dixon of J&L Composition Ltd

Contact Lenses A–Z

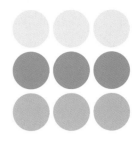

Nathan Efron

BScOptom PhD (Melbourne) DSc (UMIST) MCOptom
FAAO (Dip CL) FIACLE FCLSA FVCO ILTM

Professor of Clinical Optometry and Dean of Graduate Studies
Director, European Centre for Contact Lens Research, Department of Optometry and
Neuroscience, University of Manchester Institute of Science and Technology,
Manchester, United Kingdom

Honorary Professor, Department of Ophthalmology, The University of Manchester, Manchester,
United Kingdom

Adjunct Professor, School of Optometry, Queensland University of Technology, Brisbane, Australia

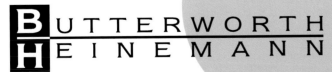
BUTTERWORTH
HEINEMANN

OXFORD AUCKLAND BOSTON JOHANNESBURG MELBOURNE NEW DELHI

BUTTERWORTH-HEINEMANN
An imprint of Elsevier Science

First published 2002

ISBN 0 7506 5302 7

British Library Cataloguing in Publication Data
A catalogue record for this book is available from the British Library

Library of Congress Cataloging in Publication Data
A catalog record for this book is available from the Library of Congress

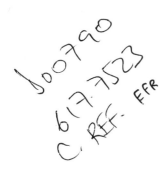

Typesetting and page design by J&L Composition Ltd, Filey, North Yorkshire
Printed in Italy

The
Publisher's
Policy is to use
**paper manufactured
from sustainable forests**

II

Contents

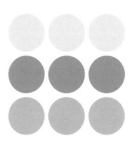

Preface

Numerous textbooks are available on the topic of contact lenses. These typically provide a thorough account of the field, and are generally broken up into chapters that offer a discursive overview of different topics and themes, supplemented by numerous illustrations, pictures, tables and reference sources. This work is designed to supplement conventional books by providing an easily accessible ready-reference source for information about contact lenses. Entries are set out alphabetically in what is more of an encyclopedic than a dictionary approach. Thus, in comparison to a dictionary of the same size and covering the same material, *Contact Lenses A–Z* contains less entries, but each entry is of greater length. Therefore, there are few narrow 'technical definitions' in this book; rather, the entries tend to cover more general themes.

It is hoped that this book will be a useful aid to students who need a quick explanation of a key term during a lecture or period of study, and to practitioners who require rapid access to material in the course of their clinical work. Thus this is a true reference text that is not really designed to be read from cover to cover.

As with any reference book of this kind, decisions have had to be made concerning which entries to include and which to leave out, how extensive the various entries should be, and what terminology should be used to describe a given concept, idea or technique. I have tried to give appropriate weighting to entries to reflect their current importance in the field, and to adopt the terminology that is most widely used. Extensive cross-referencing and the incorporation of alternative terminology (cited alphabetically with cross-references to the primary entry) will hopefully allow readers to find the information they are seeking.

The layout of the book is straightforward. Each term is set in green typeface, and the descriptive text follows in plain text. Words or phrases highlighted in **bold** within the text indicate that a separate entry can be found for that word/phrase (albeit sometimes in a different grammatical form or word order). Useful cross-references are sometimes given at the conclusion of an entry, as well as key synonyms and antonyms.

It is intended that this title will have a long life, necessitating the publication of revised editions in the future. To that end, I would be pleased to receive comments and criticism, and indications as to what should be included or removed. I can be contacted at n.efron@umist.ac.uk.

I hope that students and practitioners will find this to be a valuable reference source.

Nathan Efron

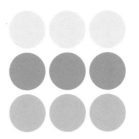

Acknowledgements

Having recently edited a major book in the field – *Contact Lens Practice* – it made sense to me to use information from that book as the core material for *Contact Lenses A–Z*. In that regard, I wish to acknowledge all the authors of *Contact Lens Practice*, who kindly gave me permission to use extracts from their respective chapters; so, thanks to Joe Barr, Noel Brennan, Adrian Bruce, Roger Buckley, Leo Carney, Pat Caroline, Neil Charman, Chantal Coles, Keith Edwards, Nizar Hirji, Sharon Ho, Milton Hom, Tony Hough, Lyndon Jones, John Lawrenson, Dick Lindsay, John Meyler, Phil and Sarah Morgan, Clare O'Donnell, Sudi Patel, Ken Pullum, Loretta Szczotka, Joe Tanner, Brian Tighe, Cindy Tromans, Barry Weissman, Craig Woods, Graeme Young and Karla Zadnik.

I have continued to receive tremendous support from my publisher, Caroline Makepeace, and her hard-working team at Butterworth-Heinemann. Book production really is a team effort, and the help and advice I receive from the Butterworth-Heinemann team has made the writing of this and other books a pleasurable experience.

My university – the University of Manchester Institute of Science and Technology (UMIST) – was very gracious in allowing me take a 12-month academic sabbatical leave in Australia to work on this and other books. I would also like to acknowledge and thank my academic host institution in Australia during this sabbatical leave, the Queensland University of Technology (QUT), and in particular the Head of the School of Optometry, Professor Leo Carney, with whom I have enjoyed comradeship and friendship for over a quarter of a century.

My family – Suzanne, Zoe and Bruce – have, as always, provided wonderful support. Suzanne offered constant encouragement while I was writing this book, and Zoe and Bruce were ever so understanding when it came to intense periods of writing and thinking.

I have been fortunate over the years to have had unrestricted access to the magnificent Bausch & Lomb Contact Lens Slide Collection, which was assembled in the course of a contact lens slide competition run by Bausch and Lomb from 1987 to 1994 at the European Symposium on Contact Lenses, which they sponsor. I spent many enjoyable hours with Rob Rosenbrand cataloguing this fabulous collection, and I wish to thank Rob, together with Keith Edwards of Bausch & Lomb, for giving me permission to publish from this resource. I wish more specifically to thank and acknowledge those listed below who either directly or indirectly (via my permission to use the Bausch & Lomb Slide Collection) contributed their clinical photographs for publication in this book. Extraordinary clinical insights and technical skills are required to take photographs of such outstanding quality, and I salute the makers of all the images displayed herein. The clinical photographers I refer to, and the images that they captured, are as follows:

Joe Barr, Figures H.5 and H.6; Biocompatibles-Hydron, Figure S.19; Adrian Bruce, Figures I.4–7, K.5 and V.5; Hilmar Bussaker, Figures P.21, I.6 and I.7; Leo Carney, Figure R.9; Patrick Caroline, Figures D.4*, L.6*, N.1* and O.2*; W. Neil Charman, Figures A.1, D.5, E.4, F.3, H.2, O.5 and S.10; Suzanne Fleiszig, Figures O.1 and P.22; Des Fonn, Figures F.7*, P.23* and S.16*; Andrew Gasson, Figure K.4*; Tim Grant, Figure S.5*; Nizar Hirji, Figure F.1; Brien Holden, Figure W.3*; Debbie Jones, Figures B.2* and C.9*; Lyndon Jones, Figures I.1–3, M.1*, N.2, N.3, O.3, O.4, P.1, P.2, P.8, S.7, S.8, S.12 and S.19*; Jan Kok, Figure P.16*; John Lawrenson, Figures C.6, C.11, C.13, E.13, G.1, L.2, L.5 and O.6; Richard Lindsay, Figures S.14 and S.15; Ron Loveridge, Figure D.3; Philip B. Morgan, Figures B.4, E.5, F.8, H.3, H.7, M.7, R.10, S.2, S.11, T.2 and T.7; Sarah Morgan, Figure P.9; John Mountford, Figure O.7; Eric Papas, Figure L.7; RD Parashar, Figure P.12*; Sudi Patel, Figures I.9, K.6, R.3 and S.1; Richard Pearson, Figure M.6; Frank Pettigrew, Figure E.12*;

Ken Pullum, Figures T.4 and T.5; Trevor Rowley, Figure P.17; Ralph Salazar, Figure R.1*; Maki Shiobara, Figure P.7*; Sarita Soni, Figure R.4*; Luigina Sorbara, Figure K.3*; Debbie Sweeney (CCLRU/CRCERT), Figure Y.1; Joe Tanner, Figures L.4 and P.13; Rob Terry, Figure V.2*; Brian Tighe, Figures P.14 and S.4; Brian Tompkins, Figures M.5 and V.1; Cindy Tromans, Figures P.3–5; C Vervaet, Figure P.10*; Rients Visser, Figure S.3*; Barry Weissman, Figures K.2 and P.15; Craig Woods, Figure M.2*; Graeme Young, Figures D.8, E.1, E.2, F.4, F.7, F.9 and F.10; and Steve Zantos, Figures E.6 and E.7.

(*Courtesy of the Bausch & Lomb Contact Lens Slide Collection)

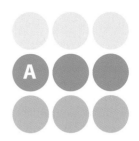

aberration, chromatic

Since the **refractive indices** of all the ocular media vary with wavelength, the eye suffers a defect due to the unequal refraction of light of different wavelengths; this may manifest as longitudinal and transverse chromatic aberration. At the fovea, the former is more important – the amount of aberration approximating to that which would occur if the eye media were all water. Unlike the **monochromatic aberrations**, longitudinal chromatic aberration varies very little between individuals and equals about 2.00 D across the visible spectrum. Since the visual axis is usually displaced from the nominal optical axis of the eye by about 5°, some transverse chromatic aberration is found at the fovea, amounting to about 36 sec arc; this further degrades foveal image quality.

aberration control, rigid lens

The steep surface curvature of **rigid lenses** means that their major aberration in relation to foveal imagery ought to be spherical aberration. Although a well-centred **aspheric contact lens** might reduce the overall spherical aberration with respect to a lens with spherical surfaces, this advantage could break down if the lens decentred by more than about 1 mm, when substantial amounts of coma and defocus could be introduced (depending upon the exact lens parameters involved). Image quality with a **spherical lens** is generally more robust against decentration. Although the effects of rigid lens spherical aberration on visual performance at photopic levels are generally small, there is some evidence that asphericities that optimize vision for the individual are appreciated by the wearer.

aberration control, soft lens

For foveal vision and well-centred contact lenses having steeply curved surfaces, the classical aberration of greatest potential importance is spherical aberration, in which the power of the contact lens varies with distance from its axis. This is in contrast to spectacle lenses where, since the eye moves with respect to the lens, oblique **astigmatism**, distortion, field curvature and transverse chromatic aberration are all introduced whenever the visual axis moves away from the optical centre of the lens. Indeed, spherical aberration is of little importance in spectacle lenses, whereas control of the off-axis aberra-

tions is a major design aim. With the exception of diffractive lenses for **presbyopia**, longitudinal chromatic aberration is normally of negligible importance in either spectacle or contact lens design, since any contribution from the correcting lens is much smaller than that of the eye itself.

The benefits of **aspheric lens** surfaces need to be considered in terms of the combined aberration of the lens–eye system; a contact lens with minimal spherical aberration does not necessarily lead to the best visual performance. In principle, the aberration of the lens should balance that of the eye so that the combined system has minimal aberration.

With soft lenses, the draping of the lens to conform to the conicoidal corneal surface results in the anterior surface of the flexed lens retaining the natural benefit of peripheral corneal flattening in reducing spherical aberration. It is only if lenses are of high power (outside the range −6.00 D – +3.00 D) and pupils are large that amounts of spherical aberration will have a detectable impact on visual performance.

In the light of developments in our understanding of the wide variations in corneal contour and aberration found among different individuals, it is reasonable to suggest that the interaction of the optical aberrations of any particular design of soft lens with those of the eye is likely to vary with the individual, rather than being the same across all the population.

Although the concept of neutralizing the spherical aberration of the eye by that of the contact lens is attractive, the realities of the situation should be borne in mind. Most eyes do not suffer only from primary spherical aberration but have a complex mixture of regular and irregular aberrations. Movement and flexure of the **soft lenses** on the eyes may introduce additional asymmetric aberrations. Thus, correction of the spherical aberration component will still leave substantial uncorrected monochromatic aberration, together with **chromatic aberration.** It may be that the ocular aberration of a minority of eyes is amenable to correction; such patients may be identifiable in the future if simple routine measurement of individual ocular aberration becomes possible.

aberration, correction of ocular

Until recently, the irregular nature of the monochromatic wavefront aberration of the eye has made it impossible to correct fully, although some reduction can be achieved with appropriately **aspheric contact lenses.** Longitudinal chromatic aberration can be corrected by a suitable achromatizing doublet lens, but the improvement in retinal image quality in white light is small and occurs mainly at intermediate spatial frequencies; no improvement in conventional high contrast, white-light visual acuity is normally detectable. More recently, however, real progress has been made in correcting **monochromatic aberration** using either adaptive optics or liquid crystal phase plates. While all these corrections are at present only feasible in the laboratory, they do show that marked improvements in spatial vision can be achieved over the uncorrected eye, particularly if both monochromatic and **chromatic aberrations** are corrected. If only monochromatic aberrations are corrected, performance in white light only improves modestly.

In theory, having measured the wave aberrations of the individual eye, the form of the cornea could be appropriately shaped (e.g. by a computer-controlled scanning-spot excimer laser) to compensate for the aberrations – although currently our limited knowledge of regression effects would make this difficult to achieve exactly. Alternatively, a **tight-fitting contact lens** with minimal transverse and rotational movement might be engineered to play the same role. At best, however, such approaches would only reduce the monochromatic aberrations, which in any case may change with the level of accommodation. The blur effects due to chromatic aberrations would remain uncorrected. Moreover, the worst **monochromatic aberration** occurs in the periphery of the dilated pupil, and pupil dilation only occurs when light levels are low and visual performance is largely limited by neural, rather than optical, factors. For these reasons, correction of aberration only seems likely to be profitable in the case of individuals whose monochromatic aberration is particularly high.

aberration, monochromatic

Aberration acts to introduce additional blur into both in-focus and out-of-focus images. Monochromatic aberration can arise from a variety of causes. The eye would be expected to display the classical Seidel aberrations (spherical aberrations, coma, oblique **astigmatism**, field curvature and distortion) inherent in any system of spherical centred surfaces but, due to the various asphericities, tilts, decentrations and irregularities that may occur in its optical surfaces, its aberrational behaviour is much more complex than that which would be expected on the basis of simple schematic eye models.

Aberration is most commonly expressed in terms of the wavefront aberration. The behaviour of a 'perfect' optical system, according to geometrical optics, can either be visualized as involving rays radiating from an object point to be converged to a unique image point, or as spherical wavefronts diverging from the object point to converge at the image point, so that the object point is the centre of curvature of the object wavefronts and the image point that of the image wavefronts (Figure A.1A). The rays and wavefronts are everywhere perpendicular to one another. If we have aberration, the image rays fail to intersect at a single image point. Similarly, the wavefronts, which are still everywhere perpendicular to the rays, are no longer spherical (Figure A.1B). It is usual

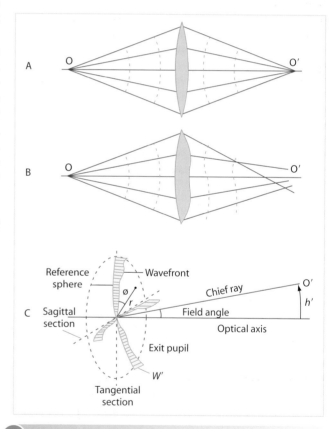

Figure A.1 (A) With a perfect lens, rays from the object converge to a single image point. Alternatively, we can visualize divergent spherical wavefronts (shown dashed) from the object point converging as spherical wavefronts to the image point. (B) If the lens suffers from aberration, the imaging rays fail to converge to a single point and the corresponding wavefronts are not spherical. (C) The wavefront aberration, W', is specified as the distance between the ideal wavefront, or reference sphere, centred on the gaussian image point, O', and the actual wavefront in the exit pupil. It is usually adjusted to be zero at the centre of this pupil.

to express the wavefront aberration at any point in the pupil as the distance between the ideal spherical wavefront, centred on the Gaussian image point, and the actual wavefront, where both are selected to coincide at the centre of the exit pupil (Figure A.1C).

abrasion
See relief of pain, therapeutic lenses for.

acanthamoeba keratitis
Acanthamoeba is a protozoa that has chameleon-like tendencies in that it is able to transform from a chemotherapeutically susceptible trophozoite to a resistant cystic form. The trophozoites are polygonal and can be up to 45 μm in diameter, and the cysts are double-walled and up to 16 μm in length. Acanthamoeba species are widely distributed in the natural environment, and have been isolated from swimming pools, hot tubs, soil, dust, reservoirs, under ice, the nasopharyngeal mucosa in healthy humans, and even the air we breathe.

A fully developed corneal ulcer may take weeks to form. Typical signs include:

- **corneal staining**
- pseudodendrites
- epithelial and anterior stromal infiltrates, which may be focal or diffuse
- radial keratoneuritis – a characteristic circular formation of opacification that becomes apparent relatively early in the disease process (Figure A.2).

Acanthamoeba keratitis has a slow time course of recovery. The condition may progress over many months with periods of apparent improvement followed by regression. Patients are inevitably left with superficial nebulae corresponding to the site of infection. *See* antimicrobial efficacy.

accessory lacrimal glands
Numerous small accessory lacrimal glands, which include the eponymous glands of Wolfring and Krause, are found within the **conjunctival stroma.** They have a particular predilection for the upper fornix and above the tarsal plate, and on the basis of proportion of total lacrimal tissue, it has been estimated that they contribute 5–10% of aqueous tear volume. Structurally, they have a similar appearance to the **lacrimal gland** proper. However, true acini are absent, and glands consist of elongated tubules that connect with ducts that open onto the conjunctival surface.

accommodation
The process of causing the crystalline lens of the eye to change shape so that it has greater plus power, thus

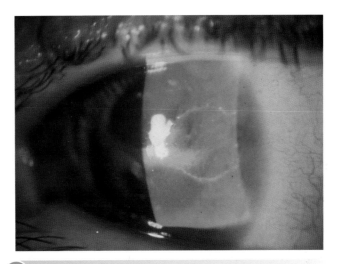

Figure A.2 Characteristic pattern of radial keratoneuritis in a soft lens wearer with Acanthamoeba keratitis.

allowing near objects to become clear. The amplitude of accommodation declines with age (Figure A.3). Few everyday tasks require accommodation in excess of about 4.00 D, so it is normally only as individuals approach 40 years of age that marked problems with near vision start to appear. It is, however, important to recognize that, even for objects lying

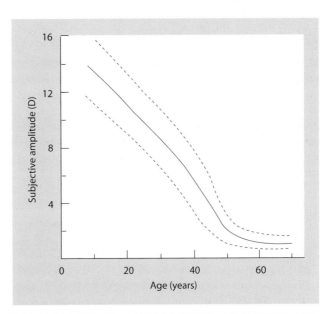

Figure A.3 The decline in monocular amplitude of accommodation, referenced to the spectacle plane, with age. After A. Duane (1922) Studies in monocular and binocular accommodation with their clinical implications. *Am. J. Ophthalmol.,* **5**, 865–877.

within the available range of accommodation, accommodation is rarely precise. 'Lags' of accommodation usually occur in near vision, and 'leads' for distance vision. Since the accommodation system is driven via the retinal cones, these lags increase if the environmental illumination is reduced to mesopic levels and the accommodation system is inoperative at scotopic light levels. *See* presbyopia.

accommodation demand

Just as the position of the correcting lens affects the correcting power required and the **spectacle magnification**, so it also influences the **accommodation** required to view a near object. The accommodation necessary with any particular correction can easily be calculated for any given object distance, lens position and correcting power by determining the difference between the vergence of the light striking the **cornea** when viewing a near object and that for a distant object. However, an adequate approximation for most purposes is that the accommodation demand, *A* dioptres is given by:

$$A \approx -L(1 + 2\,aK)$$

where *L* is the object vergence (negative for real objects), *a* is the vertex distance and *K* is the ocular refraction. In this approximation, *a* is zero for a contact lens, so that it can be seen that for a **myope** (negative K) the accommodation demand is higher with contact lenses than with spectacles lenses, whereas the reverse is true for **hypermetropes**. For an object at 33 cm ($L = -3.00$ D) and a spectacle vertex distance $a = 14$ mm, the difference in demand with the two types of correction becomes significant (> 0.25 D) when the magnitude of the refractive error, *K*, is larger than about 3.00 D. Thus, higher myopes approaching **presbyopia** might slightly delay the need for a reading addition by wearing spectacles, whereas hypermetropes would find near vision easier with a contact lens correction.

ACLM

See Association of Contact Lens Manufacturers.

acne rosacea

See systemic disease, contact lens wear in.

acoustic neuroma

See eyelid pathology, therapeutic lenses for.

acute red eye reaction

See contact lens induced acute red eye (CLARE).

aerosol saline

See saline solutions.

aesthesiometry, contact

See Cochet–Bonnet aesthesiometer.

aesthesiometry, non-contact

See non-contact aesthesiometry.

aftercare, contact lens

Contact lenses are generally very well tolerated by the majority of patients; however, appropriate aftercare of the contact lens patient is essential to ensure that long-term success is maintained. Aftercare procedures are as important as the original lens fitting, because the lenses that were fitted initially may develop unanticipated complications that require correction at any time during post-fitting patient care. In fact, it is commonly held that contact lens aftercare represents a continuum and as such can never be considered to be complete.

Aftercare schedules will vary based on lens type, mode of wear, and underlying corneal physiology (Table A.1). For example, patients wearing **rigid lenses** should be examined more frequently during the first few months of lens wear. Patients using lenses for **extended wear** must be monitored more frequently, with the initial visits in the early morning hours to assess lens adherence or excessive overnight corneal swelling. Additionally, the following groups of patients generally require more frequent aftercare as part of their management compared with uncomplicated cosmetic lens wearers: those with corneal pathology such as **keratoconus** or corneal dystrophy; those **post-keratoplasty** or **post-refractive surgery**; those using contact lenses for other **therapeutic** applications such as **aphakia** or high ametropia; and also **paediatric patients**.

The general strategy adopted for aftercare visits is to consider the procedures in two phases: those conducted with the patient wearing lenses (assuming that the patient presented wearing lenses), and those conducted following lens removal. Certainly, patients should present to all aftercare visits while wearing lenses, unless a complication warrants lens discontinuation. It is rarely necessary to conduct all possible aftercare procedures at every follow-up visit. Essential procedures (such as those outlined below) generally should be performed; these can be supplemented with ancillary testing to solve specific problems. The aftercare visit may on occasions be very brief; for example, if a patient presents with a minor problem soon after a having been given a full aftercare examination, and the solution is straightforward, it may only be necessary to see the patient for a few minutes. The only caveat here is that, for medico-legal reasons, **vision** should always be measured if the patient enters the consulting

Table A.1 Suggested aftercare schedules

soft lens daily wear	soft lens extended wear	rigid lens daily wear	rigid lens extended wear	therapeutic use
1–2 weeks	1 day (a.m. visit)	1–2 weeks	1 day (a.m. visit)	1 week
1 month	1 week	1 month	1 week	3–4 weeks
3 months	1 month	2 months	2 weeks	2 months
6 months	3 months	3 months	1 month	3 months
every 6–12 months thereafter	every 3 months thereafter	6 months	3 months	6 months
		every 6–12 months thereafter	every 3 months thereafter	every 6 months thereafter

room, no matter how brief the visit. The procedures conducted during the two phases of an aftercare examination are as follows.

1. Procedures conducted with the patient wearing lenses:
   - history taking
   - visual acuity
   - **over-refraction**
   - over-**keratometry**
   - external examination
   - **slit-lamp biomicroscopy**
   - lens surface assessment
   - lens fitting characteristics
   - lens–eye interactions.
2. Procedures conducted following lens removal:
   - uncorrected vision
   - refraction
   - keratometry and corneal topography
   - **slit-lamp biomicroscopy**
   - lens inspection and verification
   - additional procedures, which may not be readily available to all contact lens clinicians, include corneal thickness measurements (**pachometry**) and endothelial **specular microscopy**; digital slit-lamp imaging is a valuable method of recording clinical information
   - other procedures as required, including visual fields, ophthalmoscopy, tonometry, gonioscopy, binocular vision assessment, **corneal sensitivity**, **tearscope** evaluation, colour vision assessment etc.
   - concluding discussion with patient.

ageing, contact lens

The pre-insertion **water content** of all soft lenses decreases significantly over time. This ageing process is different from the well-known phenomenon of lens dehydration over the course of a number of hours throughout a day. The extent of ageing must be considered in the context of the intended **life** of the lens; thus, adverse ageing-related effects of a lens that occur at a constant rate over a 1-month period can be minimized or avoided if the lens is replaced weekly instead of monthly.

It is clear that a combination of physical and/or physiological factors cause this irreversible reduction in **water content** of the hydrogel lenses over time. It follows that some change to the lens appears to have caused a progressive reduction in water uptake by the lens each night during storage, in what amounts to a 'lens ageing' effect. The most likely explanation for this ageing effect is that lens spoilation acts either to displace water from the lens, or it alters the nature of the lens material in such a way that less water is absorbed by it. This phenomenon occurs more in some patients than in others. A negative clinical ramification of this phenomenon is that there is an associated loss of oxygen performance with dehydration. Thus, the corneas of patients wearing lenses that display significant cyclic ageing will be generally more prone to chronic hypoxic complications, as well as specific acute hypoxic complications in the period immediately preceding lens replacement.

Alcon Laboratories

The company traces its inception to 1945, when two pharmacists pooled their meagre resources to open a small pharmacy in Fort Worth, Texas. Combining the first syllable of each man's last name, Robert D. Alexander and William C. Conner christened their fledgling enterprise the Alcon Prescription Laboratory. This was the beginning of Alcon Laboratories – today a US $2 billion international pharmaceutical company specializing in the discovery, development, manufacture and marketing of ophthalmic products and instrumentation.

In 1997, the company was acquired by Nestlé – an international company headquartered in Switzerland. In the ensuing years, Alcon expanded its scope into the ophthalmic surgical marketplace. Today, Alcon operates in over 170 countries and employs over 10 000 staff world-wide, with international headquarters in Fort Worth, Texas, USA. Website: www.alconlabs.com

alignment rigid bitoric lenses
See cylindrical power equivalent rigid toric lenses.

alkali burns
See chemical injuries, therapeutic lenses for.

Allergan
International company based in California, USA. Allergan, Inc., headquartered in Irvine, California, is a technology-driven, global health care company providing eye care and specialty pharmaceutical products world-wide. Allergan develops and commercializes products in the eye care pharmaceutical, ophthalmic surgical device, over-the-counter contact lens care, movement disorder, and dermatological markets.

Allergan targets its products and research and development to specific disease areas. These include glaucoma and retinal disease, cataracts, dry eye, psoriasis, acne, photo-damage, movement disorders, pain, metabolic disease and various types of cancer. Leading edge technologies in which the company has established leadership positions include second-generation alpha-2 agonist compounds, receptor-selective retinoids, foldable intraocular lenses, injectable neurotoxin, and convenient contact lens care products.

Allergan markets products in more than 100 countries. Founded in 1950, Allergan became a public company in 1970, merged with SmithKline Beckman in 1980, and was re-established as an independent entity in 1989. In 2002, Allergan's optical medical device business, which includes contact lens solutions, was formed into a new company called Advanced Medical Optics. Website: www.allergan.com

alternating vision lenses for presbyopia
These lenses have distance and near powered portions, set out in a similar way to that observed in a bifocal spectacle lens. Although soft alternating bifocals have been available in the form of concentric and crescent segment designs, they have not generally proved successful due to ineffective translation. Translating designs are therefore almost exclusively available as rigid lenses. During primary gaze, the distance portion of the contact lens is positioned over the pupil. When gaze is directed downwards during reading, the near portion translates upwards to allow near vision correction (Figure A.4). Segment position and lens translation are the keys to success, and the lower lid has an important role in positioning and stabilizing the lens against the globe. The position of the lower lid should be no lower than the inferior limbus, otherwise translation is less effective and often inadequate. Upper lid movement also plays an important role in lens translation, as the upward movement of the lower lid is restricted to about 0.8 mm. It may be more challenging to fit patients with ambient pupil sizes greater than 3 mm, as the segment has to be positioned lower to avoid the pupil margin and consequently requires greater translation to achieve adequate pupil coverage of the near portion.

The two distinct portions that make up an alternating lens may be either fused or solid, and a range of alternative segment shapes are available. Lens stability, position and translation can be controlled by introducing prism onto the lens, truncating the lens, or both. Regardless of lens design, the success of alternating vision contact lenses is made possible by adequate lower lid tone, which facilitates upward translation of the lens during downgaze. This positions the near portion of the lens over the pupil and allows near vision. The truncated edge should be finished in such a way to encourage comfortable effective translation and minimize the risk of the lens slipping beneath the lower lid.

Solid designs can be cut from a single piece of material, and the segment shape and design can vary. If the optical centres of the distance and near portion do not coincide, image jump will occur with down gaze, and lenses of 3.00 D or greater frequently result in intolerable diplopia for the wearer. For this reason, it is better to avoid solid construction lenses in these powers unless using a monocentric design. In these designs optical centres of both distance and near portions of the lens are coincident, which produces a straight top segment bifocal contact lens with the same properties as an 'executive' bifocal spectacle lens.

Fused-segment rigid lenses use a fused insert of higher refractive index than the rest of the lens to generate the add power, whilst the front surface curvature remains continuous. There is minimal image jump and blanks are supplied to laboratories, allowing individual lens specifications to be made to order, including more complex front and back surface geometries. Care must be taken not to fit these lenses with the segment position too high as this increases the risk of reflections being noticed from the top of the segment. The fused segment is fluorescent, allowing easy observation using a **Burton lamp**.

Alternating lenses are generally fitted on alignment or with minimal apical corneal touch. The truncation should rest on the lower lid. The lens should have a vertical diameter at least 2 mm smaller than the horizontal visible iris diameter; this encourages the required inferior centration and rapid recovery of lens position following blink as well as upward movement during depressed gaze. Translation over the corneal surface is more likely if there is unimpeded vertical movement, so a steep fitting approach should be avoided. In general, a lens fitted too steeply will tend to swing nasally and show poor translation, unlike a flat lens fit, which decentres temporally.

Most alternating bifocal contact lenses are fitted so that the segment is positioned in line with the inferior pupil margin during primary gaze in ambient illumination. Alternatively, some solid designs are such that the segment should be fitted higher to occupy approximately 20% of the pupil area. More importantly, the near segment should occupy at least 75% of the pupil diameter during depressed gaze to allow adequate near vision. An exception is when fitting fused rigid lens designs, as the segment position should be positioned approximately 0.4–0.7 mm below the pupil margin when observed under **slit-lamp** illumination. This minimizes light reflections from the segment line interfering with distance vision performance. As a general rule, it is best to err on setting the segment top a little high, as this can subsequently be lowered by increasing truncation. A near horizontal segment line position is preferred; however, a small amount of nasal rotation is acceptable because the natural convergence of the eyes at near helps offset this rotation.

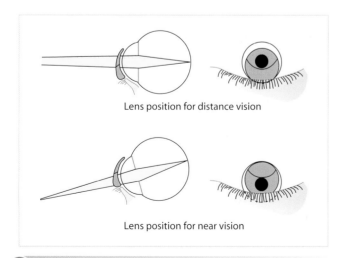

Lens position for distance vision

Lens position for near vision

Figure A.4 Rigid bifocal lens positions for distance and near vision.

Observing segment positions under slit-lamp illumination can be deceptive due to the resultant pupil miosis. A better assessment can be made using an ophthalmoscope focused on the lens surface. If an optimal alignment fit shows significant rotation away from the desired position, the lens can be re-ordered with prism offset by the angle through which the lens mislocates to compensate for the rotation. For example, if the lens persists in rotating by 15° nasally in the right eye, ordering the prism base at 285° rather than 270° orientates the lens correctly. Increasing the amount of prism can also be useful in reducing superior centration.

ametropia
General term for all forms of refractive defects of the eye whereby light from a distant object is not focused on the retina when **accommodation** is relaxed, resulting in blurred distance vision. *Antonym*: emmetropia.

aniseikonia
A binocular perceptual distortion of space that is induced when corresponding retinal images of the two eyes are unequal. This occurs when **anisometropia** is corrected by spectacle lenses, causing marked differences in **spectacle magnification** between the two eyes. This condition can be disturbing and disorientating to the patient. A small amount of aniseikonia can also be induced when the magnitude and/or axis of cylinder correction is changed. The effect is usually transient, and patients adapt within hours of receiving a new or changed optical correction. These distortions are much reduced in the case of contact lenses, which therefore minimize the possibility of aniseikonic symptoms. *See* spectacle magnification.

anisometropia
Difference in refractive status between the two eyes, whereby a different optical correction is required for each eye. Correction of anisometropia can result in **aneisekonia**.

anoxia
Absence of oxygen. *Adj*: anoxic

anterior limiting lamina of the cornea
This second layer of the **cornea** is also known as Bowman's layer. It varies in thickness between 8 and 14 μm. With the light microscope, it appears as an acellular homogeneous zone. Ultrastructurally, it is composed of a randomly orientated array of fine collagen fibrils, which merge with the fibrils of the anterior stroma. Fibrils are composed primarily of collagen types I, III and V. Collagen type

VII associated with anchoring fibrils is also present. There is evidence that the anterior limiting lamina is formed and maintained primarily by the epithelium, although its function is unclear. The absence of this lamina from the cornea of most mammals, and the fact that corneas devoid of this lamina over the central cornea following photorefractive keratectomy apparently function normally, suggest that it is not critical to corneal integrity.

antimicrobial efficacy

The capacity of a lens care product to eradicate or minimize microbial organisms. An important consideration for the contact lens practitioner when dispensing a care product is its performance in terms of cleaning and – perhaps more importantly in terms of wearer safety – antimicrobial efficacy.

The first safeguard for the practitioner is that, in many parts of the world, contact lens disinfectants are required to meet a number of criteria before they can be labelled and sold as such. For example, in the European Union all such products are required to display the 'CE mark', which indicates that the product has displayed a minimum level of disinfecting performance and that a number of other criteria (such as satisfactory manufacturing conditions) have been met. The CE mark requires a contact lens disinfectant to meet the performance requirements of the international standard EN ISO 14729:3 (Microbiological requirements for products and regimens for hygienic management of contact lenses). To achieve this, the product must show activity against three bacteria (*Pseudomonas aeruginosa*, *Staphylococcus aureus* and *Serratia marcescens*) and two forms of yeast (*Candida albicans* and *Fusarium solani*).

Products are first tested on a 'stand-alone' basis. Here, the disinfectant must be able to reduce the population of each of the bacteria by 99.9% (or a three log reduction) and the yeasts by 90% (a one log reduction). This testing is performed in laboratory conditions without the use of contact lenses – that is, there is a mixing of the test organisms with a fixed quantity of the solution under test.

If the product fails to meet the stand-alone criteria the 'regimen procedure' can be invoked, whereby the performance of the product in a more 'real world' situation is analysed. However, to proceed to this stage, solutions must at least have demonstrated that they are able to achieve stasis for yeast in the stand-alone test, and an overall combined five log reduction for the three bacteria, with at least one log reduction for each of the bacteria. In the regimen procedure, contact lenses are inoculated with the panel of test organisms, and then treated according to the instructions provided by the manufacturer for cleaning, rinsing and soaking. To satisfy the criteria, there must be at least a four log reduction for all the test organisms.

In order to reach the marketplace, therefore, contact lens solutions are required to achieve a set standard of performance. However, of further interest is the relative performance of the various products that are available. Although this might seem to require simply generating comparative data for a range of care products, this area is fraught with problems. For example, an approach that has been used in the past to demonstrate the disinfection capabilities of disinfectant systems is the 'D-value'. This parameter denotes the time taken for a disinfectant product to reduce the population of an organism to 10% of its original level (a one log reduction).

Although this appears to be a useful indication of solution performance, there are a number of problems with its use. The D-value assumes a linear relationship between the logarithm of the number of survivors and time. However, the action of contact lens disinfectants tends to be non-linear, which suggests that the use of D-values is inappropriate and can lead to misleading representations of product performance. Another drawback to the D-value approach is that no account is made of the minimum recommended disinfection time (MRDT) recommended by the manufacturer. For example, a product may offer a one log reduction in 20 minutes and a three log reduction in 1 hour; the clinical success of this product, however, must depend to some extent on the MRDT, which could be 10 minutes or 6 hours. A new measure of solution potency – solution 'power' – overcomes this problem. This parameter is defined as the MRDT divided by the D-value.

A difficulty with this sort of approach is that no account is made of any cleaning or rinsing (as distinct from disinfecting) that may be employed as part of the overall care system. Some wearers might tend to omit these steps with some systems and not with others; this must impact on the overall disinfecting capabilities of the regimen.

Another significant problem when assessing differences between products is that different laboratory conditions and techniques can be employed. A relevant example here is the effectivity of disinfectants against Acanthamoeba. A number of variables exist when analysing the performance of products against **Acanthamoeba**, including the strain of Acanthamoeba used, growth conditions, and contact time of the disinfectant. Indeed the results in this area are highly dependent on methodology, which has led, in part, to the efficacy of contact lens disinfectants against Acanthamoeba being omitted from ISO 14729:3.

Despite this, the effectiveness of contact lens disinfectants against Acanthamoeba is of considerable interest to contact lens practitioners. On a stand-alone basis, **hydrogen peroxide** is effective at killing both Acanthamoeba trophozoites and cysts, with overnight storage in 3% hydrogen peroxide providing better performance in this regard than the shorter contact time with a one-step system. **Multipurpose solutions** have poor anti-Acanthamoebal efficacy, although the combination of MAPD and polyquad may improve this. In a clinical setting, cleaning and rinsing is likely to remove some Acanthamoebae. Furthermore, Acanthamoeba is thought to require the presence of bacteria to survive and grow, so the antibacterial efficacy of a contact lens disinfectant will have an effect on Acanthamoebal contamination.

aphakia, contact lens correction of
Aphakia – the absence of the crystalline lens – is now rare in adults due to the high success rate of intra-ocular lenses. However, in cases where intra-ocular lens implantation is impossible – for example when the patient has ancilliary pathology such as aniridia, chronic uveitis or glaucoma – contact lenses may be indicated. Such lenses typically have high plus power (i.e. > 10.00 D). **Hydrogel** lenses may be used with close monitoring, but **silicone elastomer**, **silicone hydrogel** or high-*Dk* **rigid lenses** are preferred to ensure adequate corneal oxygenation. **Extended wear** is desired to minimize frequent lens handling. Patients wearing lenses on an extended wear basis may, with proper monitoring, wear their lenses for a month at a time. High **water content** hydrogel lenses may be preferred for comfort, and should be selected to maximize **oxygen transmissibility** for extended wear. Low water content lenses may be preferred due to durability for daily wear, but the risk of **hypoxic** problems is high. Interestingly, the aphakic eye may swell less than an unoperated eye.

Handling will typically be difficult in bilateral aphakic patients due to poor uncorrected vision and reduced manual dexterity in the elderly. Some aphakes may prefer to handle **soft lenses** due to their large size, and some may prefer rigid lenses because of their stiffness. Corrections for residual **astigmatism** and near work can be placed in spectacles to be worn over the contact lenses. Patients with conjunctival filtering blebs should be monitored closely, and contact lenses should not impinge on these blebs excessively. Preferably, topical ocular medication is instilled before and after lens wear and only under close supervision during contact lens wear. *See* high plus power contact lens design.

apparent eye size
A cosmetic disadvantage of spectacle lenses is that they alter the apparent size of the eyes of the wearer as seen by other people; the eyes appear larger with positive spectacle corrections and smaller with negative ones. Using a thin lens approximation, where the power of the correcting lens is F_c and the eye is at a distance l from the lens, it is easy to show that the paraxial magnification, M, of the anterior eye is given by:

$$M = 1/(1 + F_c l)$$

Since l is small (< 0.02 m), this can be approximated by:

$$M = 1 - F_c l$$

Thus, if l is -20 mm and F_c is -10.00 D, the eyes nominally appear only 80% of their true size. In fact, for the viewer, the apparent size will vary depending upon the viewing direction, since conditions will not necessarily be paraxial. Clearly, with contact lenses this cosmetic disadvantage is absent.

aqueous leak
See post-trauma or post-surgery, therapeutic lenses for.

aspheric rigid lens designs
A surface that is not spherical (i.e. progressively flattening or steepening) is said to be aspheric. Aspheric **rigid lenses** have two important disadvantages compared with **spherical lenses**: first, they are more difficult to manufacture, particularly using conventional lathes; and secondly, they cannot easily be checked using a **radiuscope** or **keratometer**. Nevertheless, they offer a number of advantages that arguably outweigh their disadvantages. The main advantages of aspheric designs relate to comfort. Aspheric designs tend to show less **edge clearance** and therefore induce less edge sensation from contact with the palpebral conjunctiva. Poor blending of back surface junctions in spherical lenses can cause irritation on version when the lens moves off centre and the peripheral zones come into contact with the cornea. This is generally avoided with aspheric lenses unless the periphery is poorly blended. The gradual flattening of aspheric lens surfaces results in a thinner periphery, which may also help reduce edge sensation.

Optically, aspheric designs can both improve and degrade image quality. When not aligned with the visual axis, aspheric lenses will induce **astigmatism**. On the other hand, with higher power lenses, aspheric optics can reduce spherical aberration. In **myopic** early **presbyopes**, the reduced minus power in the periphery of aspheric lenses can help with near vision and delay the need for a presbyopic correction.

Aspheric designs take different forms, but these differences are usually so subtle as to be evident only from the manufacturer's product literature. The simplest aspheric design is an elliptical shape selected to be close to (or slightly flatter than) the average cornea. More complex aspheric designs change their degree of flattening (or eccentricity) from centre to edge. Some designs are spherical in the centre and change to an aspheric geometry towards the periphery. Most aspheric designs incorporate a much flatter, often spherical, peripheral zone about 0.2 mm wide. This peripheral zone helps to avoid mechanical irritation when the lens decentres to the peripheral cornea.

Association of Contact Lens Manufacturers (ACLM)
UK-based association of companies involved in the contact lens field. Its mission statement is: 'Promoting and growing contact lens wear'. Website: www.aclm.org.uk

astigmatism
Refractive defect of the eye in which light from a distant object is focused as two orthogonal focal lines rather than a single focal point. The focal lines may straddle the retina (simple astigmatism), or form largely in front of the retina (myopic astigmatism) or behind the retina (hyperopic astigmatism). Astigmatism is corrected with toric lens forms.

asymptomatic infiltrates (AI)
This condition refers to the presence of infiltrates in the **cornea** in the absence of significant patient symptoms or epithelial compromise. In some cases AI may be a precursor to a **culture-negative peripheral ulcer**. Ocular discomfort, conjunctival hyperaemia and anterior chamber reaction are minimal or absent.

atopic eczema
See systemic disease, contact lens wear in.

atopic keratoconjunctivitis
See degenerations of the corneal epithelium, therapeutic lenses for.

average thickness of a lens
See lens thickness.

axial edge lift
See edge lift.

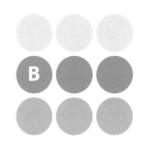

babies

See paediatric contact lenses; paediatric contact lens examination; paediatric contact lens fitting.

back optic zone diameter (BOZD)

The diameter of the optic zone on the back of the lens as measured through the lens centre (Figure B.1). The back optic zone diameter (BOZD) of a rigid lens is generally fixed for a given design in a given **total diameter** (TD), and is generally 1–1.5 mm smaller than the TD. The BOZD should be large enough to cover the pupil in most conditions, including low illumination.

With toroidal corneas, using a smaller BOZD can increase the area of alignment and therefore improve the fit. However, if the BOZD is reduced while maintaining the same TD, this results in a wider periphery, and flatter peripheral curves are required in order to maintain edge clearance.

If the BOZD is changed, it is usually necessary to change the **BOZR** in order to maintain a clinically equivalent fit. Reducing the BOZD without reducing the BOZR results in a sagittal depth that is more shallow, and therefore a flatter fit. As a rule of thumb, an increase in BOZD of 0.5 mm requires an increase in BOZR of 0.05 mm.

back optic zone radius (BOZR)

The back optic zone radius (BOZR, or 'base curve'), is the radius of curvature of the back surface of a contact lens (*see* Figure B.1). It is the main parameter to be modified when attempting to optimize the fit of a **soft lens**, a steepening of BOZR being required to tighten a soft lens fit and *vice versa*. However, even with lenses that are relatively inflexible, such as thick, low **water content** lenses, large changes in BOZR are required in order to have a significant effect on lens movement. With more flexible, thinner, high water content lenses, changes in BOZR have even less effect. The labelled BOZR is therefore of little help in soft lens fitting.

Knowledge of soft lens BOZR is not necessarily helpful when comparing different brands of lens. Lenses of similar BOZR can show widely differing sagittal depths because of differences in back surface design. This phenomenon, and differences in material mechanical properties, means that widely differing fitting characteristics can be observed on a given cornea with different brands of lenses of the same nominal BOZR.

back surface rigid toric lenses

See cylindrical power equivalent rigid toric lenses.

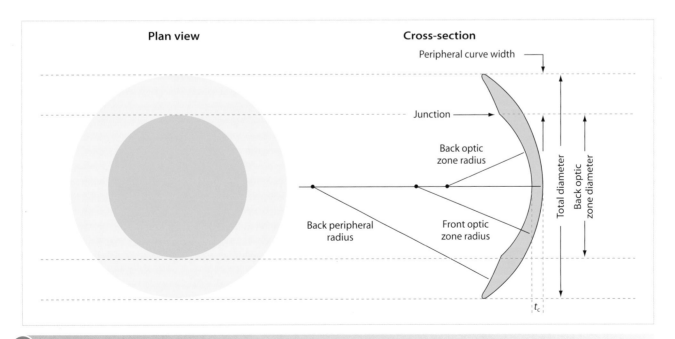

Figure B.1 Plan and cross-sectional view of a minus-powered contact lens with a single curve front surface and bicurve back surface.

back vertex power (BVP)

This is the optical power of the lens measured in dioptres. Modifications are often made to the design of **soft lenses** at the extremes of the power range. At the lower end of the minus power range (< -1.50 D), **lens centre thickness** is usually increased to improve lens handling. At the higher end of the power range, lens centre thickness is often reduced and the optic zone diameter kept to a minimum in order to reduce lens bulk and maximize **oxygen transmission**.

The thickness of high minus lenses can be further reduced, and the optical performance improved, by incorporating aspheric optics in order to overcome lens spherical aberration. With plus power lenses, the optic zone diameter is again minimized in order to minimize centre thickness. Some manufacturers have utilized a larger diameter in order to counterbalance the anticipated greater movement of plus-power lenses; however, **hyperopic** eyes tend to be smaller in diameter and therefore this is of doubtful benefit.

There tends to be little difference in lens fit between low minus and higher minus lenses of similar design. However, plus power lenses tend to show significantly more post-blink movement than minus power lenses of the same dioptric power, probably due to their greater thickness, leading to increased interaction with the upper lid.

bandage lens

See relief of pain, therapeutic lenses for; therapeutic contact lenses.

basal cells of the epithelium

See corneal epithelium.

basal lamina of the corneal epithelium

This is the basement membrane of the **corneal epithelium**, and is synthesized by basal epithelial cells. It varies in thickness between 0.5 and 1.0 μm, and under the electron microscope can be differentiated into an anterior clear zone (lamina lucida) and a posterior darker zone (lamina densa). The basal lamina is part of a complex adhesion system, which mediates the attachment of the epithelium to the underlying **stroma**. Hemidesmosomes link the cytoskeleton, via a series of anchoring fibrils, to anchoring plaques in the anterior stroma. The molecular components of this adhesion complex include type VII collagen, integrins, laminin and bullous phemphigoid antigen.

base curve

See back optic zone radius (BOZR).

basement membrane dystrophy

See recurrent erosion syndrome, therapeutic lenses for.

Bausch & Lomb

Bausch & Lomb is a global eye care company. Founded in 1853, the company has annual revenues of approximately US $2 billion and employs approximately 12 000 people in 35 countries. Bausch & Lomb products are available in more than 100 countries around the world. The global headquarters are in Rochester, New York, USA.

Bausch & Lomb has three product lines: Vision Care, Surgical, and Pharmaceuticals. Bausch & Lomb's Vision Care business manufactures and markets **soft and rigid contact lenses**, lens care products for soft and rigid lenses, eye care products such as eye drops and ointments, and vision accessories such as magnifiers and eyeglass accessories.

Bausch & Lomb offers a comprehensive line of products for ophthalmic surgery, including aberration-controlled laser refractive surgery equipment. The company also develops and markets prescription and over-the-counter drugs used to treat a wide range of eye conditions, including glaucoma, eye allergies, conjunctivitis, and dry eye. Website: www.bausch.com

BCLA

See British Contact Lens Association.

bedewing

See endothelial bedewing.

bifocal and multifocal contact lenses

Bifocal and multifocal contact lenses can be **simultaneous** or **alternating** vision designs. Simultaneous designs generally require the lens to be relatively stable on the eye, and will be associated with some form of visual compromise because objects at both distance and near are imaged simultaneously on the retina. Alternating vision bifocal lenses require significant lens movement so that the distance and near portions of the lens can be positioned over the pupil by interaction with the lids. *See* alternating vision lenses for presbyopia; monovision correction for presbyopia; simultaneous vision lenses for presbyopia.

Biocompatibles–Hydron

Biocompatibles is an international biomaterials group focused on the development and commercial exploitation of its biocompatible technology in health care and other markets. Established in 1984, the company was floated on the London Stock Exchange in 1995 and purchased the Hydron contact lens company in 2000. It is headquartered in the UK (in Farnham, Surrey), with manufacturing facilities in the UK (Farnborough), USA (Norfolk, Virginia), Ireland (Galway), Australia (Adelaide), Spain (Madrid) and Germany (Bruckmühl). Its turnover in 2000 was around US $80 million.

Biocompatibles' core technology is based on phosphorylcholine (PC), a chemical group found in the membrane of living cells. PC is the primary natural material responsible for biocompatibility. Devices coated with PC materials developed by Biocompatibles significantly reduce the incidence of adverse interactions with body fluids such as blood, tear film and urine. Through its two divisions – Eye Care and Cardiovascular – the company has been commercializing contact lenses and coronary stents. The Eye Care division of Biocompatibles–Hydron was purchased by **CooperVision** in 2002.

biomicroscope

See slit-lamp biomicroscope.

blebs

See endothelial blebs.

blepharitis

This condition is classified as being either anterior or posterior. Posterior blepharitis is a disorder of the meibomian glands (*see* meibomian gland dysfunction).

Anterior blepharitis is directly related to infections of the base of the eyelashes and manifests in two forms; staphylococcal and seborrhoeic. Staphylococcal anterior blepharitis is caused by a chronic staphylococcal infection of the eyelash follicles. The lid margins are covered in shiny brittle scales (Figure B.2), and patients may complain of:

- burning
- **dryness**
- itching
- foreign body sensations
- mild photophobia.

Management strategies include:

- antibiotic ointment
- promoting lid hygiene
- application of weak topical steroids
- artificial tears.

Seborrhoeic anterior blepharitis is due to a disorder of the glands of **Zeis** and **Moll**. The signs and symptoms are similar but less severe than for staphylococcal anterior blepharitis. Contact lens wear is generally contraindicated during an acute phase of anterior blepharitis, especially if the **cornea** is compromised. Attention to lens cleaning is critical to prevent continued recontamination of the eye. **Daily disposable contact lenses** will eliminate the problem of recontamination by contact lenses.

blinking

Contact lenses elicit reflex blinking during lens **insertion**, **removal** and other instances of manual manipulation. Also, as a result of a reflex blink, contact lenses may mislocate or become dislodged from the eye. Both **soft and rigid lens** wear cause the spontaneous blink rate to increase. In rigid lens wear this change may be more related to reflex blinking rather than spontaneous blinking; that is, the increased blink rate may be a result of continual irritation caused by the lens edge buffeting against the lid margin. Such alterations to blink rate are not thought to be permanent. Contact lenses can also affect the pattern of blinking. A decrease in the frequency of occurrence of long duration interblink periods occurs in association with rigid lens wear but not with soft lens wear. Neither rigid nor soft lens wear alters the proportion of complete, incomplete, twitch and forced blinks (Figure B.3). Infrequent or incomplete blinking with contact lenses can cause a number of problems, including lens surface drying and deposition, epithelial desiccation, post-lens tear stagnation, **hypoxia** and **hypercapnia**, and 3 and 9 o'clock staining. Faults in lens design and fitting can interfere with proper blink-mediated lid–lens interaction.

There are essentially two options when faced with a clinical problem relating to non-pathologic disorders of spontaneous blinking activity associated with contact lens wear, such as incomplete and/or infrequent blinking. These options are to train patients to modify their blinking activity, and/or to alter the lens type or lens fit.

Practitioners should remain alert to the possibility that apparent anomalies in the type or pattern of blinking activity in a contact lens wearer may be attributable to unrelated disease states. Interruptions to the neural input and/or muscular systems of the eyelids can adversely affect normal spontaneous

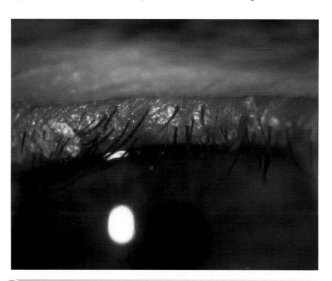

Figure B.2 Staphylococcal anterior blepharitis.

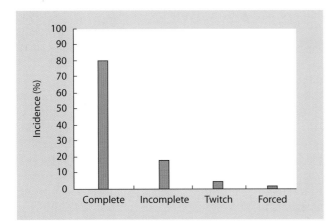

blinking activity. For example, patients with Parkinson's disease exhibit a low blink rate. Increased mechanical resistance to eyelid movement, as in Grave's disease, can also reduce blink frequency. Local pathology of the **eyelids**, such as ptosis, chalazia and carcinomas, can alter eyelid function and movement, and hence interfere with normal blinking activity. It is therefore essential to rule out the possibility of unrelated pathology before ascribing blinking dysfunction to contact lens wear.

Bowman's layer
See anterior limiting lamina of the cornea.

BOZD
See back optic zone diameter.

BOZR
See back optic zone radius.

British Contact Lens Association (BCLA)
The BCLA's mission is 'to promote excellence in contact lens research, manufacturing and clinical practice'. Membership is drawn from all sectors involved in the field of contact lenses, including optometrists, ophthalmologists, dispensing opticians, and professionals working in the contact lens and contact lens care product industry. The BCLA hosts a major conference and exhibition in May/June each year, runs numerous lectures and courses, and publishes the journal Contact Lens & Anterior Eye quarterly. Website: www.bcla.org.uk

British Universities Committee of Contact Lens Educators (BUCCLE)
This is an association of contact lens educators from university-based teaching institutions in the United Kingdom. Its aim is to nurture high standards of contact lens education in British universities. There are two full members from each institution, plus associ-

ate members. BUCCLE meets three times each year to discuss and share ideas and developments in UK contact lens education. It is sponsored by the contact lens industry. Website: www.buccle.org.uk

BUCCLE
See British Universities Committee of Contact Lens Educators.

bullous keratopathy
See dystrophies of the corneal epithelium, therapeutic lenses for; degenerations of the corneal epithelium, therapeutic lenses for.

bundling
See lens delivery systems.

Burton lamp
A number of manufacturers make a special handheld magnifying device for contact lens work. This device is usually referred to as a 'Burton lamp' (Figure B.4), after the company that manufactured the original version (Burton Manufacturing Co., USA). The Burton lamp is essentially a large magnifying lens of about +5.00 D housed in a broad frame, within which are mounted a combination of 4-W white-light and ultraviolet-light fluorescent tubes, each about 11 cm long. The operator can switch between the two light sources for white-light and **fluorescein**-stain examinations. A key advantage of this instrument is that both eyes of the patient can be viewed simultaneously, which facilitates interocular comparisons in the course of contact lens fitting. The Burton lamp is also useful for conducting an initial screening examination.

BVP
See back vertex power.

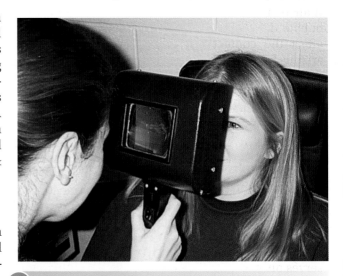

Figure B.4 Burton lamp.

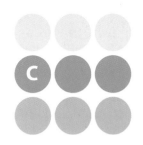

CAB
See celluluse acetate butyrate.

calcium deposition
See deposits, lens.

canaliculus
See lacrimal drainage system.

captive bubble measurement
This is one of three key techniques for measuring lens **surface wettability**; the other two are the **sessile drop** and **Wilhelmy plate** techniques (Figure C.1). The captive bubble method of measuring surface wettability is often preferred to the sessile drop measurement when assessing contact lenses because the lens does not undergo dehydration during the procedure. When contact lenses are examined the probe liquid is usually water, which has led to the method often being referred to as the 'air-in-water' technique.

With the lens immersed in water, a droplet of a second liquid (or air) is introduced at the lower (submerged) sample surface. The contact angle is then measured in the same way as described for the sessile drop technique, i.e. by direct measurement or calculated from the dimensions of the bubble. The contact angle measured is conceptually similar to that obtained when a receding angle is measured with the sessile method.

This method, however, like all methods used for contact angle analysis, is not without its difficulties. If air is introduced, care needs to be taken to avoid bubble distortion. The size of the bubble will also affect the contact angle obtained. Optical effects arising from a multiple layer optical path make it difficult to locate the precise point where the air bubble meets the solid surface. As a result, the exact determination of the tangent to the droplet at its point of contact with the lens is as problematic as for the sessile method, and will inevitably introduce a level of variability into the results.

Manufacturers have been known to quote contact angles using this method, but instead of water they use wetting or soaking solutions. The contact angle produced, however, has no fundamental significance either to surface characterization or to the prediction of eye–lens wettability. Its use in this way serves only to lower the contact angle obtained, presumably for marketing purposes.

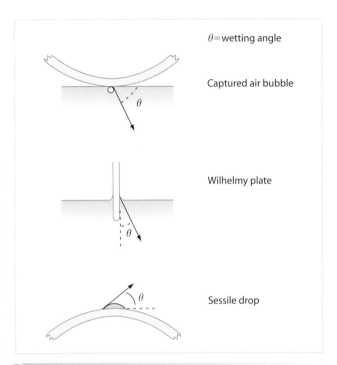

Figure C.1 Techniques for assessing lens wetting angles.

carbon dioxide permeability
This term describes the ease with which carbon dioxide may pass through a particular material under standard conditions. It is thus a property of a material, and not of a finished contact lens. Carbon dioxide permeability of a material is a function of the diffusivity (D) and solubility (k) of carbon dioxide in that material, and is represented by the term Dk. Since this term is usually associated with oxygen permeability, $Dk(CO_2)$ is used to denote permeability to carbon dioxide. The diffusivity (D) refers to the speed at which carbon dioxide molecules can pass through the material, and the solubility (k) refers to the number of carbon dioxide molecules that can be absorbed into a given volume of material.

In order to determine the carbon dioxide permeability of a material at a given temperature, it is necessary to measure the rate (volume per unit time) at which carbon dioxide passes through a sample of membrane of given dimensions (area and thickness) for a given gas pressure. The units of Dk take these variables into account, and are quite complex. It is common therefore to quote the value in 'Fatt units' (after Irving Fatt, who pioneered contact lens carbon dioxide permeability measurement) or, more formally, 'Barrer', whereby:

$$Dk(CO_2) \text{ in Barrer (or 'Fatt units')}$$
$$= 10^{-11} \, (cm^2 \cdot mlCO_2)/(s \cdot ml \cdot mmHg)$$

The international standard unit for pressure is the pascal (Pa). Because the term mmHg is now becoming obsolete internationally, it is being advocated that the closest accepted metric unit of pressure – 100 Pa, or hectopascal (hPa) – should replace the term mmHg. This approach is specified in the international standard ISO 8321-2 (2000). When hPa is used, $Dk(CO_2)$ is quoted as:

$$Dk(CO_2) = 10^{-11} \, (cm^2 \cdot mlCO_2)/(s \cdot ml \cdot hPa)$$

The difficulty here is that converting from the traditional Barrer or Fatt units to ISO units involves multiplying $Dk(CO_2)$ by the constant 0.75. Thus a lens quoted with a traditional $Dk(CO_2)$ of 40×10^{-11} $(cm^2 \cdot mlCO_2)/(s \cdot ml \cdot mmHg)$, for example, will have a revised ISO $Dk(CO_2)$ of 30×10^{-11} $(cm^2 \cdot mlCO_2)/(s \cdot ml \cdot hPa)$.

For **hydrogels**, the ratio of $Dk(CO_2) : Dk(O_2)$ is 21 : 1; that is, CO_2 is able to permeate through hydrogels 21 times more easily than O_2. The ratio of $Dk(CO_2) : Dk(O_2)$ is 7 : 1 for **rigid lens** materials and 8 : 1 for **silicone elastomer**.

carbon dioxide transmissibility

The term 'carbon dioxide transmissibility' describes the ease with which carbon dioxide may pass through a particular material of given thickness. The carbon dioxide transmissibility of a lens is a function of the **carbon dioxide permeability** (*Dk*) of the material from which the lens is made, divided by the thickness of the lens (*t*). Thus, 'carbon dioxide transmissibility' is represented by the term $Dk/t(CO_2)$, and describes the passage of carbon dioxide through a finished contact lens.

The units of $Dk/t(CO_2)$ are as follows:

$$Dk/t(CO_2) \text{ in Barrer/cm}$$
$$= 10^{-9} \, (cm \cdot mlCO_2)/(s \cdot ml \cdot mmHg)$$

When hPa is used, $Dk/t(CO_2)$ is quoted as:

$$Dk/t(CO_2) \text{ in Barrer/cm}$$
$$= 10^{-9} \, (cm \cdot mlCO_2)/(s \cdot hPa)$$

To convert from the traditional Barrer or Fatt units to ISO units, Dk/t must be multiplied by the constant 0.75.

Contact lens carbon dioxide transmissibility can be expressed in terms of either central or average transmissibility. The central lens $Dk/t(CO_2)$ is derived by dividing $Dk(CO_2)$ by the centre thickness of the lens. The average lens $Dk/t(CO_2)$ is derived by dividing $Dk(CO_2)$ by the average thickness of the lens over a defined lens radius. The average $Dk/t(CO_2)$ is always less than the central $Dk/t(CO_2)$ for minus powered lenses (which become progressively thicker from the centre to the edge of the lens), and the converse is true for plus powered lenses.

Because the ratio of $Dk(CO_2) : Dk(O_2)$ is 21 : 1 for **hydrogels** and 7 : 1 for **rigid lenses**, the $Dk/t(CO_2)$ of a hydrogel contact lens will be about three times that of a rigid lens of the same $Dk/t(O_2)$ as the hydrogel lens.

carrier, minus lens

See high plus power contact lens design.

case history, non-lens wearer

A full ocular history, including age of first optical correction and spectacle wearing habits, will help to gauge general suitability in patients who have never previously worn contact lenses ('neophytes'; see Table C.1). For example, a prospective wearer who only wears spectacles intermittently may not be an obvious choice for contact lens wear. However, if that intermittent wear is driven by a dislike for the cosmetic effect of spectacles, then contact lenses become a more obvious choice. Existing use of spectacles for distance and near vision may give some indication of whether the patient will have to adapt to significant changes in accommodation and convergence once contact lens wear is initiated. This may be particularly relevant to early **presbyopic myopes** who may either take their spectacles off to read or have insufficient reserves of accommodation to cope with the additional accommodative demands in contact lenses compared to spectacles.

Previous ophthalmologic, orthoptic or general practitioner eye treatment will give clues about past ocular status that might influence the clinical decision-making process. General health and use of medication are also significant. A positive family ocular or general health history also gives additional information about future potential risks that may relate to contact lens wear or more general patient management. It may be appropriate to ask whether the patient is a smoker, since this seems to be associated with a higher risk of **microbial keratitis**. Questioning about specific allergies will help to guide choice of lens modality, the **frequency of replacement** and the care system.

Symptoms with the present spectacles will also give information that may in future help to differentiate specific contact lens symptoms from pre-existing problems.

Contact lens-specific questions will include why the patient wants contact lenses, what he or she knows about contact lenses, and what is expected from lens wear. Questions regarding leisure activities and occupation will help to determine the most suitable type of lens, and will also provide an opportunity to offer advice on eye protection if appropriate. With more complex fittings, such as **bifocal** or **toric lenses**, it may also help to determine whether an acceptable visual outcome is likely to result from a particular lens type.

This information, when taken in conjunction with observed ocular health, refraction and binocular vision findings obtained during the initial examination, will lead to informed advice being offered to the patient on suitability for lenses generally, and on the most appropriate lens type, wearing modality and care system.

case history, previous or existing lens wearer

When the patient is a previous or existing contact lens wearer, the questioning used for the non-wearer is still appropriate (*see* **case history, non-lens wearer**; also Table C.1). However, additional lens-specific information is also required. The type of lens worn, the time since fitting and changes in lens type (e.g. from **rigid** to **soft lenses** or from **spherical** to **toric lenses**) all start to build a picture of the lens-wearing history. When such changes have been made, it is useful to determine the patient's understanding as to why they were necessary. It is important to determine what modality of wear, frequency of replacement and choice of care system was recommended by the previous practitioner, and whether the patient actually complied with those recommendations.

Average daily wearing time, the number of nights of overnight wear and the number of hours wear at the time of consultation all help to determine the significance of any clinical signs seen during the present and subsequent ocular examination. In particular, it is important to understand the primary complaint of the patient (if any) and any other symptoms that are present at the first consultation. It may also be instructive to inquire as to the reasons why care is no longer being provided by the original practitioner. Knowing the length of time since the last contact lens assessment will help in the judgement of the severity of any ocular changes as well as indicating likely future patient **compliance**; however, patients are notoriously poor at estimating the time course of previous management.

As with all history taking, it is important to use follow-up questions so as to extract as much information as possible relevant to understanding the

Table C.1 Initial history taking for the previous or existing lens wearer and non-lens wearer	
patient new to contact lenses	**previous or existing contact lens wearer**
age at first correction	as new patient plus:
use of spectacles	date of first contact lens correction
full time/part time	type of lens worn
current or present prescription	at initial fitting
ocular history	currently
medical treatment	modality recommended
hospital treatment	daily or overnight wear
orthoptic treatment	replacement frequency recommended
general health history	care system recommended
medication	compliance with recommendations
prescribed or 'over the counter'	average/maximum wearing time
family ocular history	number of nights worn without removal
family general health history	hours of continuous wear at time of visit
smoker – yes/no	primary complaint
allergies	other symptoms/signs
motivation for lens wear	reason for discontinuation of previous care
expectations of lens wear	date of last appointment
occupational/recreational activities	

patient history and making informed clinical decisions. This is particularly true where there are presenting patient problems, whereby history taking will follow the same pattern as for a general aftercare examination.

cast moulding

This has become the dominant technology in high volume **soft lens** manufacture. As with **spin casting**, a series of highly polished steel tools is used to fabricate polypropylene moulds. The steel master tools are used to make millions of matching male and female moulds, typically in groups of six or eight (Figure C.2).

Cast moulding generally takes place in a continuous, automated production line. Monomer in liquid form is introduced into a concave female mould, which defines the shape of the lens front surface. An ultraviolet-transparent male mould is mated to the female mould, and the two are clamped together in a carefully controlled environment. The contact lens edge is formed when the two sides of the mould come together. There is considerable science and art in the control of the polymerization process and the pressure applied to the mould to form the lens. The crucial part is to arrange for the excess **polymer** (so-called 'flash') to be squeezed out while leaving the edge intact.

Once the polymer is encapsulated in the mould, it is 'cured' – a process in which the assembled moulds are irradiated with ultraviolet light to effect polymerization so as to form the dry contact lens. Most cast moulding processes are designed so that when the dry lens is removed from the mould there is no need to polish the edge. The moulds are disassembled and discarded, and the lens that is released – still in rigid form – is hydrated in **saline**. Inspection is undertaken either manually or using automated video-based, computer-controlled image analysis. Finally, the lens is packaged and autoclaved.

It should be recognized that the above description is a highly simplified account of a sophisticated engineering process. Various manufacturers have introduced a number of unique variations, such as wet-state polymerization, the employment of reusable glass moulds, and use of the male half of the mould for final lens packaging. **Toric** and **bifocal lenses** can be manufactured using cast moulding technology by engineering the master tools to contain the desired lens forms; these design elements are faithfully transposed to the moulds and then to the final lens.

CCLRU grading scales
See grading scales.

celluluse acetate butyrate

This was one of the original gas-permeable **rigid contact lens** materials. Celluluse acetate butyrate (CAB) is a cellulose ester that is less rigid and less brittle (i.e. 'tougher') than polymethyl methacrylate (PMMA). The **oxygen permeability** of CAB is about 20 times greater than that of PMMA (which is still very low), and is capable of being fabricated by moulding techniques. Because CAB lacks the dimensional stability of other rigid lens materials, it is seldom used for making contact lenses.

CE mark
See antimicrobial efficacy; Medical Devices Directive.

centration, soft lens
See fitting soft lenses.

centre thickness of a lens
See lens thickness.

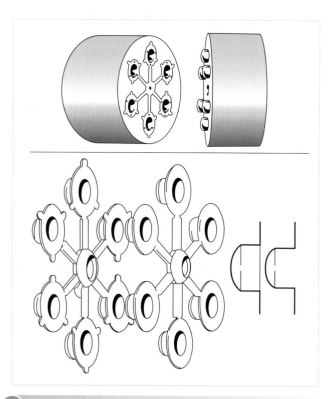

Figure C.2 Matching male and female steel tools (top) are filled with liquid polypropylene and fitted together. Once the polypropylene has set, the tools are pulled apart to leave a 'flower' of six identical female moulds. An identical procedure (with opposite-shaped tools) is used to make the male moulds. The male and female moulds are filled with the contact lens polymer and brought together (bottom) until polymerization is complete.

charges, contact lens
See fees and charges, contact lens.

chemical bond tinting
In this **soft lens** tinting process, a strong covalent chemical bond is formed between the dye chromophore and the polymer. The technique involves soaking the lens in a dye solution, in the presence of a catalyst, for a fixed time at a specified temperature. The lens then needs to be put through a series of extraction processes to remove any residual unreacted agents. The result, as with **vat dye tinting**, is a stable, uniform translucent tint. *See* tinted lenses.

chemical injuries, therapeutic lenses for
Much has been written about the use of contact lenses in the management of chemical injuries, especially alkali burns. However, research into the role of the limbal stem cells in the genesis of the **corneal epithelium** indicates that contact lens coverage of the chronic epithelial defect cannot prevent the colonization of the **cornea** by conjunctivally-derived epithelial cells. There are, however, some situations in which a contact lens can assist healing, supported by topical medications, although intensive care is required.

children
See paediatric contact lenses; paediatric contact lens examination; paediatric contact lens fitting.

chlorhexidine-thimerosal-preserved disinfecting solution
Chlorhexidine is probably the most widely used biocide in antiseptics, especially for hand-washing and oral products. Its action has been closely studied, and it is believed that its uptake by both bacteria and yeast is extremely rapid. Chlorhexidine damages cell walls and subsequently attacks the bacterial cytoplasmic or inner membrane, or the yeast plasma membrane.

Thimerosal is considered to be a less effective antimicrobial agent overall, although its action against fungi is better than that of chlorhexidine. Due to this, a combination of chlorhexidine gluconate and thimerosal became common in disinfectants for **soft contact lenses**. However, owing to the absorption of these agents onto soft lenses, toxic and hypersensitivity reactions were reported when they were used clinically. The build-up of these preservatives, and the subsequent leeching onto the ocular surface over time, had the potential to cause discomfort and discontinuation of lens wear. These products were ultimately superseded by others that offered a similar level of convenience and **antimicrobial efficacy**, but a lower adverse reaction rate.

A novel approach for a chlorhexidine system, known as OptimEyes, involved dissolving a tablet in tap water to provided a solution with a chlorhexidine concentration of 0.004%. The solution was shown to be effective against a panel of challenge micro-organisms, and also against most of the micro-organisms found in tap water. The use of tap water as part of the lens care process was controversial. Although this product was specifically designed for use with tap water, practitioners were concerned that contact lens wearers would consider standard tap water as an acceptable component of lens care generally. The product was simple and cheap to use, and it provided action against **Acanthamoeba**. Its disadvantages included the reliance on a supply of rising mains tap water and, importantly, it was contraindicated for use with FDA Group IV lenses. This was because the action of chlorhexidine is reduced with ionic lenses. With the increasing popularity of Group IV lenses throughout the 1990s, the OptimEyes product did not become a mainstream soft lens care product.

chlorine disinfecting solution
Chlorine-releasing agents have long been established as disinfection systems for swimming pools, baby-feeding equipment and medical instrumentation. In the 1980s, chlorine-releasing systems were developed for the disinfection of **soft contact lenses**. These were seen as being highly convenient because of their ease of use, portability and low adverse reaction rate. In markets that did not have access to multipurpose solutions when planned replacement lenses were introduced at the end of the 1980s, these systems became very popular.

Two chlorine-releasing systems achieved market success. **Alcon** introduced the Softab product in the early 1980s. This was a tablet of sodium dichloroisocyanurate, which was dissolved in saline to form three parts per million (ppm) chlorine. **Sauflon** developed the Aerotab product in the mid-1980s which released 8 ppm chlorine. These solutions were effective at killing a range of micro-organisms, including bacteria and fungi; the killing action was thought to be due to the direct effect of the chlorine on some vital constituent of the cell of the micro-organism, such as its protoplasm or enzyme system. However, these products became associated with an increase in contact lens-related microbial keratitis – for example, the 'optimal' use of a chlorine system was associated an approximately 15-fold increase in the likelihood of **Acanthamoeba keratitis** compared with **hydrogen peroxide** or other solutions.

The association of ocular infections with chlorine solutions, despite satisfactory laboratory performance, suggests that there were problems with the efficacy of these systems with normal day-to-day usage. One issue was that the overnight dissipation of chlorine resulted in a loss of disinfecting power, so prolonged storage was not appropriate with these products. There was also evidence that the antimicrobial performance was severely reduced when lenses were soiled. The negative publicity generated by the high incidence of **microbial keratitis** among users of chlorine disinfection systems, and the widespread availability of **multipurpose solutions** which were also very easy to use, led to a great reduction in the use of chlorine-releasing systems throughout the 1990s.

ChromaGen lenses

The ChromaGen lens is available in the form of a **soft contact lens** or as sunglasses. The contact lens is prescribed for either one or both eyes, depending on the type and severity of the defect. A variety of tints are available, and a trial and error method is used to determine the combination that gives the best subjective response in terms of an apparent enhancement of colour vision. The precise mechanism that allows colour perception to be changed by ChromaGen lenses in those suffering from colour vision deficiency is not certain. It is claimed that the difference in images produced by the different ChromaGen filters produces what is known as a haploscopic effect, which may change the way that the brain interprets coloured images from the eye. It is also claimed that these lenses cure dyslexia and migraine. Most of these claims have been challenged and/or rejected, and a great deal of further research is necessary in order to prove the efficacy of this product. *See* X-Chrom lens.

CIBA Vision

CIBA Vision was established in 1980 as a diversification effort of Ciba-Geigy's US Pharmaceutical Division. In 1996, Ciba-Geigy merged with Sandoz to form Novartis, the world's leading life sciences company, and CIBA Vision became the eye care unit of Novartis. Today CIBA Vision is the world's third largest company in the combined optics segment (lenses and lens care products), and the world's sixth largest company in the ophthalmic pharmaceuticals segment. With headquarters in Atlanta, Georgia, USA, CIBA Vision manufactures **soft** and **rigid contact lenses** and solutions. The company acquired the Wesley Jessen Pilkington Barnes Hind group of companies in 2000. Website: www.cibavision.co.uk

cicatricial conjunctivitis, therapeutic lenses for

No type of contact lens can prevent conjunctival shrinkage, but a **scleral lens** or ring can support the fornices during the healing process following mucous membrane transplantation. More usually, contact lenses are fitted to protect the **cornea** from the hostile environment created by the disease. *See* eyelid pathology, therapeutic lenses for.

cilia
See eyelids.

CJD
See trial lens set disinfection.

cleaning
See surfactant cleaning.

clinical records
See record keeping.

Cochet–Bonnet aesthesiometer

Measurement of **corneal sensitivity** in the clinical setting has traditionally been achieved by using a Cochet–Bonnet aesthesiometer (Figure C.3). This device can be hand held or mounted on a slit lamp, and uses a single nylon thread to produce various forces by varying its length in 0.5-cm steps (the longer the thread, the lighter the force). The filament is placed lightly onto the **cornea** by the clinician, using a support that allows manipulation in the x–y–z planes, whilst being viewed through the **slit-lamp biomicroscope**. The subject reports when the thread can be felt on the ocular surface, and the length of thread at which this occurs is recorded. The corneal touch threshold is defined as the length of the nylon filament at which the subject responds to 50% of the number of stimulations. This length is converted into pressure using a calibration curve, and the reciprocal of this value gives the corneal sensitivity. Using this technique it has been demonstrated that corneal sensitivity varies with surface location and is altered by age, iris colour, ambient temperature, time of day, contact lens wear and pregnancy.

A number of factors complicate the use of such a device and can result in variations in the results obtained. These include physical aversion to the

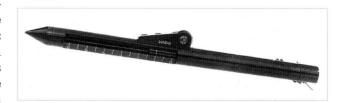

Figure C.3 Cochet–Bonnet aesthesiometer.

approach of the device, problems with mounting the device accurately in the slit lamp, and the impact of ambient humidity on the stiffness of the thread.

Cogan's microcystic dystrophy
See recurrent erosion syndrome, therapeutic lenses for.

collagen fibrils
See corneal stroma.

collagen lamellae
See corneal stroma.

coloured lenses
See ChromaGen lenses; tinted lenses; X-Chrom lens.

comfort drops
See re-wetting solutions, soft lens; wetting solutions, rigid lens.

comfort, soft lens
See fitting soft lenses.

compensated rigid bitoric lens
These are lenses that, like **spherical lenses**, do not correct for any residual **astigmatism**. They are bitoric because the front surface contains a cylinder solely for the correction of the induced astigmatism. A compensated bitoric can be thought of as a lens designed to correct all of the refractive cylinder created due to the corneal toricity. If the corneal toricity is equal to the spectacle astigmatism, then the cylinder will be fully corrected when a compensated bitoric lens is worn. A compensated bitoric lens can rotate on the eye without visual disturbance because the effect of the rotation is counteracted by an equal change in the cylinder power of the tear lens. *See* cylindrical power equivalent rigid toric lenses; induced astigmatism with rigid toric lenses; residual astigmatism with rigid toric lenses; stabilization of rigid toric lenses; toric lens design, rigid; toric lens, rigid.

compliance
See non-compliance.

compliance enhancement
The general principles of enhancing patient compliance with instructions and guidelines issued by an eye care practitioner are encapsulated in the following guidelines:

1. *The clinic.* The clinic must have the following qualities:
   - staff should be informed and aware of key issues
   - advice given should be consistent over time and between personnel
   - appointment times should be individualized (as opposed to 'block booking')
   - waiting times should be minimal
   - there should be continuity of care wherever possible
   - the clinical environment should be warm and friendly.

2. *The practitioner.* Important qualities of the practitioner are to:
   - project (rather than internalize) a devotion to eye care
   - listen effectively to what the patient has to say
   - use minimum jargon
   - emphasize key points, especially following delivery of a long and perhaps complex set of instructions
   - set specific and realistic goals for patients to aim at
   - adopt strategies to motivate patients.

3. *Aftercare.* Strategies for optimizing the effectiveness of the **aftercare** visit include:
   - sending appointment reminders
   - advising patients of the importance of regular check-ups
   - providing feedback and reward to patients
   - repetition of key information
   - stimulating the patient's interest in vision
   - providing in-practice information via leaflets and posters, videos etc.

4. *The patient.* A valuable approach to learning patient attitudes is to explore the health beliefs using a compliance 'decision tree' (*see* Figure C.4). The answers to the sequence of questions posed in the decision tree will indicate whether or not the patient is likely to be compliant with a contact lens system. If it is determined that the health beliefs of the patient are likely to lead to non-compliance, steps should be taken to modify the erroneous beliefs. This can be achieved via a variety of strategies, such as talking persuasively, supplying pertinent information, or utilizing a health care contract that emphasizes the responsibilities of the patient for achieving safe and comfortable ocular health during lens wear.

5. *The advice.* Care systems should be simple and easy to understand, tailored for the individual, ritualized, and not too expensive. Advice given to patients should be verbal and written. Printed material should be readable and well illustrated. Clearly illustrated sequential steps with minimum wording will aid understanding and interpretation. Written material should also contain warnings; obviously, a balance must be found

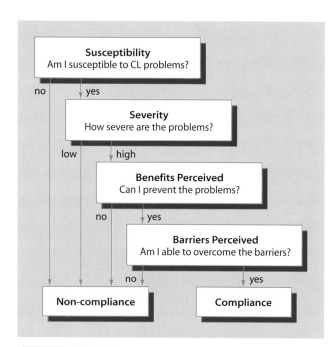

Figure C.4 'Decision tree' for exploring patient health beliefs.

whereby patients are alerted to possible dangers but are not frightened away from wearing lenses.

6. *The contact lens industry.* An important role is played by the contact lens industry in compliance enhancement, and this role falls into three broad categories:

- pricing policy – it is self-evident that prohibitive **pricing** will produce a general disincentive to purchase all of the required products and to use them as required, and the contact lens care industry thus has an obligation to contain prices as far as economically possible

- product support – clear and unambiguous packaging and simple instructions are thought to be important contributing factors to compliance enhancement, and such issues are the sole responsibility of the contact lens industry; many companies also provide attractive 'starter packs' which motivate patients

- research and development – contact lens care systems should be designed to be effective, as distinct from the usual practice of designing systems that are merely efficacious. An efficacious system is one that can be demonstrated to work under ideal situations – that is, assuming full patient compliance – whereas an efficient system is one that will work in a 'real world' scenario, allowing for a certain

level of inevitable non-compliance. Full compliance does not exist; all patients will be at least partially non-compliant in some aspect of their care regimen. If this argument is accepted, then it behoves the contact lens industry to develop effective contact lens care systems. *See* non-compliance.

conditioning solutions
See wetting solutions, rigid lens.

confocal microscope
The confocal microscope (Figure C.5) is unlike conventional microscopes because defocus causes the image to disappear rather than appear as a blurred image. The properties of the confocal microscope stem from its ability to focus the illuminating light and the focal plane of the microscope objective on precisely the same point. In most modern clinical confocal microscopes a point light source is focused onto a small volume within the specimen and a confocal point detector is used to collect the resulting signal. This results in a reduction of the amount of out-of-focus signal from above and below the focal plane, producing a marked increase in both lateral (x, y) and axial (z) resolution. Because only one tiny area of the specimen is observed by each point source, a useful full field of view must be gained by mechanically scanning the area of interest. By varying the plane of focus of both the source and detector within the tissue, the specimen can be optically 'sectioned' non-invasively and detailed information on corneal structure determined.

The microscope objectives most commonly used are non-applanating water immersion objectives that are optically coupled to the **cornea** using a methyl-

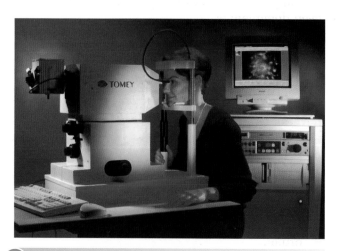

Figure C.5 Confocal microscope.

cellulose gel. To obtain the maximum axial resolution (and hence optical sectioning), it is necessary to use a microscope objective with a large numerical aperture (which describes the light-gathering ability of the objective). However, there is a compromise in that such devices have a reduced field of view and shorter free working distances, which reduces the distance that the microscope can focus into the specimen from the surface.

The variable-slit, real-time, scanning confocal microscope has two independently adjustable slits that are located in conjugate planes. A rapidly oscillating two-sided mirror is used to scan the image of the slit over the plane of the cornea to produce optical sectioning in real time. This design has the advantages of optimal image contrast, enhanced clarity and decreased scan time, but it is more expensive than Nipkow-based systems, and z-axis quantification is not currently possible.

An adaptation of this technique, known as confocal microscopy through focusing (CMTF), rapidly moves the focal plane of the objective lens through the entire cornea at a speed of approximately 80 µm/s while x–y images are acquired at the focal plane. This means that approximately 450 sequential images (which are separated by approximately 1 µm) are acquired over the time taken to traverse the cornea (approximately 15 s). The cornea is then reconstructed using image-processing techniques and an image is produced that is similar to a histological section, albeit in three-dimensions in a living cornea. Using such techniques confocal microscopy has provided valuable data on the structure and appearance of the cornea in many disease processes, including dystrophies, keratitis and endothelial disease. In addition, corneal changes following refractive surgery, keratoplasty and contact lens wear have been documented.

conjunctiva

The conjunctiva is a thin, transparent mucous membrane that extends from the **eyelid** margins anteriorly, providing a lining to the inside of the lids before turning sharply upon itself to form the fornices, from where it is reflected onto the globe, covering the sclera up to its junction with the **cornea**. It thus forms a sac that opens anteriorly through the palpebral fissure. The conjunctiva is conventionally divided into the following regions (Figure C.6):

- marginal
- tarsal
- orbital
- bulbar
- limbal.

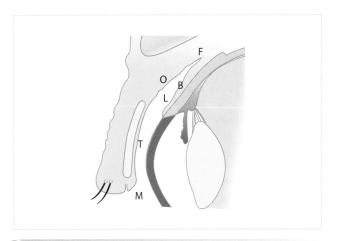

Figure C.6 Schematic representation of cross-section through the eyelid and conjunctival sac, showing the following regions: M = marginal, T = tarsal, O = orbital, B = bulbar, L = limbal, F = fornical.

The marginal, tarsal and orbital conjunctiva collectively form the palpebral conjunctiva.

The marginal zone extends from a line immediately posterior to the openings of the tarsal glands and passes around the eyelid margin, from where it continues on the inner surface of the lid as far as the sub-tarsal fold (a shallow groove that marks the marginal edge of the tarsal plate). The tarsal conjunctiva is highly vascular and is firmly attached to the underlying fibrous connective tissue. From the convex border of the tarsal plate, the orbital zone extends as far as the fornices. Over this region the conjunctiva is more loosely attached to underlying tissues, and so readily folds. Elevations of the conjunctival surface in the form of papillae and lymphoid follicles are commonly observed here.

The transparency of the bulbar conjunctiva readily permits the visualization of conjunctival and episcleral blood vessels. Here, the conjunctiva is freely movable due to its loose attachment to Tenon's capsule (the fascial sheath of the globe). As the bulbar conjunctiva approaches the cornea, its surface becomes smoother and its attachment to the sclera increases. The limbal conjunctiva extends approximately 1–1.5 mm around the cornea. Its junction with the cornea is ill defined, particularly in the vertical meridian, due to a variable degree of conjunctival/scleral overlap. The limbus has a rich blood supply, and in the majority of individuals a radial array of connective tissue elevations – the palisades of Vogt – can be seen adjacent to the corneal margin. The palisades are most prominent in the vertical meridian, and their visibility is enhanced in pigmented eyes.

The conjunctiva contributes the mucin component of the pre-ocular **tear film**, and plays an important role in the defence of the ocular surface against microbial infection. Mucins are a family of high molecular weight glycoproteins, which includes membrane-bound and secretory varieties. **Conjunctival goblet cells** are the primary source of secretory mucin, whilst surface epithelial cells of both the conjunctiva and cornea possess mucin-like molecules within their glycocalyx. The conjunctiva also forms part of a common mucosal defence system, which is an important component of the defence of the human body against micro-organisms. The conjunctiva possesses the immunological capacity for antigen processing, and cell-mediated and humoral immunity. Humoral immunity is provided by specific antibody (particularly IgA) produced by transformed B-cells (plasma cells) in the stroma. T-lymphocytes form the basis of cell-mediated immunity.

conjunctival blood vessels

The arterial supply of the **conjunctiva** derives from two sources; palpebral branches of the nasal and lacrimal arteries, and the anterior ciliary arteries. Palpebral vessels serve two vascular arcades within the eyelid. The inferior (marginal) arcade sends branches through the tarsal plate to the eyelid margin and tarsal conjunctiva. The superior (palpebral) arcade supplies the tarsal, orbital, fornix, and bulbar conjunctiva. The limbal zone, in contrast, is served by anterior ciliary arteries. The anterior ciliary arteries travel along the tendons of the rectus muscles and give off branches at the episcleral level prior to dipping down into the sclera to link with the major iridic circle. Episcleral branches pass forward and loop back a few millimetres short of the **cornea** to become conjunctival vessels. Forward extensions of these vessels form the limbal arcades (limbal loops), which is a complex network of fine capillaries. Conjunctival veins are more numerous than arteries. They can be readily differentiated from arteries due to their larger calibre, darker colour and more tortuous path.

conjunctival epithelium

The superficial layer of the **conjunctiva**. In the marginal zone, the conjunctival epithelium is stratified and squamous with few goblet cells. A subpopulation of these cells, which lie close to the mucocutaneous junction, may be acting as stem cells for the palpebral conjunctiva. Approaching the tarsus, the epithelium thins to two to three layers of cuboidal cells with scattered goblet cells. The epithelium of the orbital zone is slightly thicker (two to four cells), with more numerous goblet cells. The number of goblet cells declines over the bulbar conjunctiva, and at the limbus the epithelium is again stratified squamous, and goblet cells are absent. The limbus contains a unique array of connective tissue ridges (the palisades of Vogt) that project into the overlying epithelium. The palisades are the repositories of stem cells, and therefore act as the regenerative organ of the corneal epithelium. The conjunctival epithelium additionally contains several non-native cells, including dendritic cells, melanocytes and lymphocytes.

conjunctival goblet cells

These cells provide the mucus component of the **tear film**. They arise in the basal cell layers and migrate to the surface, becoming fully differentiated. Mature goblet cells are larger than the surrounding epithelial cells and contain a peripherally placed nucleus. The cytoplasm is packed with membrane-bound secretory granules, which discharge from the apical surface in an apocrine manner. The number of goblet cells shows a marked regional variation in density (Figure C.7), and they are occasionally seen lining intra-epithelial crypts (of Henle).

The apices of many surface epithelial cells of the **conjunctiva** contain numerous carbohydrate-containing secretory vesicles, which are seen to migrate to the cell surface where they fuse with the plasma membrane. It is likely that this represents a mechanism for recycling the cell-surface glycocalyx rather than a secondary source of secretory mucin.

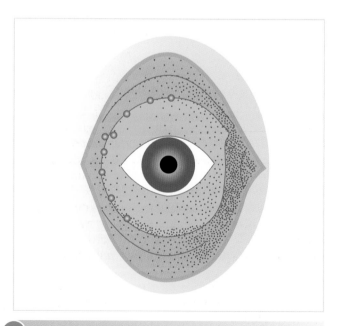

Figure C.7 Regional variation in goblet cell density in the conjunctiva.

conjunctival nerves

The **conjunctiva** receives nerves from sensory, sympathetic, and parasympathetic sources. Sensory nerves, which are trigeminal in origin, reach the conjunctiva via branches of the ophthalmic nerve. The principal function of these fibres is to equip the conjunctiva with the ability to detect a variety of sensations – for example, touch, pain, warmth and cold. Sensory nerve terminals include both free (unspecialized) nerve endings and the more complex corpuscular endings (classically referred to as Krause end bulbs). **Conjunctival blood vessels** receive a dual autonomic innervation. Parasympathetic fibres (issuing from the pterygopalatine ganglion) and sympathetic fibres (from the superior cervical ganglion) are responsible for vasodilation and vasoconstriction, respectively.

conjunctival redness

The clinical presentation of a 'red eye' can be one of the most difficult cases to solve due to the numerous possible known causes. This problem may be even more complex in a contact lens wearer because of the wide variety of causes of contact lens-related red eye. Conjunctival redness in lens wearers is generally asymptomatic, but patients may complain of itchiness, congestion, non-specific mild irritation, or a warm or cold feeling. The existence of pain usually indicates corneal involvement or other tissue pathology (e.g. uveitis or scleritis).

The **conjunctiva** contains a rich plexus of arterioles, which comprise of a thick layer of smooth muscle that is richly enervated with sympathetic nerve fibres. The smooth muscle, as well as being under central autonomic control, can be influenced by numerous local changes. Vasodilation refers to enlargement in the circumference of a vessel due to relaxation of its smooth muscle layer, which leads to decreased resistance and increased blood flow through the vessel (active hyperaemia). Since blood vessels can be observed directly through the transparent conjunctiva; this leads to an appearance of increased redness (less white sclera is visible).

A contact lens can have a local mechanical effect on the conjunctiva, resulting in increased redness. A contact lens is a device that a) can interfere with normal metabolic processes of the cornea and conjunctiva, and b) is used in association with various solutions, and can therefore affect the level of conjunctival redness via a local chemical or toxic effect. Local infection and inflammation can cause eye redness. Accordingly, treatment options fall into four broad categories:

1. Alterations to the type, design and modality of lens wear
2. Alterations to care systems
3. Improving ocular hygiene
4. Prescription of pharmaceutical agents.

In general, removal of any noxious stimulus (including a contact lens) will lead to a very rapid recovery of eye redness to normal levels. Recovery from chronic contact lens-induced redness after removal of lenses and cessation of wear takes about 2 days. *Syn.* conjunctival hyperaemia, conjunctival injection.

conjunctival staining

This manifests as areas or spots of increased fluorescence observed following the instillation of **fluorescein** into the eye and observation using cobalt blue light. About 60% of contact lens wearers exhibit conjunctival staining greater than Grade 1, versus about 10% of non-lens wearers. Small streaks of linear staining parallel to the limbus are a normal finding; this is due to pooling of fluorescein in natural conjunctival folds. The symptom of dryness is associated with increased conjunctival staining.

An imprint can be created on the **conjunctiva** as a result of chafing or physical compression by the edge of a soft lens. Chafing may be due to a lens edge design that causes the edge to 'dig in' to the conjunctiva. **Defects** in the lens edge can cause increased conjunctival staining (Figure C.8). Fitting a lens with a different edge design and a 'defect-free' edge will alleviate this problem.

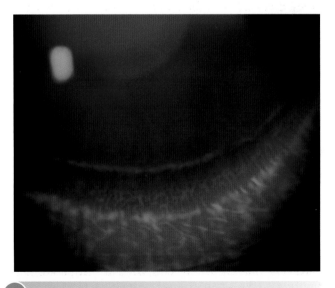

Figure C.8 Conjunctival and corneal ring staining caused by defects in the edge and periphery of a soft lens.

Compression staining will usually be accompanied by a tight fitting and/or a decentred lens, and manifests as a broad ring of heavy conjunctival staining corresponding to the lens edge, which is clearly evident following lens removal. Conjunctival vessels distal to the lens edge may be engorged. The patient is usually asymptomatic. This condition can be solved by refitting the patient with a lens of greater back optic zone radius.

Instillation of fluorescein in a **dry-eye** patient may reveal the presence of desiccation staining on the conjunctiva, which manifests as a series of diffuse punctate lesions within the interpalpebral zone. The condition will return to normal soon after removing the lens, but long-term resolution may require a combination of treating the underlying cause of the dry eye and refitting the patient with lenses that will facilitate complete conjunctival wetting.

Compromise to the conjunctiva as revealed by fluorescein staining is of concern because of recent demonstrations of morphologic changes to the conjunctival epithelium associated with lens wear. These changes include alterations to conjunctival cell shape, nuclear morphology and chromatin condensation, and are reported to be more prevalent in symptomatic lens wearers. **Soft lens** wear is also associated with a reduction in goblet cell density; this could lead to a reduction in mucus production, which in turn could explain and perhaps further exacerbate pre-existing symptoms of dryness.

conjunctival stroma

The conjunctival stroma (substantia propria) lies beneath the **conjunctival epithelium**, and is variable in thickness. It can be resolved into two distinct layers; a superficial adenoid layer and a deeper fibrous layer. The adenoid layer contains numerous lymphocytes with local accumulations in the form of lymphoid follicles. Follicles represent aggregates of predominantly B-cells, which form part of the so-called 'conjunctiva-associated lymphoid tissue' (CALT). The adenoid layer also contains a large number of mast cells, which play a major role in ocular allergy. The deep fibrous layer is generally thicker than the adenoid layer, and contains the majority of **conjunctival blood vessels** and **nerves**.

contact aesthesiometry

See Cochet–Bonnet aesthesiometer.

contact lens

A transparent optical device with dioptric power that is applied directly to the surface of the eye for the purpose of correcting defects of vision.

contact lens hygienist

See patient education.

contact lens induced acute red eye (CLARE)

Previously referred to as 'acute red eye reaction' and 'tight lens syndrome', CLARE is an acute complication of **extended soft lens wear**. In its mild form the patient notices problems upon waking naturally; when severe the patient may be awakened by the symptoms, which include ocular pain, tearing and photophobia. The patient then quickly discovers that he or she has a red eye (Figure C.9). Clinical signs include conjunctival and limbal hyperaemia, and small corneal infiltrates near the limbus.

The lens may display little or no movement upon initial examination of a patient suffering from CLARE, and debris can sometimes be seen trapped beneath the lens. **Corneal epithelial staining** may be detected following lens removal. Other transient clinical signs include anterior chamber flare, **endothelial bedewing** and guttata, low-grade corneal **neovascularization**, foci of swollen epithelium, and small non-staining areas on the corneal surface (dry spots). About 10% of cases of CLARE are bilateral, and the mean time to the first occurrence of CLARE after being fitted with extended wear soft lenses is about 10 months.

contact lens peripheral ulcer (CLPU)

This condition, which is typically seen in hydrogel **extended-wear** lens patients, is characterized by the presence of one or two small, round, full-thickness epithelial lesions (without raised edges) in the peripheral or paracentral **cornea** (Figure C.10). There is an absence of severe ocular pain, mucopurulent discharge or anterior chamber reaction. However, the patient may experience mild to moderate

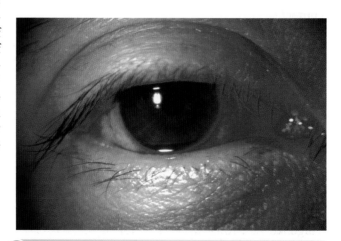

Figure C.9 Contact lens acute red eye (CLARE) with the causative bound soft lens still in place.

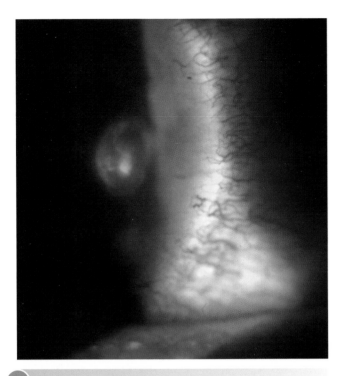

Figure C.10 Contact lens peripheral ulcer.

ocular discomfort or foreign body sensation, mild photophobia and increased tearing. Associated signs may include conjunctival and limbal hyperaemia, and infiltrates beneath or surrounding the epithelial lesion. This condition is typically uniocular, and the mean time to the first occurrence of CLPU after being fitted with extended-wear soft lenses is 26 ± 22 months. If a culture from a scraping of the ulcer fails to reveal the presence of micro-organisms, the condition may be termed a culture-negative peripheral ulcer (CNPU).

contact shell
A transparent optical device without dioptric power that is applied directly to the surface of the eye for the purpose of correcting defects of vision by neutralizing an abnormal corneal shape (e.g. as in **keratoconus**).

continuous wear
See extended wear.

conventional lenses
See non-planned lens replacement.

convergence demand
Contact lenses move with the eyes, and hence convergence demands when viewing near objects are identical to those applying in the uncorrected state. In contrast, **myopes** with a negative spectacle correction for distance observe near objects through base-in prisms, since they are no longer looking through the optical centres of their lenses. The base-in prismatic effects reduce the convergence requirement, as compared to the naked eye or contact lens situation. Spectacle-corrected **hypermetropes**, however, experience a base-out effect at near, which increases the convergence demand. Allowing for a typical interpupillary distance of 65 mm and the centre of rotation of each eye being about 12 mm behind the **cornea**, application of Prentice's rule shows that, for an object distance of 33 cm, the convergence demand for each eye is reduced by about (0.25 × lens power) prism dioptres for a negative spectacle correction and similarly increased for a positive correction. In most cases, then, the change in convergence demand is small as compared with the fusion reserves. Since both **accommodation** and convergence demands are higher for **myopes** with contact lenses, and lower for hypermetropes, the accommodation-convergence links are minimally disturbed.

CooperVision
Cooper Laboratories was founded by Parker Montgomery in 1958. In 1979, Cooper Laboratories was renamed CooperVision, went public on the New York stock exchange, and launched Permalens™, the first lens approved by the USA Food and Drug Administration for 30-day continuous wear. In 1986 CooperVision changed the name of its public company to the Cooper Companies and moved its eye care assets to a subsidiary, which became known as CooperVision. CooperVision purchased England-based Aspect Vision Care in 1997, and **Biocompatibles–Hydron** in 2002.

Headquartered in Irvine, California, CooperVision has several manufacturing facilities throughout the world, and has direct sales operations in the key markets of the UK, Italy, Germany, Sweden, Norway, Spain, Australia, the USA and Canada, plus an extensive distribution network in over 40 countries. Its Rochester-based facility manufactures soft toric and spherical lenses. Custom soft toric and spherical lenses are produced at Huntington Beach, USA. Planned replacement lenses are manufactured in Hampshire, UK. Throughout Europe, CooperVision UK also has a substantial private label business. Website: www.coopervision.co.uk

co-polymers
See polymers.

cornea
The cornea is the transparent structure at the front of the eyeball that allows light to enter the eye. It is

elliptical when viewed from in front, with its long axis in the horizontal meridian. This asymmetry is produced by a greater degree of overlap of the peripheral cornea by opaque limbal tissue in the vertical meridian. The surface area of the cornea is a 1.1 cm², which represents about 7% of the surface area of the globe. Topographically, the cornea is conventionally divided into four zones; central, paracentral, peripheral and limbal. The central zone, which covers the entrance pupil of the eye, is spherical, approximately 4 mm wide, and principally determines high-resolution image formation on the fovea. The paracentral zone, which lies outside the central zone, is flatter and becomes optically important in dim illumination, when the pupil dilates. The peripheral zone is where the cornea is flattest and most aspheric. Owing to differences in curvature between its posterior and anterior surfaces, the cornea shows a regional variation in thickness. Centrally the thickness is approximately 0.52 mm, increasing towards the periphery to 0.67 mm.

The cornea consists of the following layers (Figure C.11), working from the outermost layer: **epithelium**, **anterior limiting lamina** (also referred to as Bowman's membrane), **stroma**, **posterior limiting lamina** (also referred to as Descemet's membrane) and **endothelium**.

corneal abrasion
See relief of pain, therapeutic lenses for.

corneal distortion
See corneal warpage.

corneal dystrophy
See recurrent erosion syndrome, therapeutic lenses for.

corneal endothelium
The endothelium is a monolayer of squamous cells that lines the posterior surface of the **cornea** (Figure C.12). As it has a limited capacity for mitosis to replace damaged or effete cells, there is a progressive reduction in the number of endothelial cells with age. At birth the cornea contains a total of approximately 500 000 cells, which represents a mean density of 4500 cells/mm². During infancy cell loss is particularly marked, and a 26% reduction occurs in the first year. Thereafter the rate of loss progressively declines into old age. Since grafted corneas appear to maintain transparency and functional normality with an endothelial cell density of less than 1000 cells/mm², it would seem that the normal cell density represents a considerable 'physiological reserve'. The endothelium appears as a mosaic of polygonal (typically hexagonal) cells. In

Figure C.11 Transverse section through the cornea. The stroma, which represents 90% of the thickness of the cornea, is bounded by the epithelium (asterisk) and endothelium (arrow).

response to ocular and systemic pathology, trauma, age and prolonged contact lens wear, the endothelial mosaic becomes less regular, and shows a greater variation in cell size (**polymegethism**) and shape (pleomorphism), as cells spread to fill gaps caused by cell loss. The lateral borders of the cells are markedly convoluted, and adjacent cells are linked by tight junctions (with less frequent gap junctions). The complement of organelles seen in endothelial cells reflects their high metabolic activity, with numerous mitochondria and a prominent rough endoplasmic reticulum.

corneal epithelial wound healing
A smooth and intact **corneal epithelium** is necessary in order for the cornea to maintain clear vision. However, due to its exposed position the **cornea** is potentially vulnerable to a variety of external insults, including contact lens wear. The cornea possesses several protective mechanisms to avoid injury, but

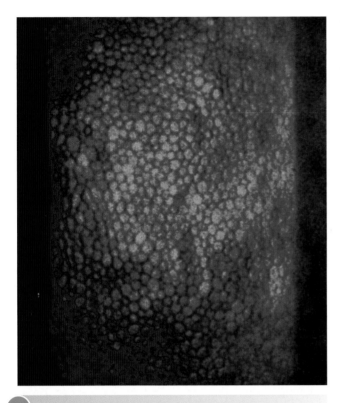

Figure C.12 Normal human corneal endothelium.

should tissue damage occur it is capable of an effective wound healing response. Corneal epithelial repair is a complex process involving an orchestrated interaction between cells and extracellular matrix, which is co-ordinated by a variety of growth factors. The process can be divided into three phases:

1. Initial covering of the denuded area by cell migration
2. Cell proliferation to replace lost cells
3. Epithelial differentiation to reform the normal stratified epithelial architecture.

Following a full-thickness epithelial defect, fibronectin, an adhesive glycoprotein, is synthesized and covers the surface of the bared stroma, where it serves as a temporary matrix for cell migration. The adhesion between fibronectin and the epithelium is mediated by integrin–matrix interactions (integrins are a family of cell surface receptors which bind to certain extracellular matrix proteins). Several growth factors have been implicated in the control of the wound healing response, including epidermal growth factor (EGF), transforming growth factor beta (TGFβ), platelet-derived growth factor (PDGF) and fibroblast growth factor (FGF). Growth factors, which are produced by a variety of sources (e.g. ocular surface epithelia and the lacrimal gland), are able

to regulate the process of epithelial migration, proliferation and differentiation. Epithelial–stromal interactions play an important role in corneal wound healing. Epithelial injury triggers keratocyte apoptosis (programmed cell death) in the anterior stroma via the release of apoptosis-inducing cytokines from epithelial cells. Keratocyte apoptosis subsequently triggers a wound healing cascade, which influences epithelial repair.

Regeneration of the corneal epithelium is highly dependent on the integrity of the limbus. A proportion of limbal basal epithelial cells possess the properties of stem cells, which are ultimately responsible for corneal epithelial replacement. Stem cells have several unique characteristics – they are poorly differentiated, long-lived, and have a high capacity for self-renewal. When these cells divide, one of the daughter cells replenishes the stem cell pool whilst the other is destined to undergo further cell divisions before differentiating. Such a cell is referred to as a 'transient amplifying' (TA) cell. Transient amplifying cells undergo several rounds of cell division before fully differentiating. These cells play an important role in epithelial wound healing, where their proliferative capacity is increased by shortening cycle times and increasing the number of times that the TAC cells can divide before maturation.

corneal epithelium

The epithelium is the outermost layer of the **cornea**, and represents approximately 10% of the thickness of the cornea (50 μm). It is a stratified squamous non-keratinized epithelium, consisting of five to six layers of cells. Three distinct epithelial cell types are recognized (Figure C.13); a single row of basal cells,

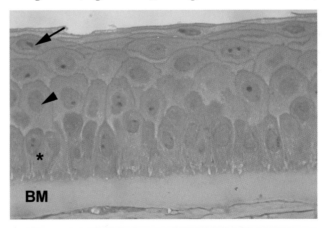

Figure C.13 Corneal epithelium in cross-section. Three cell types can be distinguished: basal cells (asterisk), wing cells (arrowhead) and squamous cells (arrow). BM = Bowman's membrane.

two to three rows of wing cells and two to three layers of superficial (squamous) cells. In addition, several non-epithelial cells are present (e.g. lymphocytes, macrophages and Langerhans cells). The epithelium forms a permeability barrier to small molecules, water and ions, as well as forming an effective barrier to the entry of pathogens. Further epithelial specialization enhances adhesion between cells, to withstand shearing and abrasive forces.

Superficial cells are structurally modified for their barrier function and interaction with the tear film. Scanning electron microscopy of surface cells shows extensive finger-like and ridge-like projections (microvilli and microplicae). Light, medium and dark cells can be distinguished, depending on the number and pattern of surface projections. It has been suggested that dark cells, which are relatively free of these surface features, are close to being desquamated into the **tear film**. By contrast, the newly arrived light cells possess a more extensive array of surface projections. In high power transmission electron micrographs, microvilli and microplicae show an extensive filamentous covering known as the glycocalyx. The glycocalyx is formed from membrane-bound glycoconjugates, and is important for the spreading and attachment of the pre-corneal **tear film**. In accordance with their barrier function, a complex network of tight junctions links superficial cells.

Wing cells are so named because of their characteristic shape, with lateral extensions and a concave inferior surface to accommodate the apices of the basal cells. Their nuclei tend to be spherical or elongated in the plane of the cornea. The cell borders of the polygonal wing cells show prominent infoldings, which interdigitate with adjacent cells, and numerous desmosomes. This arrangement results in a strong intercellular adhesion. The cytoplasm contains prominent cytoskeletal elements (predominantly actin and cytokeratin intermediate filaments), and although the usual complement of organelles is present, they are few in number.

Basal cells consist of single layer columnar cells with a vertically orientated oval nucleus. Ultrastructurally, they are similar in appearance to wing cells. The plasma membrane similarly shows pronounced infolding, and the cytoplasm contains prominent intermediate filaments. A variety of cell junctions are present, including: desmosomes, which mediate adhesion between cells; hemi-desmosomes, which are involved in the attachment of basal cells to the underlying stroma; and gap junctions, which allow for intercellular metabolic coupling. Basal cells form the germative layer of the cornea, and mitotic cells are often seen at this level.

corneal erosion
See recurrent erosion syndrome, therapeutic lenses for.

corneal exhaustion syndrome
This is a condition in which patients who have worn contact lenses for many years suddenly develop a severe intolerance to lens wear, and is characterized by:

- ocular **discomfort**
- reduced vision
- photophobia
- excessive **oedema**
- distorted endothelial mosaic
- moderate to severe polymegethism.

The suggested aetiology of this condition is that the corneal endothelium has become 'exhausted'; that is, it has suffered a reduced capacity to keep excess fluid from entering the corneal stroma. The evidence to support this concept is that patients with corneal exhaustion syndrome display marked **endothelial polymegethism**, which is in turn associated with an impaired capacity of the cornea to recover from excess stromal oedema (the endothelium being responsible for **corneal hydration control**).

corneal graft, lens fitting following
See post-keratoplasty, contact lens fitting.

corneal hydration control
The state of corneal hydration is an important determinant of corneal transparency. The hydrophilic properties of the **stroma** are to a large part determined by proteoglycans, which contribute to the fixed negative charge of the stroma and produce a passive gel swelling pressure through electrostatic repulsion. Physiologically, corneal hydration is maintained at approximately 78%. If the **cornea** is allowed to swell by ± 5% of this value, it begins to scatter significant quantities of light.

Mechanisms for the maintenance of physiological corneal hydration are located in the **corneal endothelium**; these mechanisms comprise a barrier function and a metabolically driven pump. The endothelial barrier to the free passage of molecules from the aqueous is formed principally by focal tight junctions between adjacent endothelial cells. However, in contrast to other barrier epithelia, these junctions are of low electrical resistance and allow the passage of ions and small molecules. This 'leak' is offset by the metabolically-driven pumping of ions out of the stroma by the endothelium, which maintains a transcellular potential difference (aqueous side negative) to balance stromal swelling pressure. Disruption of this osmotic gradient will result in stromal fluid imbibition.

A flux of bicarbonate ions is the predominant component of the endothelial ion transport system. The bicarbonate is generated either by a Na^+/HCO_3^- co-transporter located on the basolateral plasma membrane, or via the intercellular conversion of carbon dioxide by the enzyme carbonic anhydrase. Bicarbonate leaves the cell via an apical bicarbonate ion channel. The driving force for the bicarbonate flux is generated by a sodium-potassium ATPase, which resides on the basolateral endothelial membrane. The energy associated with subsequent sodium re-entry (via Na^+/H^+ and Na/HCO_3^- transporters) is coupled to active HCO_3^- flux.

The epithelium also contributes to corneal hydration control. The tight junctions between superficial epithelial cells form an effective permeability barrier to ions and polar solutes. For example, the anionic molecule sodium fluorescein does not penetrate an intact epithelium. Damage to the **superficial epithelial cells** allows **fluorescein** to enter the epithelium, with resulting **corneal staining**. In addition to its barrier properties, the epithelium also possesses active ion transport systems for Na^+ and Cl^-. Since these pumps contribute to the tonicity of the tear film, it is likely that they are involved in the maintenance of stromal hydration.

corneal metabolism

In order to perform its vital functions, the **cornea** requires a constant supply of oxygen and other essential metabolites (e.g. glucose, vitamins and amino acids). However, its avascularity dictates that alternative routes must exist for the provision of its metabolic needs. There are three possibilities:

1. Perilimbal vasculature
2. **Tear film**
3. Aqueous humour.

In open-eye conditions, the bulk of the oxygen required for the cornea is obtained from the atmosphere via diffusion across the pre-corneal tear film. Under steady state conditions it can be assumed that the tears are saturated with oxygen, and are therefore at an oxygen tension corresponding to the atmosphere (155 mmHg at sea level). The oxygen tension of the aqueous lies between 30 and 40 mmHg. The cornea depends on tear-side oxygen to avoid **oedema** and maintain normal function. During eye closure the oxygen level in the tears is in equilibrium with the palpebral vasculature (55 mmHg).

Significantly, corneal thickness increases by approximately 2–4% during sleep, and returns to baseline levels within 1 hour of eye opening. This is due primarily to reduced oxygen availability, but is also related to changes in tear film tonicity, temperature, humidity and pH. The oxygen flux into the cornea as a whole is in the region of 6 µl/cm^2 per hour, although the consumption rate for its composite layers is not equal. Consumption rates have been estimated as 40 : 39 : 21 for the epithelium, stroma and endothelium respectively.

The aqueous is the primary source of glucose and essential amino acids for the cornea. The glucose concentration of the tears is low compared to that of the aqueous, and the insertion of nutrient impermeable implants into the stroma results in degeneration of the tissue lying anterior to the implant. Although exogenous glucose is primarily utilized, glycogen stores are present in all corneal cells to provide glucose in conditions of metabolic stress. The role of the perilimbal vasculature in the provision of oxygen and nutrients is limited, and is only significant for the corneal periphery.

The cornea derives its energy principally from the oxidative breakdown of carbohydrates (Figure C.14). Glucose, which is the primary substrate for the generation of adenosine triphosphate (ATP), is catabolized by three metabolic pathways:

1. Glycolysis
2. Tricarboxylic acid TCA (Krebs) cycle
3. Hexose monophosphate shunt.

Anaerobic glycolysis accounts for the majority of glucose metabolism. In this pathway, glucose is first oxidized to pyruvate and then subsequently reduced to lactate, with a net yield of two molecules of ATP. The TCA cycle results in a greater energy yield (36 ATP). This pathway is most active in the corneal endothelium, which has the greatest energy requirement.

Metabolic waste products can be potentially damaging if allowed to accumulate. Although carbon dioxide can readily diffuse out of the cornea across its limiting layers, lactate is less easily eliminated. Under normoxic conditions, lactate is able to slowly diffuse across the endothelium into the anterior chamber. However, during periods of **hypoxia** the proportion of glucose that is metabolized anaerobically increases. The resulting accumulation of lactate causes stromal oedema via an increased osmotic load and localized tissue acidosis.

The hexose monophosphate shunt (also known as the pentose phosphate shunt) plays a significant role in the epithelium and endothelium, where it

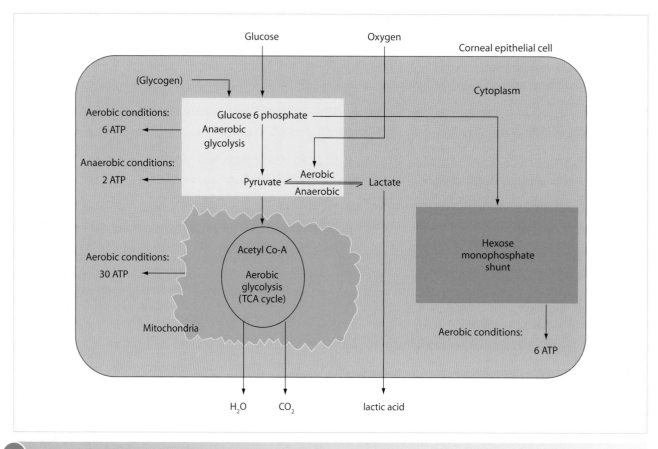

Figure C.14 Metabolic processes in a corneal epithelial cell.

accounts for 35–65% of glucose utilization. It fulfils several important functions, including the generation of intermediates for biosynthetic reactions and the prevention of oxidative damage by free radicals.

corneal moulding
See corneal warpage.

corneal nerves
The **cornea** is the most richly innervated surface tissue in the body, and it receives its predominantly sensory nerve supply from the nasociliary branch of the trigeminal nerve. There is also evidence for the existence of a modest sympathetic innervation from the superior cervical ganglion. Branches from the nasociliary nerve either pass directly to the eye as long ciliary nerves, or traverse the ciliary ganglion, leaving as short ciliary nerves that enter the eye close to the optic nerve. Nerves destined for the cornea travel initially in the suprachoroidal space, before crossing the sclera to advance radially towards the cornea.

Most of the 50–80 precorneal nerve trunks, which contain a mixture of myelinated and unmyelinated fibre bundles, enter the cornea at mid-stromal level.

Myelin is soon lost, and the unmyelinated nerve fibre bundles divide repeatedly and move anteriorly to form a rich plexiform network in the anterior one-third of the stroma (Figure C.15). Axons

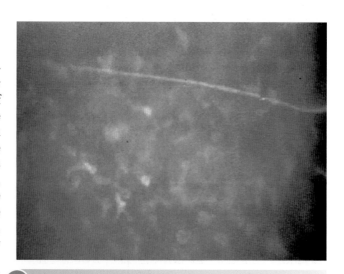

Figure C.15 Corneal nerve in a living human eye viewed with a confocal microscope.

are particularly dense immediately beneath the **anterior limiting lamina** (Bowman's layer). From this sub-epithelial plexus, axons pass vertically through the anterior limiting lamina, losing their Schwann cell sheath in the process. Upon entering the epithelium, axons turn through 90° and divide into a series of fine branches that course between the basal cells. Some branches pass into the more superficial layers before terminating. Corneal nerves display a complex neurochemistry. A variety of neurotransmitters and neuromodulators have been identified, including acetyl choline, substance P, and calcitonin gene-related peptide (CGRP). However, it is unclear how these particular neurochemicals correlate with function.

Corneal nerves serve important sensory, reflex and trophic functions. Damage to corneal sensory nerves by surgery, trauma or infection produces neuroparalytic keratitis – a condition that is characterized by progressive epithelial cell loss and oedema. The mechanism of this trophic role is not fully understood, although the release of neuropeptides (e.g. substance P and CGRP) may be a factor. Sympathetic nerves also play a role in epithelial maintenance by regulating ion transport processes, and cell proliferation and migration during wound healing.

corneal sensitivity

Carefully controlled corneal stimulation with a variety of mechanical, chemical and thermal stimuli evokes only sensations of irritation or pain. By contrast, electrophysiological studies of corneal afferent neurones have identified neurones that respond to mechanical, chemical and thermal stimulation. However, since the conscious perception of these sensations has not been demonstrated, it is likely that such specificity of modality is lost during central nervous system processing. Electrophysiological recording also allows for the mapping of receptive fields. These are often large and overlapping, which explains the inability of the **cornea** to localize a stimulus accurately. The sensitivity of the cornea to mechanical stimulation is particularly acute, and acts as a trigger for the protective blink and lacrimal reflexes. Cold receptors may be important in signalling evaporative cooling, which is a major determinant of spontaneous eye blink frequency.

Corneal sensitivity is measured as its touch threshold, and the classic technique for determining corneal touch threshold is with the **Cochet–Bonnet aesthesiometer**. Corneal sensitivity varies according to corneal location, with the central cornea being the most sensitive. The corneal touch threshold has proven to be a very sensitive measure of corneal health, with the cornea being perhaps the most sensitive organ (to touch) in the body. This has been shown to be a particularly useful measurement in contact lens wear, where the touch threshold may increase by over 100% when a non-gas permeable **polymethyl methacrylate** (PMMA) lens is worn.

corneal staining

Strictly speaking, 'corneal staining' is not a condition in itself; rather, it is a general term that refers to the appearance of tissue disruption and other pathophysiological changes in the anterior eye as revealed with the aid of one or more of a number of dyes, such as **fluorescein**, **rose bengal**, **lissamine green**, fluorexon or alcian blue. Fluorescein has by far the greatest utility in contact lens practice, so the term 'corneal staining' is generally taken to mean staining with fluorescein unless stated otherwise.

Corneal staining following instillation of fluorescein is observed under cobalt blue light as a bright green fluorescence, which can be described as 'punctate' (spot-like), 'diffuse' (spots merging together) and 'coalescent' (large regions of confluence) (Figure C.16). The staining pattern may be described according to the following groups of type descriptors:

- arcuate, linear or dimpled
- superior, inferior, temporal, nasal or central
- deep or superficial.

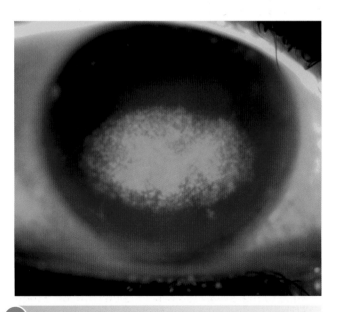

Figure C.16 Confluent corneal staining.

Staining 'syndromes' include:

- 'inferior epithelial arcuate lesion' ('smile stain')
- 'superior epithelial arcuate lesion' (SEAL; otherwise known as 'epithelial splitting')
- 'exposure keratitis'
- 'epithelial plug' – a large, coalescent field of full-thickness epithelial loss.

Observed areas of fluorescence indicates one of three phenomena:

1. Fluorescein entering damaged cells
2. Fluorescein entering intercellular spaces
3. Fluorescein filling the gaps in the epithelial surface that are created when epithelial cells are displaced.

Depending on the cause of the problem, severe staining (Grades 3 and 4) may be accompanied by:

- bulbar **conjunctival redness** and chemosis
- **limbal redness**
- excessive lacrimation
- stromal infiltrates.

Visual acuity is generally unaffected by corneal staining, although a slight loss might be expected in extreme cases (Grade 4). There is no clear relationship between the severity of staining and the degree of ocular discomfort.

There are numerous contact lens-related causes of corneal staining, which can be broadly classified into six aetiological categories:

1. Mechanical
2. Exposure
3. Metabolic
4. Toxic
5. Allergic
6. Infectious.

In many cases the pattern of staining, and whether the condition presents in one or both eyes, can provide a clue to the cause. Low level staining (less than Grade 2) does not necessarily require action to be taken. Such staining is commonly observed in contact lens wearers; it is typically transient, and in a daily lens wearer will have disappeared by the following morning. However, persistent minor staining forming a characteristic or repeatable pattern, as well as staining greater than Grade 2, may require intervention.

Management strategies are generally self-evident if the cause can be discerned. For example, mechanical trauma due to a foreign body trapped beneath a **rigid lens** can be resolved by removing and rinsing the lens and rinsing the eye; exposure keratitis causing 3 and

9 o'clock staining in a rigid lens wearer can be resolved by fitting **soft lenses**; epitheliopathy due to metabolic disturbance can be solved by fitting a lens of higher **oxygen transmissibility**; staining due to toxicity or allergy can be resolved by eliminating the toxic or allergic agent; and staining associated with an infection is treated by applying the appropriate antimicrobial therapy. Recovery from **corneal staining** generally occurs within hours or days of removal of the offending source, but will be more prolonged if lenses are worn during the recovery period.

corneal stroma

This structure is approximately 500 μm thick, and accounts for 90% of the thickness of the **cornea**. It is composed predominantly of collagen fibrils (68% dry weight) embedded in a highly hydrated matrix of proteoglycans. A variety of different collagen types have been identified. Type I is the major stromal collagen, and there are lesser amounts of types III, V and VI. Collagen fibrils are arranged in 200–250 layers (lamellae) running parallel to the surface. Lamellae are approximately 2 μm thick and 9–260 μm wide, and extend from limbus to limbus. Fibrils of adjacent lamellae make large angles with each other. In the superficial stroma angles are less than 90°, but they become orthogonal in the deeper stroma. This particular arrangement of collagen imparts a high tensile strength for corneal protection, which is important given its exposed position. Within lamellae, all collagen fibrils are parallel, with uniform size and separation. The mean fibril diameter in the human cornea is 31 nm, with an interfibrillar spacing of 55.3 nm. This narrow fibril diameter and constant separation, which is a characteristic of corneal collagen, is a necessary prerequisite for transparency.

The interfibrillar space contains a matrix of proteoglycans (approximately 10% of dry weight). Keratan sulphate and dermatan sulphate are the major corneal proteoglycans. These molecules are highly sulphated and, along with bound chloride ions, create a polyanionic stromal interfibrillar matrix, which induces osmotic swelling. As well as playing a major role in the maintenance of fixed levels of corneal hydration, collagen–proteoglycan interactions are important in determining the spatial arrangement of collagen fibrils.

Collagen and proteoglycans are maintained by keratocytes (Figure C.17). These cells occupy 3–5% of stromal volume and lie between collagen lamellae, flattened in the plane of the cornea. Keratocyte density is non-uniform; density decreases from superficial to deep stroma and increases from the centre to

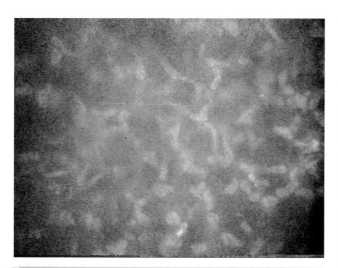

Figure C.17 Stromal keratocytes appear as irregular white spicular shapes when viewed with a confocal microscope (only the cell nuclei are visible).

the periphery. Keratocytes display a large central nucleus, and long slender processes extend from the cell body. Processes from adjacent cells sometimes make tight junctions with each other. Cell organelles are not numerous but comprise the usual complement of organelles, including, endoplasmic reticulum, Golgi apparatus and mitochondria.

corneal topographic analysis

The aim of corneal topography (also termed 'keratoscopy' or 'videokeratography') is to describe accurately the shape of the corneal surface in all meridians. In most cases the technique uses a similar principle to **keratometry**, in that it determines the size of the image of a target reflected in the corneal surface, the primary difference relating to the fact that for keratoscopy a series of circular concentric targets are used (a **Placido-disc** image; see below). This arrangement allows both central and peripheral curvature to be determined. The topographer captures the image electronically on a computer, and uses sophisticated image-processing software to provide immediate analysis of the reflected image (videokeratoscopy). Using this technique it has been clearly demonstrated that the **cornea** is aspheric, and can best be described as a flattening ellipse whose rate of flattening is asymmetrical about its centre.

Modern topographers can be categorized into two distinct forms; reflective devices and slit-scanning devices. Reflective devices measure topography based on the reflection of mires from the anterior surface tear film, which is essentially identical in shape to the corneal surface. The images are cap-

tured with a video camera, and a computational approach is adopted to analyse the data and derive a description for the corneal shape. The choice of computational method is important, as this will largely dictate the accuracy and validity of the keratoscope. The most frequently utilized computational method is the 'slope of surface' method. Basically, devices that use this technology measure slope directly as a function of distance from a central reference axis, and derive curvature from these results. It is important to note that these distance-based instruments are only estimating the average shape of the cornea, since the algorithms are based on a radially symmetric surface, which does not accurately describe the cornea. These axial or sagittal measurements result in an underestimation of the radius of curvature in areas that may be steeper than the central cornea, and an overestimation in areas that are flatter. More recently the algorithms have been modified, and are now generally based on the radius of curvature in an attempt to provide a better estimate of the local shape of the cornea.

The images (or 'maps') produced by reflective or placido-based keratoscopes display the power distribution of the corneal surface using colour-coded displays, in which greens and yellows represent powers characteristic of those found in normal corneas, blues or cooler colours represent flatter areas (low powers), and reds or hotter colours represent steep areas (high powers; Figure C.18). These maps permit recognition of corneal shape through pattern recognition, and swiftly reveal the presence of abnormal powers. All devices display simulated keratometry (SimK) values, which are analogous to standard keratometry values, and simultaneously display the power and axis of the flattest meridian. A number of manufacturers now produce hand-held topographers. These portable devices can prove very useful for examining children, the elderly and the infirm, and for 'off-site' consultations.

The Orbscan II™ device uses a slit scanning method to obtain topographic measurements of both anterior and posterior corneal surfaces, in addition to the anterior lens and iris. The instrument scans across the anterior corneal surface, obtaining 40 sequential slit images, whilst simultaneously recording eye movements and reflection data from a placido-disc device. The data are then reassembled into a three-dimensional reconstruction of the anterior and posterior corneal surfaces. The advantage of this system is that it allows for the measurement of multiple ocular surfaces. The instrument differs from traditional keratoscopes in that it uses a combination of slit scan triangulation and surface reflection to

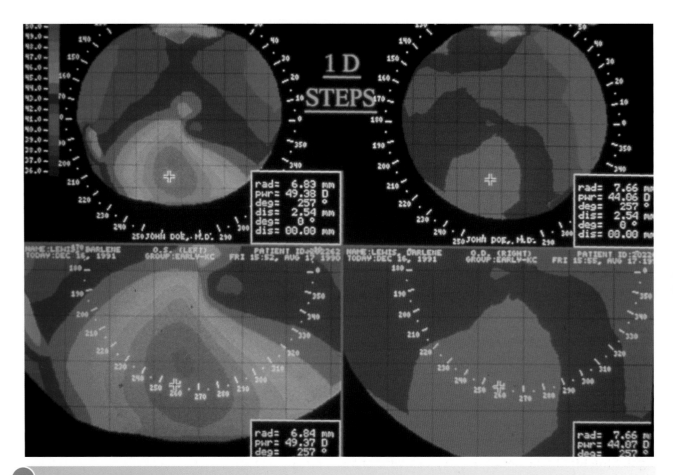

determine corneal shape. Specifically, this instrument unifies triangulated and reflective data to obtain accurate measurements of corneal elevation, slope, curvature and thickness. In addition to conventional axial and tangential maps, shape data can be displayed as an elevation map in which the relative height of the cornea is compared to a spherical reference surface. Elevations above the reference sphere are coloured red, and depressions below the reference sphere are coloured blue.

corneal topography

The topography of the anterior **cornea** is of particular interest since, as the dominant refractive surface, its form has a major influence on overall refractive error and ocular **aberration**. In contact lens work, it is of enormous importance to the fitting geometry.

The radius of curvature over the central region, as measured by conventional keratometers, shows considerable individual variation, and it has been recognized for more than a century that many corneas display marked **astigmatism**. Corneal astigmatism is not necessarily equal to the total ocular astigmatism, since additional astigmatism (residual astigmatism) may be contributed by the crystalline lens.

Earlier work on corneal topography using modifications of traditional **keratometers** concentrated on approximating the form of the corneal surface by a conicoid, in which each meridian is a conic section. In this approach the anterior corneal surface can be described by the equation:

$$x^2 + y^2 + pz^2 = 2r_0 z$$

where the coordinate system has its origin at the corneal apex, z is the axial coordinate, r_0 is the radius of curvature at the cornea apex, and the shape factor p is a constant parameter characterizing the form of the conic section for the individual eye. Values of $p < 0$ represent hyperboloids; $p = 0$, paraboloids; $0 < p < 1$, flattening (prolate) ellipsoids; $p = 1$, spheres; and $p > 1$, steepening (oblate) ellipsoids. The same equation is sometimes written in terms of the Q-factor or the eccentricity e of the conic section, where:

$$p = 1 + Q = 1 - e^2$$

Mean human r_0 and p values are 7.72 ± 0.27 mm and 0.74 ± 0.18 respectively. Thus the typical general form of the cornea is that of a flattening ellipsoid, with the curvature reducing in the periphery; however, not all corneas will have this form.

In recent years, **corneal topographic analysis** has been facilitated by the development of a range of instruments that marry optical with electronic and computer technology. These instruments show that the conicoidal model is only a first approximation to corneal shape, and that individual eyes show a wide range of individual asymmetries. In particular, the rate of corneal flattening is often different in different meridians, while the corneal cap of steepest curvature may be displaced with respect to the visual axis, on average lying about 0.8 mm below. Currently the most popular form of output for the topographic data is the colour-coded map of the cornea, showing regions of different power. This may be a little misleading, since each local area of the cornea is toroidal rather than spherical.

corneal transparency

Under normal conditions the **cornea** is highly transparent, transmitting more than 90% of incident light. Structurally the cornea is a typical connective tissue, consisting principally of a matrix of collagen and proteoglycans. Under normal circumstances such an arrangement would favour light scatter, with consequent loss of transparency. However, corneal transparency can be explained on the basis of the small diameter and regular separation of the stromal collagen – the collagen fibrils of the stroma are disposed in a regular crystalline lattice, and light scattered by the fibrils is eliminated by destructive interference in all directions other than the forward direction. This situation holds as long as the axes of the collagen fibrils are arranged in a regular lattice with a separation less than the wavelength of light (Figure C.19).

The factors involved in the maintenance of collagen fibril size and spatial order are not fully understood. It has been proposed that collagen fibril diameters may be controlled by the incorporation of minor collagens (e.g. type V) into the predominantly type I fibrils, and that their spatial separation is a function of proteoglycan–collagen interactions. Proteoglycans are a family of glycoproteins that consist of a protein core to which are attached sugar chains of repeating disaccharide units termed glycosaminoglycans (GAG). In the **corneal stroma** two major proteoglycans have been identified; keratan sulphate

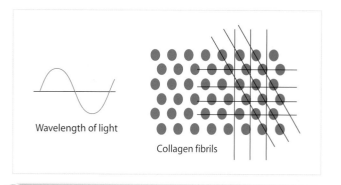

Figure C.19 Collagen fibrils have an orderly structure and a spacing that is less than the wavelength of light.

and dermatan sulphate. Several keratan sulphate isoforms have been described in the cornea of different species. In the human cornea an isoform predominates that has been termed lumican. There appears to be a link between the keratan sulphate content of the cornea and transparency; transgenic mice that lack the gene for lumican fail to develop a clear cornea.

corneal transplantation, lens fitting following
See post-keratoplasty, contact lens fitting.

corneal warpage

Videokeratographic corneal mapping techniques reveal that all forms of contact lens wear are capable of inducing small changes in **corneal topography**. These shape changes, which are generally referred to as 'warpage', are primarily mediated by the **stroma**, which is the main structural entity of the cornea (the epithelium and endothelium offering little mechanical resistance to deforming forces).

The degree of irregularity of corneal surface shape can be expressed by various mathematical indices. For example, the surface asymmetry index (SAI) provides a quantitative measure of the radial symmetry of the four central videokeratoscope mires surrounding the vertex of the **cornea**. The higher the degree of central corneal symmetry, the lower the SAI. Mean SAI values (± standard error of mean) associated with various forms of lens wear are as follows: non-lens wear, 0.35 ± 0.03; PMMA, 0.86 ± 0.22; daily wear rigid, 0.48 ± 0.09; daily wear soft, 0.48 ± 0.11; extended wear soft, 0.46 ± 0.08.

The surface regularity index (SRI) is a measure of central and paracentral corneal irregularity derived from the summation of fluctuations in corneal power that occur along semi-meridians of the 10 central photokeratoscope mires. The more regular the anterior surface of the central cornea, the lower the SRI. The SRI is highly correlated with best spectacle-corrected visual acuity. Mean SRI values (± standard error of mean) associated with various forms of lens wear are as follows: non-lens wear, 0.41 ± 0.04; PMMA, 1.17 ± 0.34; daily wear **rigid**, 0.93 ± 0.18; daily wear **soft**, 0.52 ± 0.08; **extended wear** soft, 0.51 ± 0.06.

All known forms of contact lens-induced warpage can be explained in terms of three underlying pathological mechanisms that primarily act on the stroma. These mechanisms are:

1. Physical pressure on the cornea exerted either by the lens and/or eyelids
2. Contact lens-induced stromal **oedema**
3. Mucus binding beneath rigid lenses.

The relative contributions of these factors will govern the type and extent of topographical alteration.

Rigid lenses can induce clinically significant warpage, which may be especially evident in patients with higher prescriptions requiring thicker lenses or unusual lens designs. Such lenses will impart greater physical and **hypoxic** stress on the cornea compared with thinner lenses made of the same material. Altering the parameters of a rigid lens can reduce the physical impact of the lens on the cornea and thus minimize corneal shape changes. Of course in any case of rigid contact lens-induced warpage refitting into soft lenses will usually provide a cure, because soft lenses are known to have little or no effect on corneal topography.

The prognosis for recovery of normal corneal topography is highly variable and is dependent upon the cause, magnitude and duration of the lens-induced deformation. The time course of recovery from physical forces on the cornea is difficult to predict. Recovery from chronic lens-induced oedema is known to occur within 7 days of cessation of lens wear, and thus recovery from oedema-mediated warpage would be expected to follow a similar time course.

corneal wrinkling
See wrinkling.

cornea plana
See distorted corneal shape, therapeutic lenses for.

cosmetic tinted lenses
A cosmetic tinted lens can be defined as a lens that is designed to beautify an otherwise normal appearance. This can amount to enhancing eye colour with translucent tints, modifying eye colour with a combination of translucent and opaque tints, or com-

pletely changing eye colour with opaque tints. Cosmetic tinted lenses are considered to be a fashion accessory, and as such they are often worn by **emmetropes**. Indeed, most tinted lenses are produced for their cosmetic effect. The most frequently used tints are aquamarine, blue, green and amber. As is the case with handling tints, cosmetic tints do not appreciably affect vision or colour perception, although patients may report an initial transient effect. The light transmission through cosmetic tinted lenses is usually in the range of 75–85%.

Selective distribution of a tint across the surface of lenses designed for cosmetic use allows four basic combinations (Figure C.20). The variables are whether or not to leave a 1.5-mm band clear of tint around the lens edge, and whether or not to have a clear pupil. A full tint covering the pupil appears more natural; however, this creates a small but constant tinting effect on vision. A clear pupil eliminates the visual effect but introduces problems of obtaining good alignment and size-matching between the clear pupillary zone of the lens and the natural pupil of the eye, which of course will vary with ambient lighting . Tints that extend to the edge of the lens are cosmetically unsatisfactory because they are visible against the white sclera at the limbus. *See* tinted lenses.

'cost per wear' (CPW) model
See pricing.

cost to patient
See pricing.

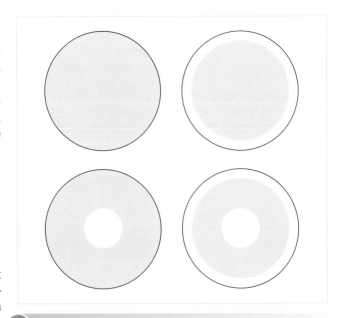

Figure C.20 Four basic combinations of cosmetic tint.

costume lenses
See theatric tinted lenses.

crazing
See surface damage, lens.

culture-negative peripheral ulcer (CNPU)
See contact lens peripheral ulcer.

cylindrical power equivalent rigid toric lenses
All types of rigid toric lenses (apart from **compensated rigid bitoric lenses**) come under this classification, and the unifying feature that these lenses have in common is that they incorporate a correction for residual **astigmatism**. This type of lens can be further categorized as follows:

1. *Alignment bitoric lenses* (also known as parallel bitoric lenses). Both the front and back surfaces are toroidal. The front surface incorporates correction for residual astigmatism as well as for the induced astigmatism. In addition, the axes of the spectacle refraction over the lens correspond with the principal meridians of corneal curvature, so the correction for the residual astigmatism will be along one of the principal meridians of the lens (hence the name 'alignment bitoric'). As such, the use of the term 'alignment bitoric' here should not be confused with alignment in regard to lens fitting.

2. *Back surface toric lenses*. These lenses have a toroidal back surface but a spherical front surface. The design principle is similar to that for alignment bitoric lenses. As with alignment bitoric lenses, the front surface incorporates correction for residual astigmatism as well as for the induced astigmatism, and the axes of the spectacle refraction over the lens correspond with the principal meridians of corneal curvature, so the correction for the residual astigmatism is along one of the principal meridians of the lens. In the case of a back surface toric lens, however, the correction for the residual astigmatism is equal and opposite to the correction for the induced astigmatism. Hence, the two required cylindrical corrections cancel each other out, meaning that the front surface can be left spherical. Very occasionally, a case of induced and residual astigmatism cancelling out one another is encountered in practice. A back surface toric design is only possible if the correction for the residual astigmatism is *equal* and *opposite* to the correction for the induced astigmatism. A back surface toric design is therefore only worth considering if the ocular astigmatism of the patient is greater than the corneal astigmatism. The residual astigmatism must also be of a magnitude such that it will be neutralized by the resultant induced astigmatism. The likelihood of both of these requirements being met is low, so only in a small percentage of cases will a back surface toric design be appropriate. Indeed, in most cases the induced astigmatism usually exaggerates the effect of the residual astigmatism.

3. *Front surface toric lenses*. Residual astigmatism frequently needs to be corrected in cases where the patient is fitted well, physically, with a lens utilizing a spherical back optic zone. Such a lens therefore requires a toroidal front surface, but lens rotation must be avoided, otherwise visual disturbance will result. When the corneal astigmatism is less than 2.00 D a toric back surface will not generally prevent lens rotation, and so other forms of lens stabilization, such as prism ballast or truncation, are required.

4. *Oblique bitoric lenses*. As with alignment bitoric lenses, oblique bitoric lenses have toroidal front and back surfaces. With oblique bitoric lenses, however, the principal meridians of the toroidal back and front surfaces are not parallel, due to a difference between the axes of the spectacle refraction and the principal meridians of corneal curvature. The specification and manufacture of these types of lenses is very difficult. One solution is to use a fitting set of lenses, all of which have a toroidal back optic zone and a spherical front surface. A refraction is performed over the appropriate trial lens and then the oblique cylinder obtained from this refraction is incorporated onto the front surface of the lens. These lenses are rarely prescribed. *See* compensated rigid bitoric lenses; induced astigmatism with rigid toric lenses; residual astigmatism with rigid toric lenses; stabilization of rigid toric lenses; toric lens design, rigid; toric lens, rigid.

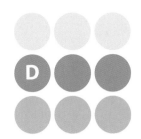

daily disposable lenses

Daily disposable lenses are one of the two versions of true, single-use only, disposable lenses, the other being disposable **extended wear** lenses. Three brands of daily disposable lenses were launched into major contact lens markets from the mid-1990s. These three brands are known today as Soflens one day (**Bausch & Lomb**), Focus Dailies (**CIBA Vision**) and 1 Day Acuvue (**Johnson and Johnson**). Unlike monthly replacement lenses, which tend to be worn on most days, daily disposable lenses tend to be worn on a part-time basis (Figure D.1).

The clinical benefits of daily disposable lenses include fewer symptoms, fewer deposits, better vision, better comfort, fewer tarsal abnormalities, fewer ocular complications, and better overall satisfaction compared with conventional lenses. The obvious advantage offered by daily lens disposal is a fresh, sterile pair of lenses for wear each day. If cost and parameter availability were not limiting factors, then it could be argued that all daily-wear **soft lens** patients should be using this modality. The expansion of available parameters and lens types is already beginning to occur, as signalled by the recent launch of Focus Dailies Progressives (CIBA Vision) – daily disposable multifocal lenses for **presbyopic** patients.

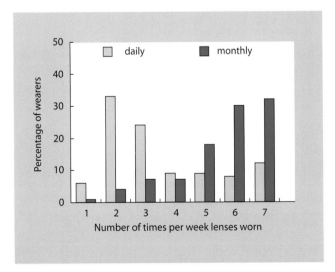

Figure D.1 Number of times per week patients wear monthly- versus daily-replacement lenses.

Specific advantages of daily disposable lenses from the standpoint of the practitioner include the following:

- less patient education time is required; virtually no advice needs to be given about lens care
- the absence of a lens storage case from the regime is beneficial, given the role that a lens case can play in the development of ocular infection
- less professional 'chair time' is required because there are no problems relating to lens care solutions (e.g. toxicity or sensitivity reactions) or to patient **non-compliance** with use of solutions
- less ancillary staff time is required because there is no need for discussions and sales relating to lens care products
- there are no disputes concerning wearing frequency (e.g. some patient might argue that a lens designed for monthly replacement, but only worn once a week, can last for 3 months)
- daily disposability is more hygienic for intermittent wearers, as long-term storage problems are eliminated (making daily disposability the replacement modality of choice for such patients).

Advantages of daily disposable lenses from the perspective of the patient include:

- there is no need to be concerned with lens care systems (although it is desirable for daily disposable lens wearers to have a supply of sterile **saline** or **multipurpose solution** for lens rinsing if there is discomfort during, or soon after, lens **insertion**)
- there are no anxieties about lost or damaged lenses
- daily disposable lenses are convenient and compact for travel; there is no need to carry bulky lens care solutions
- daily disposable lenses are highly cost effective in that lens wear is directly linked to lens cost (unlike, say, a monthly disposable lens that may, for example, only be worn five times during the month)
- daily disposable lenses are excellent for monovision correction of **presbyopia**, as it is easy to alternate between various lens combinations (e.g. two distance lenses versus **monovision**, depending on the need)

- daily disposable lenses are easy to discard ('any time, any place, without a case')
- compliance is easier because there are fewer instructions to remember.

da Vinci, Leonardo

Many contact lens historians point to Leonardo da Vinci's *Codex of the Eye, Manual D*, written in 1508, as having introduced the optical principle underlying the contact lens. Specifically, da Vinci described a method of directly altering corneal power by immersing the eye in a bowl of water (Figure D.2). Of course, a contact lens corrects vision by altering corneal power. However, da Vinci was primarily interested in learning of the mechanisms of **accommodation** of the eye, and did not refer to a mechanism or device for correcting vision.

deep stromal opacities

Apparently benign, deep stromal opacities (DSOs) are occasionally seen in the **corneas** of contact lens wearers. The opacities have been variously described as being white, grey, brown, blue and cyan in colour, and cloudy, scar-like, lattice-like and stellate in form. They are sometimes associated with folds and striae in Descemet's layer, and with deep stromal **neovascularization**. It is possible to distinguish DSOs from infiltrates (which typically reside in the anterior half of the stroma) because DSOs are invariably located deep in the **stroma** (Figure D.3). However, DSOs can take on a similar appearance to certain forms of posterior stromal dystrophy, and some of the reported cases of DSOs may have been confused with dystrophies. The aetiology of this condition is unknown but probably varied.

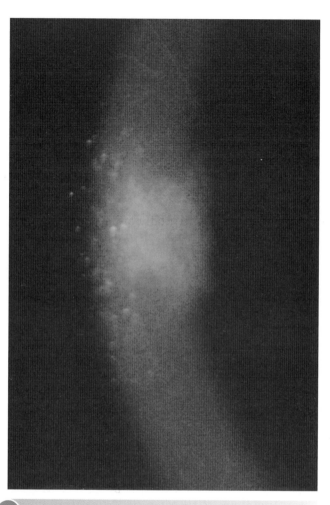

Figure D.3 Deep stromal opacities.

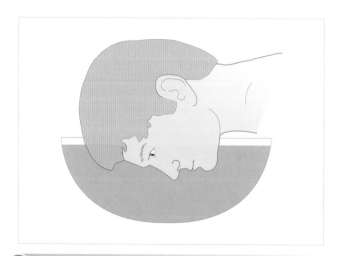

Figure D.2 Idea of Leonardo da Vinci to alter corneal power.

defects

See quality, soft lens.

degenerations of the corneal epithelium, therapeutic lenses for

Conditions such as Salzmann's nodular degeneration, rosacea keratopathy and atopic keratoconjunctivitis (with or without ectasia) can sometimes be so uncomfortable that a therapeutic contact lens is indicated. Such a lens will probably also have visual improvement potential. Concurrent conjunctival disease and tear abnormality may well benefit from the use of a **scleral lens**. Corneal trauma or surgery that has depleted endothelial functional reserves can lead to epithelial bullous keratopathy, the discomfort of which is often amenable to management with **hydrogel** lenses. In many cases, a corneal transplant will subsequently provide a cure.

denatured protein

See deposits, lens.

densitometry
See specific gravity, rigid lens.

density, contact lens
See specific gravity, contact lens.

deposits, lens
The extent of general lens deposition increases over time. Numerous factors, many of which are interactive, are involved in the formation of deposits on the front or back surface of contact lenses. These factors include:

- lens wear modality (daily or continuous wear)
- bulk chemical composition of the lens
- lens **water content**
- physico-chemical nature of the lens surface (such as ionicity)
- chemical composition of lens maintenance solutions
- adequacy of lens maintenance procedures (a measure of patient **compliance**)
- hand contamination
- proximity to environmental pollutants
- intrinsic properties of the **tears** of the patient.

The most common tear-derived components of lens deposits are proteins, which cannot be detected under normal clinical viewing conditions. A heavy deposition of protein can manifest as a general lens haze on the surface of both **soft** and **rigid lenses**, and extensive lipid formation can appear as a clear smear or smudge on the lens surface.

Visible soft lens deposits generally take months or years to form, and are thus only encountered in patients wearing lenses on a **non-planned replacement** basis. The most common form of visible deposition derived from the tear film is known as 'jelly bumps' or 'mulberry deposits', which consist of various layered combinations of mucus, lipid, protein and, sometimes, calcium. Barnacle-like calcium carbonate deposits, which are also derived from the **tear film**, can project anteriorly and be a source of discomfort. Iron deposits, which are derived from exogenous sources, appear as small red-orange spots or rings, and form when iron particles become embedded in the lens and oxidize to form ferrous salts (Figure D.4). These deposits were often seen in patients who did not replace lenses regularly and who frequently commuted on trains or trams, as there is a high probability of fine iron particles (which are thrown into the air as the vehicle moves along the steel tracks) coming to rest on the lens surface. Deposits such as those described above are rarely seen on rigid lenses because of the

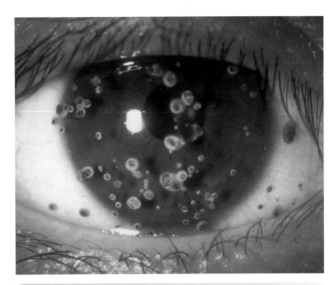

Figure D.4 Iron deposits on a soft lens worn on a non-replacement basis.

inability of contaminants to become embedded in the lens surface.

It is clear that proteins and lipids from the tears can deposit on soft lenses, and to a lesser extent on rigid lenses, within minutes of insertion; however, such deposits are thought to be innocuous over periods of less than 1 month. Lipid is easily removed with **surfactant cleaning**. A small amount of protein deposition may be beneficial to the eye, as long as it does not become denatured, because the protein forms a natural biocompatible lens coating. Although these rapidly forming deposits can not be seen and do not generally compromise vision or comfort, they can reduce lens **surface wettability**.

Long-term protein deposition can be problematic because in time it can become denatured and thus no longer be 'recognized' by the eye, leading to an adverse immunological reaction. Lens surface protein can also absorb (and concentrate) preservatives and other active ingredients in contact lens care solutions, which may be released back into the eye in noxious concentrations, leading to toxic reactions. The physical presence of excess deposits can also cause direct mechanical insult to the anterior eye.

Soft lenses can also become discoloured over time. The cause may be intrinsic or extrinsic. High levels of melanin can lead to a brown discoloration; nicotine can become absorbed into the lenses of patients who smoke or spend time in a smoky environment, leading to an orange-brown discoloration; and exposure to mercury can lead to a black/grey discoloration. Extreme lens discoloration can be cosmetically unsightly to an onlooker.

depth-of-focus

If the retinal image is gradually defocused, its quality will deteriorate due to defocus blur. Nevertheless, there is a finite range of focus over which this blur causes no appreciable deterioration in visual performance; this range is referred to as the 'depth-of-focus'. The precise value of the total depth-of-focus depends on how it is assessed (Figure D.5). For typical photopic **pupil diameters** of about 4 mm, visual performance will remain relatively unaffected provided that the spherical error of focus does not exceed about ±0.25 D.

Descartes, René

In 1636, Descartes described a glass fluid-filled tube which was to be placed in direct contact with the **cornea** (Figure D.6). The end of the tube was made of clear glass, the shape of which would determine the optical correction. Of course such a device is impractical, since blinking is not possible; nevertheless, the principle used by Descartes to neutralize corneal power directly is consistent with the principles underlying modern contact lens design.

Descemet's membrane

See posterior limiting lamina of the cornea.

design, contact lens practice

See layout, contact lens practice.

desmosomes

See corneal epithelium.

diabetes, contact lenses for

Given the alterations to the anterior segment that accompany diabetes, an important issue to be addressed is whether or not cosmetic contact lenses should be prescribed for diabetic patients. Daily-wear **soft contact lenses** can be a viable mode of vision correction for patients with diabetes. Practitioners should not expect to see adverse clinical signs in diabetic contact lens wearers that are any different from those seen in non-diabetic lens wearers. If adverse signs are detected in a diabetic lens wearer, they should not be attributed solely to the fact the patient has diabetes. However, the predisposition of the diabetic patient to corneal infection should always be borne in mind.

'Hand grooming' is especially important for the diabetic patient. Roughening of the fingertips caused by home blood-glucose monitoring could lead to damage to the lens surface during cleaning, and patients should therefore be reminded to inspect contact lenses for damage prior to lens insertion. Fingernails should be kept short and smooth to reduce the risk of corneal erosion.

diffuse wide-beam illumination, slit-lamp technique of

A ground-glass filter is placed in the focused light beam of the **slit lamp**. This will defocus and diffuse the light to give a broad, even illumination over the entire field of view and is generally used to provide low magnification views of the opaque tissues of the anterior segment, including the bulbar **conjunctiva**, sclera, iris, **eyelid** margins and the tarsal conjunctiva of the everted lids (Figure D.7).

dimensional stability, soft lens

See swell factor, soft lens.

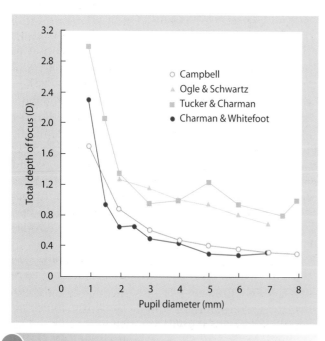

Figure D.5 Examples of experimental measurements of photopic, total monocular depth-of-focus as a function of pupil diameter.

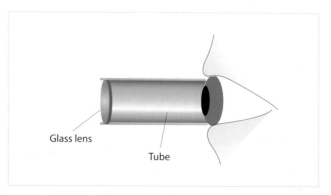

Figure D.6 Fluid-filled tube described by René Descartes.

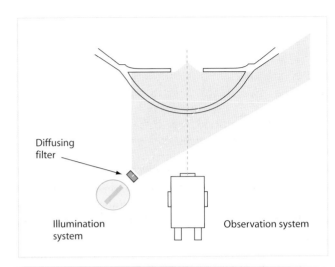

Figure D.7 Diffuse wide-beam illumination. Adapted from L. W. Jones and D.A. Jones (2001) Slit lamp biomicroscopy. In *The Cornea: its Examination in Contact Lens Practice* (N. Efron, ed.), pp.1–49, Butterworth-Heinemann.

dimensional instability, rigid lens

The ability of a **rigid lens** to maintain its shape in the presence of deforming forces is referred to as dimensional stability. The problems associated with the use of increasing quantities of siloxymethacrylates to achieve high **oxygen permeabilities** in rigid lens materials are two-fold. First, incompatibility, phase separation and deterioration in mechanical properties – particularly dimensional stability – limit the proportion of such monomers that can be incorporated. Secondly, their use requires the incorporation of hydrophilic monomers containing hydroxyl, carboxyl, amide or lactam groups to improve wettability, and these monomers tend to reduce oxygen permeability and produce low levels of water uptake, which in turn reduces dimensional stability.

In general, rigid lenses of higher oxygen permeabilities tend to suffer from mechanical instability. This manifests clinically as lens flexure (temporary bending) or warpage (permanent bending) whereby, for example, the lens tends to conform to the topography of a toric **cornea**. Such problems can be overcome by increasing the **lens thickness** and/or using a material of lower oxygen permeability, but these changes could have an adverse effect on ocular health by restricting corneal oxygenation.

The extent to which a strip of material will either extend or shorten when a force is applied to the material can be predicted from Young's modulus. This is a universally accepted method for quantifying the 'stiffness' of lens materials; a higher Young's modulus indicates a 'stiffer' or less flexible material.

direct delivery

See lens delivery systems.

direct focal illumination, slit-lamp technique of

This describes any illumination technique where the slit beam and viewing system are focused coincidentally. The illumination beam is turned up as brightly as possible (ensuring that the patient remains comfortable) and placed at a separation of 40–60° on the side of the microscope corresponding to the same side of the **cornea** to be viewed. The beam is swept smoothly over the ocular surface and the illumination system moved across to the opposite side as the beam crosses the mid-point of the cornea. Typically a beam width of 2–3 mm is chosen initially, and this may be reduced so as to bring more contrast (due to less light scatter) to an area of interest. While scanning the external ocular surface a low-to-medium magnification is initially chosen, and the magnification is increased if any area of interest needs to be examined more closely.

discharging the contact lens patient

See patient discharge.

discomfort, contact lens induced

The most common patient symptom that will be reported to a contact lens practitioner is that of discomfort, and in particular '**dryness**'. Reconciliation of patient symptoms with clinical signs is a constant challenge to all health care practitioners. There is always the potential to devote undue attention to a complaint that bears little significance to the well-being of the patient, or conversely to give token consideration to a symptom arising from a potentially serious condition. Furthermore, there are many signs that the clinician detects that will also have a major influence upon patient management, but for which the patient shows no or minimal symptoms. Conditions that may be asymptomatic, such as corneal **neovascularization**, **microcystic** oedema and **endothelial polymegethism**, are important pathophysiologic signs that require some form of management. However, the most rewarding management plans, from the perspective of the patient, are those that alleviate discomfort.

During adaptation to contact lens wear, **soft lenses** offer a greater level of comfort than **rigid lenses**. Both soft and rigid lenses are very comfortable once the patient has become adapted to lens wear, but nonetheless occasions will arise when lenses become less comfortable. The neural mechanisms by which the **conjunctiva** and **cornea** produce ocular sensibilities during contact lens wear have yet to be elucidated. Certainly, these mechanisms are somewhat imprecise. For example, ocular sensibilities are often poorly differentiated, such that the description and localization of an abnormal event in the eye by a patient is often inaccurate. It is therefore not surprising that patient reports of ocular sensations can be confusing to the practitioner. In the absence of major anomalies of the lens or eye, the comfort of the lens appears to depend upon the interaction between the lid and the lens.

The exact nature of the stimulus that gives rise to the sensation of dryness is also unclear, and the reasons for the high frequency of this symptom in contact lens wearers are a matter for speculation, given that it is the least frequently reported symptom of non-lens wearers. Since there are no specific 'dryness receptors' in human tissue, the ocular sensation of dryness must be a response to specific coding of afferent neural inputs. One may hypothesize that dryness results from an interference with tear physiology and structure by the contact lens, the particular mechanism being an increased tear evaporation and faster break-up of the tear film. The sensation may also arise from the neural misinterpretation of stimuli seemingly unrelated to dryness, such as direct mechanical interaction of the lens with the ocular tissues, lens dehydration, or vasodilation and the subsequent rise in local temperature. *See* discomfort following lens insertion; discomfort, investigation of.

discomfort following lens insertion

Soft lenses can attract debris during lens preparation prior to insertion, and wearers can experience some mild irritation. Patients should be advised that sliding the lens temporally onto the sclera can relieve this, and they can be taught the following procedure. For the right eye, the patient looks directly into the mirror and turns the head to the right whilst maintaining a straight-ahead gaze. This helps to expose a large area of temporal conjunctiva onto which the lens can be displaced. Using the right hand, the patient displaces the inferior lid slightly with the middle finger and uses the forefinger to slide the lens completely off the **cornea** onto the temporal **conjunctiva**. The patient will usually experience instant relief from any previous foreign body sensation. At this point, the patient blinks three to five times, which washes tears over the cornea, thereby displacing any unwanted debris. The lens can be manually repositioned onto the cornea, or alternatively the patient can look temporally and execute a couple of blinks, which will achieve the same result. If a foreign body sensation persists after this technique has been tried, the lens should be removed,

rinsed and inspected for any signs of damage; the lens can then be reinserted if all looks well, or replaced if it is damaged. If foreign body-type discomfort is experienced on insertion of a rigid lens, the lens should be removed, rinsed and reinserted. The above procedures can also be undertaken by a practitioner if the patient experiences discomfort following lens insertion during a fitting/evaluation examination (Figure D.8). *See* discomfort, contact lens induced; discomfort, investigation of.

discomfort, investigation of

Patients can employ one or more of a myriad of descriptions to describe symptoms of discomfort during contact lens wear. Terms that may be used include:

- scratchy
- uncomfortable
- cold
- watery
- hurting
- tired
- gritty
- painful
- hot
- **dry**
- sore
- burning
- itchy
- aching
- irritated
- stinging

A systematic approach can be applied to quantify the level of subjective discomfort experienced during lens wear. Specifically, the severity of discomfort can be described in three ways, known as:

1. Nominal – purely descriptive terms are used, such as mild or severe.
2. Ordinal – the level of severity is ranked on a scale of discrete steps, e.g. grades 0, 1, 2, 3 or 4. Descriptors may be employed for the extreme

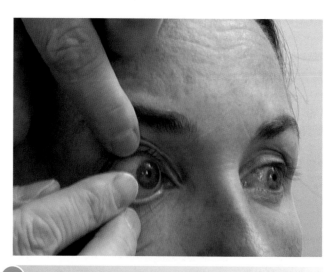

Figure D.8 Displacing a soft lens to dislodge a foreign body.

grades as a guide, e.g. grade 0 means 'no sensation' and grade 4 means 'extreme pain'.

3. Analogue – the level of comfort is indicated on a continuous scale. A popular technique employed in contact lens research is the **'vertical analogue scale'**.

The following strategies can be used to determine whether the discomfort is eye- or lens-related:

- always be on the lookout for concurrent ocular pathology that may be unrelated to lens wear (e.g. glaucoma)
- consider the laterality of the discomfort – for example, discomfort due to a toxic reaction to a contact lens solution would be expected to be bilateral, whereas discomfort due to a damaged contact lens would be expected to be unilateral
- remove the lenses – persistent discomfort following lens removal suggests an ocular problem that may or may not have been caused by the lens; relief of discomfort following lens removal suggests a lens problem
- swap the lenses between the eyes – an ocular problem is indicated if unilateral discomfort remains in the same eye after the lenses have been swapped; a lens-related problem is indicated if unilateral discomfort transfers to the other eye after the lenses have been swapped
- prescribe ocular lubricants – relief after an ocular lubricant has been instilled into the sore eye suggests a mechanical or abrasive source of the discomfort.

There are many possible causes of lens-related discomfort. These causes, and strategies for alleviating the problem, include:

- poor fitting lens – change to a better fitting lens; specifically, a lens of larger diameter and/or steeper base curve may move less and therefore be more comfortable
- physical **defects** in the lens – replace the lens and/or change to a non-defective product
- particulate matter partially embedded in the lens – replace the lens
- foreign bodies beneath the lens – rinse the lens
- higher water content lenses are generally thicker and initially less comfortable than thinner lenses – use thinner lenses
- a toric soft lens might be slightly less comfortable than its spherical equivalent because of thick stabilization zones – employ a toric design with a thinner profile
- dehydration of hyper-thin (< 0.04 mm) soft lenses can lead to epithelial drying and discomfort – re-fit the patient with standard thickness lenses (> 0.07 mm)
- older lenses tend to feel more dry – replace lenses more frequently
- lenses with surface deposits can be uncomfortable – replace lenses more frequently.

If a patient complains of lens discomfort but there is no apparent cause after having carefully examined the lens and eye, the lens should be thoroughly cleaned with a **surfactant cleaner**, rinsed in **saline** and reinserted into the eye. If the discomfort persists, the lens may contain a sub-clinical defect, or it may have a microscopic foreign body imbedded in the back surface. In either case, the lens should be replaced.

Various forms of contact lens-related ocular pathology can cause discomfort, and it should be noted that the apparent severity of the tissue pathology does not necessarily correlate with the degree of discomfort suffered by the patient. Such conditions include:

- corneal epithelial **microcysts** – may cause slight discomfort
- corneal stromal **oedema** – moderate oedema ($< 5\%$ swelling) can cause mild discomfort; severe oedema ($> 20\%$ swelling) can be very painful, although the pain may be attributed to associated pathology such as an anterior uveal reaction; oedema associated with the **corneal exhaustion syndrome** may be very uncomfortable
- acute red eye – occurs in **extended wear** patients and can be very painful; lens removal often gives immediate relief
- **superior limbic keratoconjunctivitis** – causes increased lens awareness and itching; symptoms are alleviated by ceasing lens wear
- infectious keratitis – can be extremely painful, especially **Acanthamoeba keratitis**, even leading to patients becoming suicidal
- **tear film** dysfunction – discomfort is due to lens surface drying; ocular lubricants can provide short-term relief.

Ocular discomfort during contact lens wear may be due to the use of associated lens care products. Specifically, the discomfort may be related to:

- solution pH
- solution tonicity
- solution toxicity
- solution allergy
- lens denaturation due to **heat disinfection** (rarely used today)
- residual un-neutralized **hydrogen peroxide**
- hydrogen peroxide burn.

See discomfort, contact lens induced; discomfort following lens insertion.

disinfection

See antimicrobial efficacy; trial lens set disinfection.

dispensing visit

See patient education; patient discharge.

disposable lenses

See planned soft lens replacement.

distorted corneal shape, therapeutic lenses for

Congenital abnormalities of **corneal topography**, such as **keratoconus**, keratoglobus and cornea plana (Figure D.9), typically result in vision loss that can only be corrected with **rigid** forms of **contact lenses** – usually scleral lenses. Keratoconus occurs in 5.5 out of 10 000 in the population, and keratoglobus and cornea plana are extremely rare. Patients suffering from these conditions are usually highly motivated to wear scleral lenses. *See* keratoconus, contact lens correction of.

Dk

See carbon dioxide permeability; oxygen permeability.

Dk/t

See carbon dioxide transmissibility; oxygen transmissibility.

dot matrix print tinting

This technique of making a coloured contact lens involves applying a matrix pattern of small opaque dots to the front surface of the lens (Figure D.10). The dots are created by bonding an opaquing agent (such as titanium dioxide) and a colouring agent (which may be a pigment or dye) to the lens surface. A binding polymer such as di-isocyanate is used to form a strong chemical bond between the opaque tinted agent and the lens surface. The final cosmetic effect will be a combination of dot matrix pattern and reflections from the natural iris between the opaque matrix dots. *See* tinted lenses.

drug delivery, contact lenses for

Hydrogel lenses steeped in pilocarpine solutions (e.g. 4%, unpreserved) are sometimes used in the management of acute closed angle glaucoma. This technique has also been used in the delivery of antibiotics, antiviral agents, epidermal growth factor and fibronectin.

dry eye

Of all the symptoms experienced by contact lens wearers, that of 'dryness' is reported most frequently. A major difficulty in assessing the symptom of 'dryness' is that there may be many stimuli that elicit this sensation; that is, it can not be assumed

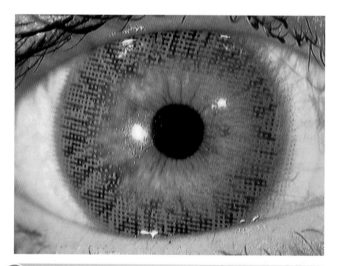

Figure D.10 Lens with a matrix of opaque blue dots.

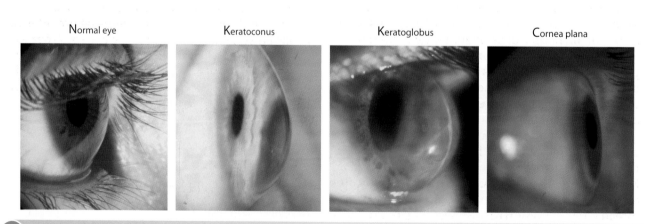

Normal eye · Keratoconus · Keratoglobus · Cornea plana

Figure D.9 Congenital abnormalities of corneal shape.

that the cause of a patient symptom of 'dryness' is necessarily due to an absence of moisture in the eye. Because there are no specific 'dryness receptors' in human tissue, ocular dryness must be a response to specific coding of afferent neural inputs. Aside from an actual dry eye, reports of 'dryness' may arise from the neural misinterpretation of stimuli that are unrelated to dry eye, such as vasodilation induced by mechanical irritation of ocular tissues by deposits on the lens surface. Thus, the condition of 'dry eye' may be related to a broad spectrum of tear film abnormalities in addition to a reduced tear volume.

A prudent initial approach in dealing with a tentative diagnosis of contact lens-induced dry eye is to apply a comprehensive **dry eye questionnaire** that attempts to identify the following:

- other systemic correlates of dryness, such as dryness of other mucous membranes of the body (e.g. mouth, vagina)
- the use of medications
- the effect of different challenging environments
- the times when dryness is noted.

Such questionnaires can help identify a true dry eye situation in prospective or current contact lens wearers, and thus form a clinical rationale for more detailed assessment.

The most fundamental test that a clinician can apply when investigating contact lens related dry eye is to observe the **tear film** using the **slit-lamp biomicroscope**. The overall integrity of the tears during lens wear can be assessed by observing the general flow of tears over the lens surface following a blink, as indicated by the movement of tear debris. A 'sluggish' movement may indicate an aqueous-deficient, mucus-rich and/or lipid-rich tear film, and the amount of debris provides an indication of the level of contamination of the tears (for example, from over-use of cosmetics). This can result in increased deposit formation, intermittent blurred vision and symptoms of dryness. Incomplete blinking in soft lens wearers can lead to lens dehydration and consequent **epithelial staining** of the inferior **cornea**, corresponding to the position of the palpebral aperture.

The volume of tears in prospective and current contact lens wearers can be assessed by observing the height of the lower lacrimal tear prism. Measurements of tear meniscus radius of curvature and height correlate well with results of the cotton thread test, non-invasive tear break-up time (NITBUT) and ocular surface staining scores, demonstrating the value of such an assessment in diagnosing contact lens associated dry eye. A wide-field, cold cathode light source, which is available as a hand-held instrument known as a **tearscope**, can be used to assess tear quality during lens wear.

Most of the strategies that are applied to alleviating signs and symptoms of dry eye of the non-lens wearing eye can also be applied to the eye during contact lens wear. The following types of lenses are most suitable for patients experiencing dry eye problems:

- **soft lenses**, for full corneal coverage (although some patients report relief from dry eye symptoms after changing from a soft lens to a rigid lens)
- high **water content** lenses, to maximize the volume of water in front of the lens
- lenses that display minimal in-eye dehydration, to prevent ocular surface desiccation
- lenses that are replaced frequently, for optimal, deposit-free surface characteristics.

Numerous other strategies have been advocated for alleviating contact lens related dry eye, including:

- avoidance of preservatives in care solutions
- avoidance of solutions altogether via the use of **daily disposable lenses**
- use of re-wetting drops
- periodic lens rehydration
- use of nutritional supplements
- control of evaporation
- prevention of excess tear drainage (with punctal plugs)
- use of tear stimulants
- reduction of wearing time, and ceasing lens wear.

dry eye questionnaire
Perhaps the most widely noted symptom of contact lens wearers is a sensation of **dryness**. Contact lenses will disrupt the normal **tear film**, and it is important to pay particular attention to both the quantity and the quality of the tears before offering advice on suitability for contact lens wear. A dry eye questionnaire can be used to identify patients who have a tendency to ocular sicca and those who might develop symptoms associated with provocative factors such as contact lens wear.

Drysdale method of surface curvature measurement
See radiuscope.

D-value
See antimicrobial efficacy.

dye dispersion tinting
This technique is used primarily to create a translucent tint in **rigid lenses**. A dye or pigment is mixed

into the polymer matrix by adding the dye to the monomer mixture prior to polymerization, or by adding the dye to the **polymer** and then mixing to disperse the colour. This results in an evenly distributed, stable dye. The disadvantages of this process are that it is not possible to vary the distribution of tint across the lens (e.g. to create a clear pupil), and that the density of tint is proportional to lens thickness. This process is unsuitable for **soft lenses** because the dye, which is non-water-soluble, can leach out from the polymer during hydration. *See* tinted lenses.

dynamic stabilization
See stabilization of soft toric lenses.

dystonia
See filamentary keratitis, therapeutic lenses for.

dystrophies of the corneal epithelium, therapeutic lenses for
Epithelial basement membrane dystrophy is by far the most common epithelial dystrophy, but other dystrophies that can involve the **corneal epithelium** are also often the cause of pain that can be relieved with **soft lenses**. They include Reis–Bückler's dystrophy, Meesmann's dystrophy, lattice dystrophy, and Fuchs's dystrophy, in which the failing **corneal endothelium** cannot prevent stromal **oedema** and bullous keratopathy in the epithelium. Thygeson's superficial punctate keratopathy is not considered to be a dystrophy, but it is appropriate to consider this condition here; this keratopathy can sometimes be managed successfully with **hydrogel** lenses, although weak topical steroid is the more usual form of management.

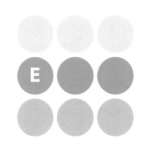

ECDP
See equivalent carbon dioxide pressure.

edema
See oedema.

edge clearance
Without a peripheral gap between the edge of a **rigid lens** and the **cornea**, known as 'edge clearance', mechanical pressure from the lens edge leads to superficial corneal damage (Figure E.1). Edge clearance is also important for tear exchange and to enable lens removal using the lids. The edge clearance can be specified axially (as shown in Figure E.1) or radially. A minimum axial edge clearance of 60–80 μm when the lens is centred is considered to be the optimal value. **Edge lift** is measured with respect to the continuation of the spherical lens back curve.

edge defects
See quality, soft lens.

edge fluting
See fluting.

edge form
The shape of the lens edge is one of the most important factors in minimizing any **discomfort**. Poor edge rounding in particular can result in greater edge awareness by the upper eyelid. Good rounding of the front surface edge is more important than rounding of the posterior edge. This suggests that the interaction of the edge of the lens with the eyelid is more important in relation to comfort than the interaction with the **cornea**. Figure E.2 shows examples of edge shapes.

edge lift
Certain lens fitting philosophies are based on the concept of edge lift. Figure E.3 summarizes the various parameters used to describe edge lift. Edge lift is the distance between a point on the edge of the lens back surface and the circular continuation of the back optic zone. This can be measured axially or radially. Unlike **edge clearance**, edge lift is not referenced to the corneal surface.

With reference to Figure E.3, the edge lift can be calculated from the basic geometry of the lens surface as follows:

$$\text{REL} = \sqrt{[(r - s_2)^2 + y^2]} - r$$

$$\text{AEL} = (s_1 - s_2), \text{ where } s_1 = r - \sqrt{(r^2 - y^2)}$$

where REL is radial edge lift and AEL is axial edge lift. Measuring the overall **sag** of a finished lens, namely s_2, allows both the axial and radial edge lift to be derived. However, the error in both derivations is dependent upon errors in r and y. The likely magnitude of the final error can be estimated using partial differential equations for the two expressions. For example, consider a lens of **BOZR** 7.7 mm and TD 10 mm. If the respective errors in r, y and s_1 were ±0.015 mm, ±0.1 mm and ±0.01 mm, then it can be shown that the errors in REL and AEL would be ±0.053 mm and ±0.071 mm. These figures represent the precision in the determination of REL and AEL.

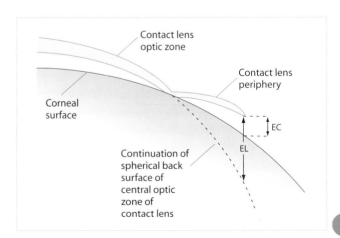

Axial edge lift (EL) and edge clearance (EC).

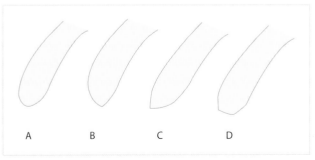

Various edge forms on rigid lenses. (A) Well rounded edge. (B) Sharp posterior edge. (C) Sharp anterior edge. (D) Flat edge.

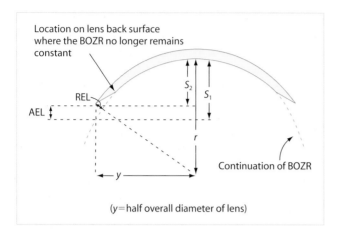

Location on lens back surface where the BOZR no longer remains constant

REL

AEL

S_2

S_1

r

Continuation of BOZR

y

(y=half overall diameter of lens)

Figure E.3 The form of the edge of a rigid lens can be defined in terms of either axial edge lift (AEL) or radial edge lift (REL).

Alternatively, for AEL, the sag of a monocurve lens of identical BOZR and TD could be used to directly measure s_1 in an attempt to improve precision. The lens may be placed on a glass plate, and by using a travelling microscope s_2 could be measured. The exact shape and dimensions of the lens edge profile will affect the estimation of edge lift.

edge shape
See edge form.

edge thickness of a lens
See lens thickness.

education of patients
See patient education.

EFCLIN
See European Federation of the Contact Lens Industry.

effectivity
The role of the distance correction is to produce an intermediate image at the far point of the particular eye. Due to the non-zero vertex distance of any spectacle correction, this far point will lie at slightly different distances from the two types of correcting lens. Thus the spectacle and contact lens powers required to correct a particular eye will differ.

From Figure E.4A it can be seen that, using a reduced eye model, if the vertex distance is a (taken as positive) and the ocular refraction is K, giving a far point distance from the **cornea** $k = 1/K$, the second focal point of the correcting lens lies at a distance $a + k$. Thus the power, F_c, of the correcting lens is:

$$F_c = 1/(a + k) = 1/(a + 1/K) = K/(1 + aK)$$

For a contact lens, a will be zero so that the required value of F_c equals the ocular refraction in this simple model. This does not apply with a spectacle lens. The result is that a **hypermetrope** will require a higher-powered contact lens than spectacle lens, the reverse occurring for a **myope**. The difference between the required powers of correction only becomes significant (i.e. greater than 0.25 D) when the magnitude of the ocular refraction exceeds about ± 4.00 D (Figure E.4B). Appendix B provides a table for vertex distance correction.

Efron Grading Scales for Contact Lens Complications
See grading scales.

electrical contact thickness gauge, soft lens
Electronic contact systems relying on the electrical conductivity of **soft lenses** can be used to measure the thickness of soft lenses. The lens is centred on a

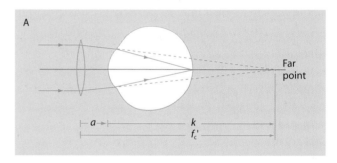

A

Far point

a

k

f_c'

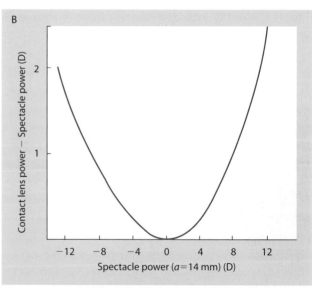

B

Contact lens power – Spectacle power (D)

2

1

−12   −8   −4   0   4   8   12

Spectacle power (a=14 mm) (D)

Figure E.4 (A) Geometry relating the far point of an ametropic eye and the correcting lens. (B) Difference between the required powers of a contact lens and spectacle corrections, as a function of the spectacle correction, assuming that the vertex distance of the spectacle lens is 14 mm.

support dome that has an electrical contact in its surface. Another contact is gradually lowered onto the lens, and its position relative to the first contact is monitored using a vernier scale. On contact with the lens, a flow of electrical current is detected and the vernier scale is read.

electrolytes in tears
See tear electrolytes.

electromechanical thickness gauge, soft lens
An electromechanical thickness gauge is operated by lowering a lightweight probe until it touches the surface of a **soft lens** sitting on a support dome (Figure E.5). The force of contact of the probe is extremely low (around 0.015 N). Using this technique, thickness can be measured to a resolution of 0.01 mm. The device still tends to compress the lens, thus the result is typically a few microns lower than the true thickness.

emmetropia
Light from a distant object is perfectly focused on the retina when **accommodation** is relaxed, resulting in clear distance vision – that is, the absence of a refractive defect of the eye. *Antonym*: ametropia.

endothelial bedewing
Contact lens associated endothelial bedewing (CLEB) is characterized by the appearance of small particles in or on the **endothelium** in the region of the inferior central **cornea**, immediately below the lower pupil margin. The area of bedewing can vary in shape. For example, CLEB may appear as an oval cluster of particles or a less discrete dispersed formation. The condition is usually bilateral. The cells

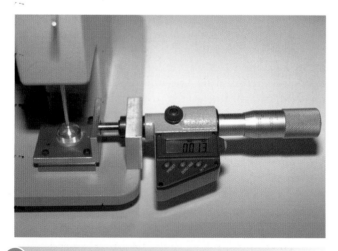

Figure E.5 Electromechanical thickness gauge modified for measuring central and peripheral lens thickness.

invariably display 'reversed illumination' (see **'microcysts'** for an explanation of this phenomenon), suggesting that bedewing represents inflammatory cells rather than intracellular endothelial oedema (which would display unreversed illumination). When viewed in direct illumination, CLEB can appear as fine white precipitates or as an orange/brown dusting of cells. The colour of the particles can give a clue regarding the length of time they have been present; newly deposited cells are often whitish in colour, but these become pigmented over time. The cells can become engulfed within the endothelium over time.

The following signs may co-exist with CLEB:

- conjunctival injection
- epithelial erosion
- epithelial oedema
- reduced corneal transparency.

The main associated feature of endothelial bedewing is either total or partial intolerance to lens wear. Some patients may present after having recently abandoned lens wear. Patients may also complain of 'fogging' of vision or of stinging.

On the assumption that CLEB represents a mild inflammatory uveal response, the origin of the inflammatory cells is likely to be the iris and/or ciliary body. During inflammation, vascular permeability is increased and inflammatory cells leave vessels in the iris and ciliary body and float around in the aqueous until they come to rest on the endothelial surface. The reason for the deposition on the inferior cornea relates to the characteristic pattern of aqueous current flow. One would therefore expect occasionally to observe mild aqueous flare in patients with CLEB, but this does not appear to have been reported. This mild inflammatory status probably causes lens intolerance.

Patient management is guided by symptomatology rather than clinical signs. Wearing time should be reduced to a level that represents the balance between the needs of the patient to wear lenses for a desired length of time each day versus the level of **discomfort** that can be tolerated. The presence of inflammatory cells on the endothelial surface should be viewed with great caution by clinicians, because the condition may not necessarily be related to lens wear. Certainly, all forms of uveitis should be considered and tests should be conducted to exclude such possibilities. In all cases of CLEB intraocular pressures should be measured, because some inflammatory cells may have migrated into the anterior angle, creating a blockage of aqueous outflow. Gonioscopy is also indicated, especially if intraocular pressure is elevated.

The pattern of recovery from CLEB is variable. In some cases bedewing will completely disappear within 4 months, and in other cases it may change little over a much longer time period. Lens intolerance may persist for many months in some patients, even after the bedewing has disappeared.

endothelial blebs

The endothelial mosaic undergoes a dramatic alteration in appearance in all lens wearers within minutes of inserting a contact lens. These changes can only just be resolved when observed under the highest magnification possible (×40) using the **slit-lamp biomicroscope**. When viewed at much greater magnification (×200), a number of black, non-reflecting areas can be seen in the endothelial mosaic corresponding to the position of individual cells or groups of cells. These are called blebs (Figure E.6). There is also an apparent increase in the separation between cells. There is a large variation in the intensity of the response between patients.

Blebs can be seen within 10 minutes of lens insertion. The number of blebs peaks in 20–30 minutes (Grade 3), then decreases to a lower level after about 45–60 minutes. A low-level bleb response (Grade 1) can be observed throughout the remainder of the wearing period. **Hydrogel** lenses cause a greater bleb

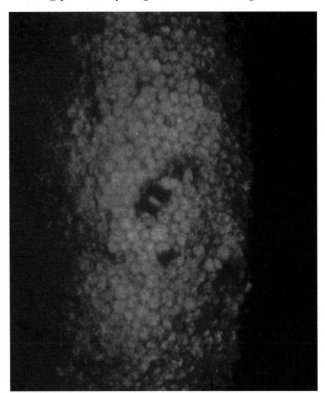

Figure E.6 Endothelial blebs.

response than **rigid lenses**, and hydrogel lenses of greater average thickness also induce a greater response than thinner lenses.

The appearance of blebs can be explained as follows. When the endothelium is viewed using specular reflection, light rays reflect from the tissue plane corresponding to the interface between the posterior surface of the **endothelium** and the aqueous humor. This interface acts as the reflective surface because it represents a significant change in tissue **refractive index**. The light rays that are reflected from this interface give rise to an observed image of an essentially flat (or slightly undulating) and featureless endothelial cell mosaic. Light rays that strike 'blebbed' endothelial cells will be deflected away from the observation path, leaving a corresponding area of darkness. Thus an endothelial bleb is simply an individual endothelial cell (or group of adjacent cells) that has become swollen and bulged in the direction of the aqueous humor, giving rise to the compelling optical illusion that the cell (or cells) has disappeared.

Endothelial blebs are caused by a local acidic pH change at the endothelium. Two separate factors induce an acidic shift in the cornea during contact lens wear:

1. An increase in carbonic acid due to retardation of carbon dioxide efflux (hypercapnia) by a contact lens
2. Increased levels of lactic acid as a result of lens-induced oxygen deprivation (hypoxia) and the consequent increase in anaerobic metabolism of epithelial tissue.

All cells in the human body function optimally when surrounded by extracellular fluid that is maintained within an acceptable range of pH, temperature, tonicity, ion balance etc. The carbonic acid and lactic acid alter the physiological status of the environment surrounding the endothelial cells by shifting the pH in the acidic direction. This induces changes in membrane permeability and/or membrane pump activity, resulting in a net movement of water into certain endothelial cells when the threshold for a change in membrane permeability is exceeded for those cells. The resultant cellular oedema in such cells is observed as 'blebbing'.

Despite their stunning clinical appearance, blebs are asymptomatic and are thought to be of little clinical significance. After removal of a contact lens, blebs disappear within minutes.

endothelial microscope

See specular microscope.

endothelial polymegethism

The human corneal **endothelium** is a single cell layer that appears as an ordered mosaic of primarily hexagonal-shaped cells. A significant variation in apparent size of cells is referred to as *endothelial polymegethism* (Figure E.7). ('Polymegethism' is derived from the Greek words *megethos*, meaning size, and *poly*, meaning many.) The extent of polymegethism increases throughout life, and consequently the degree of lens-induced polymegethism should be taken to mean the degree of change in excess of that expected for a given age.

It is difficult to assess the integrity of the endothelium using a **slit-lamp biomicroscope**, because individual endothelial cells are just beyond the limit of resolution. Thus, a normal endothelial mosaic can only be seen as a speckled or textured field. Endothelial polymegethism of a severity greater than Grade 2 can sometimes be detected because some of the larger cells can be seen. Inspection of the endothelium is best undertaken by imaging the cornea through the eyepiece of a slit-lamp biomicroscope, or using instruments designed specifically for

high magnification imaging, such as the **specular microscope** or **confocal microscope**.

An anecdotal association exists between endothelial polymegethism and a condition termed 'corneal exhaustion syndrome'. This may be related to the link between endothelial polymegethism and impairment of corneal hydration control, whereby recovery from **oedema** is significantly slower in the corneas of contact lens wearers (who have high levels of polymegethism) compared with corneas of non-lens wearers (who have lower levels of polymegethism).

It is likely that the aetiology of endothelial polymegethism – contact lens induced endothelial acidosis – is precisely the same as the aetiology of **endothelial blebs**, where the former represents a chronic response and the latter represents an acute response to the same stimuli. Endothelial acidosis may induce changes in membrane permeability and/or membrane pump activity, resulting in water movement that acts to elongate endothelial cell walls. A reconfiguration of cell shape then occurs in order to preserve cell volume, resulting in the appearance of polymegethism at the apical surface of the endothelium.

Lenses of lower oxygen performance induce higher levels of polymegethism. From a clinical perspective, it is essential to take note of the presence of significant endothelial polymegethism and to take action to minimize the metabolic stress to the cornea known to be associated with this change. Strategies for alleviating contact lens induced hypoxia and hypercapnia include the following:

- fitting lenses of higher **oxygen transmissibility**
- sleeping in **extended-wear** lenses less frequently
- changing from extended lens wear to daily lens wear
- reducing lens wearing time
- fitting **rigid lenses** with more movement and edge lift (to enhance oxygen-enriching tear exchange).

The prognosis for recovery from endothelial polymegethism is poor. Recovery from polymegethism is likely to take many years, if it occurs at all.

endothelium
See corneal endothelium.

enhancement of compliance
See compliance enhancement.

entropion
See eyelid pathology, therapeutic lenses for.

environmental impact
Concerns have been expressed regarding the possible environmental impact of **disposable contact**

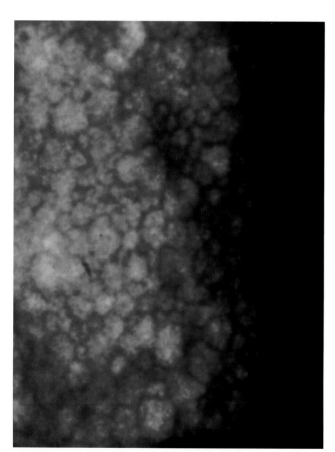

Figure E.7 Endothelial polymegethism.

lenses. Specifically, consideration needs to be given to the amount of waste glass, plastic, metal and paper involved in the consumer use of various modalities of contact lenses (solutions can be ignored because they have a negligible environmental impact). **Non-planned lens replacement** has the highest environmental impact and monthly lens replacement the lowest environmental impact, with daily disposability falling between the two (Figure E.8). It is certain that the overall level of wastage incurred in contact lens manufacture is more significant than that incurred by consumers. From a wider perspective, the environmental impact of wastage in the use of contact lenses and care systems by consumers pales into insignificance when considered against major sources of world environmental pollution (e.g. road construction, general domestic wastage, deforestation etc.).

enzyme cleaning systems
See protein removal systems.

EOP
See equivalent oxygen pressure.

epithelial degeneration
See degenerations of the corneal epithelium, therapeutic lenses for.

epithelial dystrophies
See dystrophies of the corneal epithelium, therapeutic lenses for.

epithelial microcysts
See microcysts.

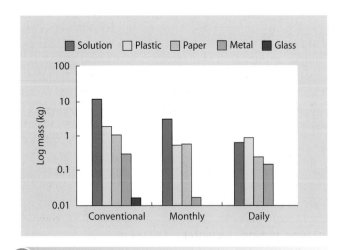

Figure E.8 Mass of various material components of daily, monthly and 'conventional' (non-replacement) systems used by a single patient over a 12-month period.

epithelial thinning
The **corneal epithelium** is normally about 50 µm thick at the corneal centre. The following contact lens-related effects can cause a reduction in epithelial thickness:

- **rigid contact lens** wear
- **reverse geometry lenses** used for **orthokeratology**
- long-term extended hydrogel contact lens wear (*see* Gothenburg Study).

In most cases the thinning is reversible, with recovery to full epithelial thickness within 1 month of cessation of lens wear.

epithelial vacuoles
See vacuoles.

epithelial wrinkling
See wrinkling.

epithelium
See corneal epithelium.

equivalent carbon dioxide percentage
See equivalent carbon dioxide pressure.

equivalent carbon dioxide pressure
This represents the partial pressure of atmospheric carbon dioxide (CO_2) at the **cornea**–contact lens interface beneath a contact lens. Equivalent carbon dioxide pressure (ECDP) values are derived from *in vivo* human experiments, whereby the efflux of CO_2 from the **cornea** after application of a contact lens is compared to that following corneal exposure to various environments of known CO_2 content for about 5 minutes (Figure E.9). Efflux of CO_2 is measured by pressing a CO_2 electrode against the cornea and monitoring the build-up of CO_2 in the electrode. A higher rate of build-up of CO_2 indicates higher pre-exposure levels of CO_2.

The pressure of CO_2 in the atmosphere is 0.3 mmHg. Because the partial pressure of carbon dioxide in the aqueous is about 40 mmHg, and because CO_2 can diffuse rapidly through the cornea, the partial pressure of CO_2 at the corneal surface will never exceed 40 mmHg. Thus the ECDP scale effectively ranges from 0–40 mmHg. If it is stated that the ECDP beneath a lens is 25 $mmHgCO_2$, it is inferred that the cornea has responded as if it was in a gaseous environment containing 25 $mmHgCO_2$.

equivalent oxygen percentage
See equivalent oxygen pressure.

equivalent oxygen pressure
This represents the partial pressure of atmospheric oxygen at the **cornea**–contact lens interface beneath

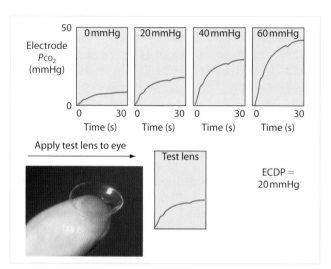

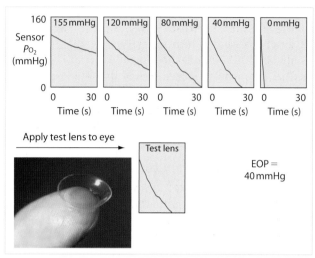

Figure E.9 Equivalent carbon dioxide pressure technique. The rate of corneal carbon dioxide efflux following lens wear is matched to that following exposure to known carbon dioxide environments.

Figure E.10 Equivalent oxygen pressure technique. The rate of corneal oxygen uptake following lens wear is matched to that following exposure to known oxygen environments.

a contact lens. Equivalent oxygen pressure (EOP) values are derived from *in vivo* human or rabbit experiments, whereby the corneal respiratory response ('hunger' for oxygen) after application of a contact lens is compared to that following corneal exposure to various gaseous oxygen environments of known oxygen content. Hunger for oxygen is taken to be the rate at which oxygen is consumed by the **cornea** from the oxygen-enriched Teflon™ membrane of a polarographic oxygen sensor when the sensor is pressed against the cornea immediately following exposure of the cornea to either a contact lens or a gaseous environment for about 5 minutes (Figure E.10). A higher rate of consumption indicates pre-exposure to a more **hypoxic** environment.

Under conditions of standard temperature and pressure at sea level, the partial pressure of oxygen in the atmosphere is 159 mmHg (or 155 mmHg allowing for water vapour pressure); this represents the theoretical maximum oxygen partial pressure at the cornea–contact lens interface beneath a contact lens. If it is stated that the EOP beneath a lens is 30 mmHg, it is inferred that the cornea has responded as if it was in a gaseous environment containing 30 mmHg O_2.

Whereas the percentage of oxygen (20.9%) remains constant under any conditions and at any altitude within the earth's atmosphere, the oxygen partial pressure falls at increasing altitudes. Some prefer to think in terms of 'equivalent oxygen percentace' rather than 'equivalent oxygen pressure' (the acronym 'EOP' of course remains the same). Thus the EOP scale ranges from 0–155 mmHg or from 0–20.9% when thinking in terms of oxygen pressure or oxygen percentage, respectively. Under conditions of standard temperature and pressure at sea level, these two scales are interchangeable; to convert mmHg to $\%O_2$, multiply by 0.1348.

erosion
See recurrent erosion syndrome, therapeutic lenses for.

ethnic variations in ocular dimensions
Ethnic variations in ocular topography may be of relevance to contact lens fitting. In the UK-resident Chinese population, **corneas** have been noted to be steeper and smaller and to show less corneal flattening than Caucasian eyes. This suggests a requirement for smaller **rigid lenses** showing less peripheral flattening for such patients. The eyes of American Japanese people show, on average, a smaller HVID but no difference in corneal curvature. It is likely that environmental factors such as nutrition, as well as cultural differences, influence **corneal topography** and probably account for the mean flattening that has been observed in corneal curvature noted in the Japanese population over a 20-year period. Oriental eyes tend to show a narrower palpebral aperture – on average, about 1.0 mm smaller than in Caucasian eyes. Corneas in Afro-Caribbean populations tend to be larger and flatter than corneas of Chinese or Japanese populations.

Eurolens Research

Established in 1990 at UMIST, Manchester, by Professor Nathan Efron, Eurolens Research (which is an abbreviation of the longer title of 'European Centre for Contact Lens Research') has developed into an international focal point for contact lens research and development. The activities of Eurolens Research include the following:

- research – undertaking both pure and applied research projects funded by both peer-reviewed and industry grants; the research is performed at postgraduate and postdoctoral levels, and is aimed at furthering our understanding, and assisting in the improvement, of contact lenses
- industry/research/practitioner interface – actively promoting growth in the contact lens market by providing a university-based research link between industry and the profession
- public awareness – acting as a voice for the profession and industry when speaking to the lay media on issues relating to contact lens practice, with the main aim of promoting contact lens wear as a natural, safe and comfortable mode of correcting vision defects
- information source – serving as the European resource centre in the field of contact lenses and related subjects
- education – educating and training students, practitioners and contact lens educators in the art and science of contact lens practice.

Eurolens Research has about eight members of staff, whose day-to-day activities are co-ordinated by Research Manager, Dr Philip Morgan.

European Centre for Contact Lens Research
See Eurolens Research.

European Federation of the Contact Lens Industry (EFCLIN)

An organization for European contact lens manufacturers and wholesalers, EFCLIN offers a platform for exchange of information on technical and marketing subjects.

extended wear

This refers to a contact lens that is worn during the day followed by at least one sleep cycle (overnight) without removal. From a cosmetic standpoint, extended wear offers convenience to patients because there is no need for routine lens cleaning and disinfection. Extended-wear lenses also have important therapeutic applications as bandage lenses for use following ocular surgery and in the treatment of a wide variety of ocular pathology.

During the early development of **soft lenses** it was suggested that it might be possible to wear contact lenses continuously for many weeks, months or even years without removal; however, it soon became clear that such a practice was not clinically viable.

Various combinations of lens removal and lens replacement have been advocated over the years, and this has been driven to some extent by directions from the USA **Food and Drug Administration** (FDA). In 1981, the FDA gave approval for certain lenses to be worn continuously for 30 days and nights, after which the lenses had to be removed and cleaned, left out overnight, and reinserted the next day for another 30 day/night cycles, and so on. This recommendation was later revised to 7 day/night cycles in view of the growing body of evidence at the time that the risk of **microbial keratitis** increased significantly the longer lenses were worn without removal. With the introduction of disposable lenses in the late 1980s, lens removal was linked to lens replacement. The Acuvue™ disposable soft lens was designed as a lens that could be worn for 7 day/night cycles and discarded thereafter. **Silicone hydrogel lenses** have both USA and European regulatory approval to be worn for up to 30 day/night cycles. At the present time, 'extended wear' is taken to mean a 7 day/night cycle of lens wear, and 'continuous wear' is taken to mean a 30 day/night cycle of lens wear.

A primary concern in prescribing lenses for extended wear is that the lenses must provide sufficient oxygen to avoid excess corneal **oedema**. The Holden–Mertz criterion for the critical lens **oxygen transmissibility** (Dk/t) to meet this 'no oedema' criterion is 87 Barrer/cm. The maximum achievable Dk/t for hydrogel lenses is about 35 Barrer/cm. It is therefore not possible for hydrogel lenses to meet this criterion; nevertheless, certain patients appear to have higher thresholds for developing excess oedema and are capable of wearing hydrogel lenses successfully overnight. 'Stress testing' has been advocated as a means of assessing suitability for sleeping in lenses; this involves measuring the oedema response to a standard 'test lens' worn for a specified period with the eyes closed. Such tests have yet to be fully validated.

Silicone hydrogel lenses have oxygen transmissibilities in excess of 100 Barrer/cm (Figure E.11); these lenses therefore satisfy the Holden–Mertz criterion and can be advocated for continuous/extended wear. The incidence of microbial keratitis with these lenses appears to be less than has been reported with hydrogel lenses (although this claim has yet to be

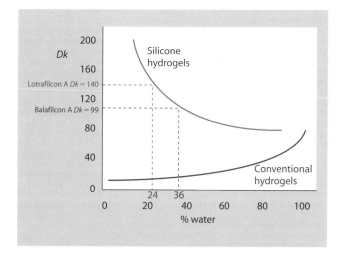

Figure E.11 Relationship between water content and oxygen permeability (*Dk*) for conventional hydrogel and silicone hydrogel materials.

scientifically validated). Non-sight threatening conditions such as **sterile keratitis** (which manifests in many forms), superior epithelial arcuate lesions and **papillary conjunctivitis** appear to be occurring at a similar rate in silicone hydrogel and conventional hydrogel lens wearers.

external hordeolum
This condition presents as a discrete, tender swelling of the anterior lid margin; specifically, it is an inflammation of the tissue lining the eyelash follicle and/or an associated **gland of Zeis** or **Moll**. Contact lenses may add to the discomfort of an external hordeolum due to various mechanical pressures exerted by the lens, and patients may prefer to cease lens wear during the acute phase of the condition. *Syn.* Stye.

eye dominance
See ocular dominance.

eyelashes
See eyelids.

eyelid pathology, therapeutic lenses for
If the lids are deficient (for example, congenitally or following trauma or surgery), or immobile (for example, following seventh (facial) nerve disease), part or all of the anterior globe may be exposed and dry. The **corneal epithelium** will be eroded and undergo dysplasia, and blood vessels will invade the previously clear **stroma**, unless protection can be given. Possibilities include a temporary or permanent tarsorrhaphy, temporary paralysis of the levator palpebrae superioris muscle using botulinum toxin, and the use of **therapeutic contact lenses**.

The lids themselves may consititute the challenge. They may be inturned (entropion) so that the lashes touch and traumatize the globe (trichiasis), or the tarsal conjunctiva – especially the area adjacent to the lid margin – may be keratinized. Both situations are found in chronic cicatrizing disease, such as Stevens–Johnson syndrome and cicatricial pemphigoid, and following chemical injury. Keratinization without entropion is a feature of atopic keratoconjunctivitis. Most soft lenses will not survive in this type of environment, rapidly becoming decentred and often falling out of the eye. There is a place for **rigid lenses** here, but the first choice will often be a scleral lens.

Ptosis results in an unsightly cosmetic appearance and can deprive the eye of vision if severe. A scleral lens with a ptosis crutch is one possible solution (Figure E.12).

When the **cornea** is insensitive – such as following surgery for acoustic neuroma, in herpes zoster ophthalmicus, and in trigeminal neuralgia – great care must be taken when fitting contact lenses. The danger is that the insensitivity of the eye will result in a situation where the patient is not alerted to otherwise painful complications such as epithelial detachment and infection. Patients with acute corneal problems due to neuroparalytic keratitis are usually best managed with lid taping, tarsorrhaphy or botulinum toxin induced ptosis.

eyelids
The eyelids are two mobile folds of skin that perform several important functions: they act as occluders, which shield the eyes from excessive light, and through their reflex closure afford protection against injury. The lids also form a pre-corneal **tear film** of uniform thickness during the upturn phase of each

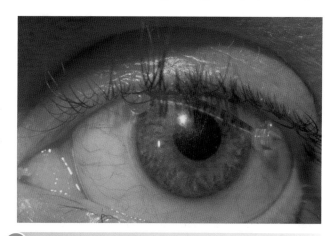

Figure E.12 Lid support lugs built into a scleral lens to act as a ptosis crutch.

blink. The action of blinking is important for tear drainage.

The eyelids are joined at their extremities, termed the canthi, and when the eye is open an elliptical space, the palpebral fissure, is formed between the lid margins. The position of various folds, or sulci, indicate to the clinician the integrity or otherwise of the anatomical configuration of the eyelids (Figure E.13). In the adult, the length of the fissure is approximately 30–31 mm, with a vertical height of 10–11 mm. In the primary position, the upper lid, which is the larger and more mobile of the two, typically covers approximately the upper third of the cornea, whilst the lower lid is level with the inferior corneal limbus. The eyelid margins are about 2 mm thick from front to back. The posterior quarter consists of conjunctival mucosa, and the anterior three-quarters is skin. The junction between the two is referred to as the mucocutaneous junction. Two or three rows of eyelashes (cilia) arise from the anterior border of the lid margins. These are longer and more numerous in the upper lid. The lashes receive a rich sensory nerve supply, and their sensitivity provides an effective alerting mechanism.

The meibomian (tarsal) gland orifices emerge just anterior to the mucocutaneous junction. About 30–40 glands open onto the upper margin, and slightly fewer (20–40) onto the lower. On eversion of the lids the yellowish meibomian acini are visible as yellow clusters through the tarsal **conjunctiva**. At the medial angle, the eyelid margins enclose a triangular space, the lacus lacrimalis, which contains the plica semilunaris and the caruncle. Lacrimal papillae are small elevations, located 5–6 mm from the medial canthal angle, which have a small aperture (punctum) that forms the opening to the lacrimal drainage system.

Movements of the eyelids occur through the co-ordinated action of several muscles – the **levator palpebrae superioris**, **tarsal muscles**, the **orbicularis oculi**, and the frontalis muscle. The elevation

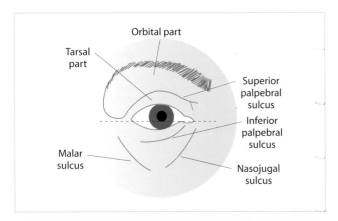

Figure E.13 Surface anatomy of the eyelids.

of the upper lid and the control of its vertical position are mediated principally by the levator. In vertical gaze, lid position and eye movements are closely linked. During elevation, the state of contraction of the levator is varied to maximize visibility. In extreme upgaze, lid retraction is augmented by the action of the frontalis, which elevates the eyebrows. In downgaze, co-ordinated lid movements similarly occur through levator relaxation. In periodic and reflex blinks the levator is spontaneously inhibited prior to orbicularis contraction in lid closure. Similarly, in lid opening the orbicularis relaxes, followed by contraction of the levator. Spontaneous eye blink activity is influenced by both central and peripheral factors.

Compared to the upper lid, the lower lid is relatively immobile and has no counterpart to the levator palpebrae superioris. The depression of the lower lid that occurs in downgaze is due to the attachment of the sheaths of the inferior oblique and inferior rectus muscles to the tarsal plate via a fibrous extension.

eye size
See apparent eye size.

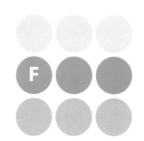

FDA
See Food and Drug Administration.

FDA soft lens classification
See water content, hydrogel.

fees and charges, contact lens
The very personal and individual nature of both services and products involved in optometry means that 'mass production' approaches cannot be applied without risking negative effects to the practice. When making pricing decisions, three elements normally need to be taken into account: the practice cost base, the patients and customers to the practice, and the competition. The fees and charges of the practice will generally be a compromise between what the business needs to cover costs, what the patients and customers expect to pay for the services and the products, and what the competition charges. Pricing issues are further confounded by the fact that not every practice owner will seek to maximize profits, and nor is detailed information about costs, competition and the potential patient/customer easily available to the practice.

The concept of the speciality–commodity continuum applies to both contact lens products and services. At one extreme is the service product, consisting of a speciality service and highly differentiated from the rest of the competition, whilst at the other extreme is a commodity. Figure F.1 illustrates this speciality–commodity continuum as a conceptual map, describing some of the characteristics of the competition, gross profits, price differentiation and image differentiation associated with the two extremes. Eye care practices would be best served by ensuring that contact lens products and services do not slide to the extreme commodity end. It is worth noting the features of a commodity, which include self-determination of need, self-management of use, being non-invasive with little (perceived) potential for harm, being non-regulated, and price determined by market forces.

Developing a fees and charges schedule is never an easy task. Once one subscribes to the need to move away from the commodity end of the market (where competition relies primarily on purchase decisions based only on price) to the speciality end, then the need for a professional model for fees and charges becomes paramount. One way to do this is to establish the expenses overhead per hour for the practice

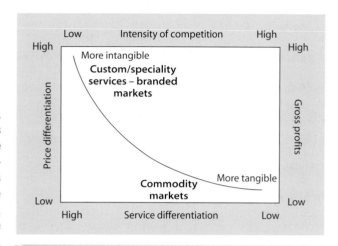

Figure F.1 The speciality–commodity continuum.

(chair time). Knowing the actual chair time required for differing types of contact lens services (e.g. **spherical rigid lenses**, **soft lenses**, daily/monthly **disposable soft lenses**, **toric and bifocal lenses** etc.), allowing for potential unscheduled visits, adding the contact lens material and care system costs (duly marked up at, say, 20–35%), and any other handling charges, this figure can then be used to calculate the fees and charges for any service-product provided by the practice. With the advent of mail-order contact lenses, Internet trading and an increasing trend for contact lenses to be considered as a commodity, it is important to adopt a transparent fees and charges schedule that is competitive on a like-for-like basis without eroding the professional fees dimension.

fenestrated lenses for optic measurement (FLOMs)
See fitting scleral lenses.

fenestration
A hole in a lens that has one or more of the following effects:

- facilitating tear exchange beneath the lens
- enhancing corneal oxygenation (alleviating hypoxia)
- alleviating the build-up of carbon dioxide (hypercapnia) beneath the lens
- modifying the extent of positive and negative force (suction pressure) beneath the lens
- allowing air bubbles to form beneath scleral lenses, which aid 'settling back'.

Fenestrations are usually only employed in scleral lens fitting. *See* fitting scleral lenses.

Fick, Adolf Eugene

There was a great deal of activity in contact lens research in the late 1880s, which has led to debate as to who should be given credit for being the first to fit a contact lens. Adolf Eugene Fick (Figure F.2), a German ophthalmologist working in Zurich, appears to have been the first to describe the process of fabricating and fitting contact lenses; specifically, he described the fitting of afocal scleral **contact shells** – first on rabbits, then on himself, and finally on a small group of volunteer patients. Fick's work was published in the journal *Archiv für Augenheilkunde* in March 1888.

field of fixation

With a spectacle lens, a prismatic effect associated with the lens periphery results when the eye is rotated to view objects away from the axis of the correction; a larger eye movement, in comparison with the uncorrected eye, is required with a negative spectacle lens and a smaller one with a positive correction. These fixation effects are absent with contact lens corrections, since the lenses follow the movements of the eyes from fixation to fixation.

field of view

With a spectacle lens a **prismatic effect** associated with the lens periphery results when the eye is stationary, whereby an annular zone of the visual field is invisible (a ring scotoma) with a positive correction and an annular zone of the visual field is seen diplopically with a negative correction (Figure F.3). The periphery of the **field of view** may be slightly affected if the lens or its optical zone is small. In the case of **rigid lenses**, **flare** or glare may occur due to discontinuities at the edge of the lens or optic zone affecting ray pencils from the periphery of the field.

filamentary keratitis, therapeutic lenses for

A 'wet' form of filamentary keratitis sometimes occurs without tear volume deficiency in herpes simplex keratitis, recurrent erosion, dystonia, and Theodore's superior limbic keratoconjunctivitis. This condition often responds well to the use of **hydrogel** lenses. The more usual 'dry' form of filamentary keratopathy occurs in tear deficiency, although contact lenses have little part to play in the management of this form of the disease. **Scleral lenses** have been used successfully in 'dry' filamentary keratitis.

financial considerations

See indications and contraindications for contact lens wear.

financial management in contact lens practice

Income to a contact lens practice will arise from patients, customers and third party payments

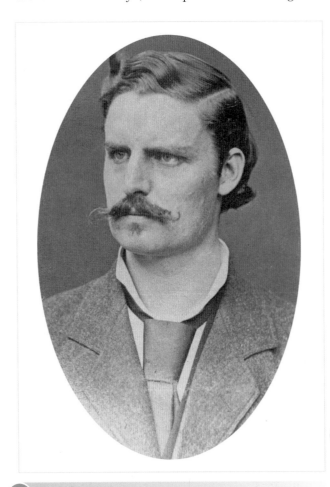

Figure F.2 Adolf Eugene Fick.

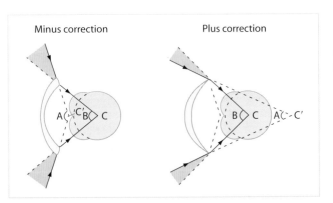

Figure F.3 Fields of view as seen through spectacle lens corrections. The centre of rotation of the eye is at C, and its image is seen through the spectacle lens at C'. B is the apparent macular field of view and A the actual field.

(national and private health insurance, driving licence authorities, employers etc.). It is therefore important that records are kept of every transaction and that there is no hindrance to receiving these payments by any method (e.g. cash, credit cards, cheques, direct debit, standing order, electronic transfer of funds etc.). Of these methods, the use of direct debits in pre-paid subscription schemes has proved to be a particularly useful option. Similarly, the practice will need to pay its vendors (e.g. laboratories, prescription houses, various forms of sales tax, telephone, printing and stationery etc.) and its staff.

The provision of contact lens services, like general ophthalmic services, is indeed a provision of professional time. The supply of products is secondary to this, and it is appropriate to adopt an accounting method that mirrors this approach.

Computers are now used almost universally in general practice management, and in particular in the management of practice finances. Many 'off-the-shelf' software options are available and adaptable, whilst others dedicated to optometric practice management and incorporating the special needs for contact lens practice are also available. *See* fees and charges, contact lens.

fitting philosophy

This term is generally applied to **rigid lens** fitting, and refers to any specified approach to achieving a satisfactory lens fit. The fitting philosophy applies primarily to the lens design, but also to desirable aspects of the lens fit, including lens positioning and movement, and appearance of the **fluorescein** pattern. The concept of 'fitting philosophy' was prominent in the days of exclusively **scleral** and rigid lens fitting (prior to the introduction of soft lenses), and perhaps related more to the 'art' rather than the 'science' of lens fitting; as such, the term 'fitting philosophy' is seldom used today.

fitting rigid lenses

The conventional method of fitting **rigid lenses** is by use of trial lenses, although there are two other options: empirical fitting and **videokeratoscopic** fitting.

Most rigid lens fitting is still undertaken using trial (or 'diagnostic') lens fitting sets in a range of **back optic zone radius** (BOZR) and **total diameter** (TD). A set of lenses in a given trial fitting set usually follows a single design concept – for instance, constant **edge clearance**.

Lenses in a 'standard' trial fitting set are usually available in a single diameter and **back vertex power** (BVP), with a range of BOZRs in 0.1-mm steps; however, it is preferable to use fitting sets that have lenses available in two diameters (e.g. 9.2 and 9.8 mm). Examples of additional useful fitting sets include:

- plus power, e.g. +3.00 D, smaller diameter
- high minus power, e.g. 8.00 D, larger diameter
- small diameter for interpalpebral fitting, e.g. 8.6 mm
- **keratoconus**, diameter varying with BOZR.

The procedure for selecting an initial fitting of **spherical lenses** using a trial fitting set is as follows:

1. Select a lens diameter based on corneal diameter, palpebral aperture and lid configuration.
2. Select the BOZR based on the flattest **keratometer** ('K') reading, adjusting the BOZR to be flatter or steeper than K depending on BOZD. Since relatively steep fitting lenses are easier to visualize with **fluorescein**, err on the steep side.
3. If more than one power is available, select a lens power closest to the refraction of the patient.

A high degree of success can be achieved by empirical fitting, i.e. ordering initial lenses based on keratometry and refraction. Most contact lens laboratories will supply lenses on a 'per case' basis – that is, a fixed cost for an unlimited number of lens exchanges for a given 'case' (patient) until a final satisfactory fit is obtained. This is an attractive option, especially in some countries, because of concerns about cross-infection. Notwithstanding such concerns, there are occasions when most practitioners would wish to use this method – for example, when wishing to fit a design not covered by an available fitting set, or when an initial trial fitting is inconvenient for the patient.

The procedure for empirical fitting of spherical lenses is as follows:

1. Select a lens diameter based on corneal diameter, palpebral aperture and lid configuration.
2. Select the BOZR based on the flattest K reading, adjusting the BOZR to be flatter or steeper than K depending on BOZD. Flatter radii tend to be used with larger BOZD and *vice versa*.
3. If the lens is an average diameter, select the BVP based on the sphere power from the refraction (minus cylinder form) corrected for vertex distance. With an average diameter lens no adjustment is necessary; however, an adjustment is necessary if the BOZR is steeper or flatter than K.
4. Order the lens and use this effectively as a trial fitting lens, being prepared to modify or exchange the lens prior to dispensing.

Most **videokeratoscopy** (VK) instruments incorporate rigid lens fitting software. This enables the practitioners to model different rigid lens designs on an accurate representation of the **cornea** of the patient. The fitting success rates are relatively low when relying solely on the default settings of the manufacturer of the VK instrument being used, but can be relatively high when a practitioner uses the software to select an appropriate lens.

The main advantages of VK contour maps in rigid lens fitting is that they:

- indicate whether the corneal apex is decentred
- show atypical corneal shapes, e.g. extremes of corneal asphericity
- allow the practitioner to monitor changes in corneal shape
- allow virtual trial fitting of rigid lenses.

The obvious limitation of VK contour maps in trial lens fitting is that they fail to take into account the influence of the lids.

The adequacy of a rigid lens fit is first assessed in white light according to the following criteria:

1. *Diameter.* The lens should appear to be an appropriate size for the eye. A relatively small lens may fail to cover the cornea through sitting high or resting on the bottom lid. It may also be less comfortable because of greater interaction between the upper lid margin and the lens edge. Alternatively, the lens may irritate the bottom lid by dropping between blinks. Lenses that are larger than the palpebral aperture can result in problems through interacting with the bottom lid as well as the top lid. In some cases the lens will be pushed into a high riding position by occasional interaction with the bottom lid, while in other cases the lens may rest on the bottom lid.

2. *Centration.* Some decentration may be acceptable if the optic zone maintains pupil coverage, but this may also indicate poor central or peripheral fit. **Flat fitting lenses** can show decentration in any direction, depending on factors such as lid tightness.

3. *Movement.* Sluggish, limited post-blink movement may indicate a relatively **steep-fitting lens**. Fast movement sometimes indicates a flat-fitting lens, but may also be due to strong interaction with the top lid, perhaps due to excessive edge clearance.

Fluorescein is instilled into the eye and the lens fit is assessed in cobalt blue light according to the following criteria:

1. *Central fit.* If the lens is half covered by the top lid, or the lens is decentred, it may not be possi-

ble to observe the central fit without retracting the lid and repositioning the lens. This is achieved by gently holding the top and bottom lids with the index finger and thumb respectively. The lids can be used to manoeuvre the lens into a central position, and can also be used to pump extra fluorescein beneath the lens. The fluorescein pattern for well-fitting lenses will vary according to corneal asphericity and astigmatism. Spherical corneas show the simplest fluorescein patterns. The optimum fit is one that shows central alignment or just a trace of fluorescein indicating minimal central clearance. With astigmatic corneas, in the steeper meridian the central fluorescein pattern will show increasing thickness towards the edge. The most recognizable fluorescein pattern is the 'dumb-bell' pattern seen with spherical lenses on **astigmatic** corneas (Figure F.4). With steep-fitting lenses, fluorescein assessment will show a central pool of fluorescein, and this pool will appear brighter the steeper the fit. In extreme cases an air bubble may be present. With flat-fitting lenses, a central touch will be visible as an area of dark blue or black. The area of touch will be smaller, the flatter the fit. Fluorescein will be present in the periphery, and may be continuous with the peripheral band of fluorescein.

2. *Mid-peripheral fit.* Spherical lenses, particularly on astigmatic eyes, make contact with the cornea at the edge of the optic zone. If the lens is poorly blended or makes contact at a sharp angle, it may be uncomfortable and cause epithelial disrup-

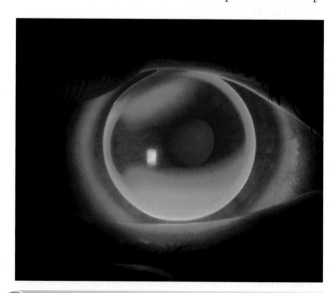

Figure F.4 Assessing central fluorescein fit having centred the lens and retracted the top lid.

tion. If a narrow line of contact between optic zones can be seen upon lens inspection, it is likely that there is a sharp junction from poor blending. A band of contact corresponding to the first peripheral zone may indicate relatively steep peripheral curves and the need for peripheral lens flattening. In the case of a flat-fitting lens, the mid-peripheral band of fluorescein may merge with that of the central zone even in the flattest meridian.

3. *Edge lift*. The width and the brightness of the peripheral band of fluorescein gives an indication of the extent of **edge clearance**. Where the edge clearance is small, the tear-film thickness may be less than the critical thickness above which the fluorescein appears a saturated yellow colour. This is generally less than the desired clearance of 80 μm or more. A less-than-bright yellow peripheral ring, therefore, indicates suboptimal edge clearance. This will be confirmed by an apparent break in the peripheral band of fluorescein when the lens decentres toward the limbus. In the case of excessive edge clearance, bubbles may be seen forming under the lens periphery. The peripheral band may also be wider than expected, and show the saturated yellow appearance over much of the peripheral band.

Once a correct-fitting lens is identified, an over-refraction is pre-formed to determine the correct lens power and lenses can be ordered for the patient.

fitting scleral lenses

Scleral lenses can be fitted by taking an eye impression or by assessing pre-formed lenses of known specifications. The objective in either case is to achieve best possible alignment over the sclera with **corneal** clearance. Different approaches are required for fitting **polymethyl methacrylate** (PMMA) versus gas-permeable scleral lenses.

A means of ventilation, most often a **fenestration**, is a prerequisite for PMMA scleral lenses, to give oxygenated tear flow. Fenestrations also admit air bubbles behind the lens and cause settling back by relieving the positive pressure in the pre-corneal fluid reservoir. These factors are problematic and contribute significantly to the unpredictable nature of scleral lens fitting. The relationship between the corneal curvature and the lens **back optic zone radius** (BOZR) is relatively unimportant with scleral lenses, where the critical feature is corneal clearance. Air bubbles greater than 0.1 mm in diameter can cause visual disturbance, while small bubbles may lead to intolerable corneal contact.

Pre-formed scleral lenses are lathe cut, which results in the optic and scleral zones being co-axial. The sclera is not symmetrical about the geometric axis, but a successful result can still be achieved in most cases. A series of lenses, each with a known back scleral radius (BSR), is tried until the optimum scleral zone appearance is achieved. If the BSR is too steep, the lens vaults from the periphery, adding to the apical clearance. If it is too flat, the periphery of the lens stands off the sclera but the apical clearance is not affected.

Having established the BSR, fenestrated lenses for optic measurement (FLOMs) are used to determine the optimum optic zone clearance by variation of the BOZR and **back optic zone diameter** (BOZD). A steeper BOZR with an unchanged BOZD, or a larger BOZD with an unchanged BOZR, increases the optic zone sagittal depth and hence the apical clearance. The BSR, BOZR and BOZD must all be varied to obtain the optimum fit. Because the typical nasal sclera is much flatter than the temporal sclera, co-axial scleral lenses tend to decentre temporally and downwards to a position of approximate symmetry, increasing the variation in the depth of the pre-corneal fluid reservoir. This may cause intractable bubbles and contact zones even when the **cornea** is reasonably regular. The spherical back surface of a pre-formed lens never matches the asymmetric corneal surface, so there can be large variations in the depth of the pre-corneal fluid reservoir. If bubbles form in the deeper areas, reducing the clearance may be the only way to reduce their size, but this may lead to compressive corneal contact.

With the impression method of scleral lens fitting, a mould of the anterior eye is made using dental alginate. This is allowed to set and plaster is then poured into the mould, giving rise to a stone cast of the eye. A PMMA sheet is thermally moulded over the stone cast, excess PMMA is cut off to the desired lens shape, the edge is polished, and substance is removed from the optic zone to give appropriate clearance between the lens and cornea. This gives a near glove-fit over the sclera irrespective of scleral topography, and enables the closest possible match to the corneal contour. Large air bubbles are therefore less likely to form beneath the lens and interfere with vision.

The great majority of eyes can be fitted, using pre-formed fitting methods, with sealed (rather than fenestrated) lenses made from gas-permeable materials. There is some disagreement as to whether sealed gas-permeable scleral lenses transmit sufficient oxygen to maintain normal corneal physiology, or whether they need to be fenestrated. The depth of the pre-corneal fluid reservoir and the quality of corneal contact zones are the key features to evaluate, as they have a bearing on both tolerance to lenses and visual performance.

The reduced 'settling back' with sealed gas-permeable scleral lenses enables precise control of corneal clearance. Assessment of corneal clearance is effected by simple observation with a thin optical section on a slit lamp; a slit width of 0.25 mm – i.e. approximately half the thickness of a normal cornea – is optimal. The extent of clearance is estimated with respect to the thickness of the cornea. The optimum corneal clearance is achieved by using combinations of the BOZR and BOZD to vary the sagittal depth, or by changing the optic zone projection (OZP) in progressive increments.

The main limitation of sealed gas-permeable scleral lens fitting is an insufficiently regular scleral zone, which leads to intrusion of bubbles into the pre-corneal fluid reservoir. This can occur immediately following lens insertion, or after a period of wear. The apical clearance can be reduced so that bubbles are displaced to the periphery of the optic zone, but the lens may be less comfortable as a result. If intrusion of bubbles is intractable, an impression is necessary. Gas-permeable scleral lenses can be produced from impressions, but the process is cumbersome compared to the pre-formed approach.

fitting soft lenses

The behaviour of a **soft lens** on the eye is determined by trial lens fitting. The selection of the first trial lens for a patient can take into account the horizontal visible iris diameter, particularly if the **cornea** appears to be unusually large or small (there should be a 1.0–1.5 mm overlap of the lens on to the white sclera; Figure F.5). The selection of back optic zone radius is a process of trial and error unless there is useful information from experience of the patient with previous lenses. For example, if the patient previously required a relatively steep lens in order to achieve a successful fit, this will suggest the need

for a similarly steep lens to obtain a good fit. The lens material and wearing regimen are also key factors in the selection of the initial trial lens. While compromises occasionally have to be made, the appropriate lens should be selected based on an assessment of the requirements of the patient rather than prescribing habits or practice policy.

The selected lens is placed on the eye, allowed to settle (*see* **settling time**), and the following assessment techniques (although not necessarily all of them) can be applied:

1. *Initial lens comfort.* The reaction of the patient to the lens in terms of comfort is the first clue to the lens fit. A well-fitting soft lens is a comfortable lens. **Tight-fitting lenses** are also usually comfortable initially, but some discomfort or lens awareness may indicate a **loose-fitting lens**. Due to the overlapping distribution of corneal nerves, it is difficult for patients precisely to locate the source of any discomfort; however, it is worth asking the patient roughly to describe the discomfort. Also, the severity of any discomfort can be gauged by observing the patient. Clearly, excessive lacrimation, blepharospam and other forms of aversion response would tend to suggest a more severe reaction.

2. *Vision.* An **over-refraction** is usually unnecessary as part of the fitting procedure. Current spherical soft lenses, because of their thinness and flexibility, rarely support a tear lens between the lens and cornea. Where an over-refraction yields an unexpected result, the labelled lens power may be incorrect; this can be checked by measuring the lens power with a focimeter. Unstable vision may indicate a loose, relatively mobile fit.

3. *Lens centration.* Some lens decentration is acceptable, provided the lens shows full corneal coverage at all times (the entire limbus is overlapped by at least 0.5 mm) and does not appear to compromise comfort. It is important to ensure that the pupil is fully covered by the optic zone of the lens. Loose-fitting lenses tend to show greater decentration, typically greater than 0.3 mm. Tight lenses show similar centration characteristics to those of well-fitting lenses.

4. *Lens movement.* Some lens movement (at least 0.3 mm) is necessary with each blink to maintain post-lens lubrication and, in turn, ensure a complete post-lens tear film. Excessive movement can cause unnecessary discomfort and disrupt vision. The absence of post-blink movement is a key indicator of lens tightness, as virtually all tight-fitting lenses show little or no movement.

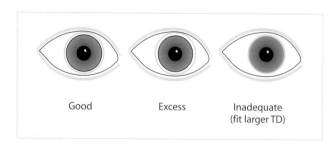

| Good | Excess | Inadequate (fit larger TD) |

Figure F.5 Diameter selection of a soft lens.

Loose-fitting lenses do not necessarily show excessive movement, so the assessment of lens movement on its own is an inadequate measure of lens fit. In a normal fit, the lens usually remains stationary when the lid moves downward during the first part of the blink (lid closure) but then moves upwards by a small amount during the second part of the blink (lid opening), returning to its original position immediately after the blink – hence the description 'post-blink movement'.

5. *Lag on upgaze and version.* The lens should decentre about 0.3 mm upon upgaze or lateral version.

6. *Push-up test.* This test is undertaken by digitally moving the lens upwards by pushing the lower lid against the lens edge. The test consists of an assessment of the amount of force necessary to dislodge the lens upwards (which should be minimal), and the speed of recentration of the lens from its dislodged position (which should not be sluggish).

7. *Peripheral fit.* A slight, barely visible edge stand-off can cause discomfort due to interaction with the lids. Excessive peripheral tightness is rarely seen with modern lenses due to their relatively thin edges; when seen, tight peripheral fits show some indentation of the bulbar conjunctiva, which may be visible on lens removal by instillation of **fluorescein** and observation of tear pooling in the indentation.

8. *Keratometry mire assessment.* The **keratometry** mires tend to distort when the lens is not aligned with the lens surface. Mire distortion tends to clear immediately after a blink with tight-fitting lenses, and between blinks with loose-fitting lenses.

9. *Videokeratoscopy.* This gives a more detailed picture than keratometry. The final contour map, however, unlike keratometry, is a static assessment.

10. *Retinoscopy.* This can be useful in confirming that the optic zone gives proper coverage of the pupil, and may be particularly useful with some bifocal designs.

Once a correct-fitting lens is identified, an over-refraction is performed to determine the correct lens power, and lenses can then be ordered for the patient.

flare

Because the overall diameter of a **rigid lens** is less than that of the **cornea**, discontinuities and flare effects may arise in the peripheral field. Flare refers to the formation of transient defocused secondary arcuate or annular images, which are observed at variable locations in the mid-periphery. This phenomenon is encountered more frequently when the pupils are enlarged, such as at night, and is due to refractive effects of the tear meniscus at the lens edge and/or the peripheral curve (Figure F.6). Patients seem to become less troubled by this phenomenon over time.

flat lens fit

A lens that has a curvature which is less than that of the anterior eye (especially the **cornea**) is deemed to be fitting flat. The degree of flatness cannot be simply predicted by comparing the back central optic radius of the lens with central corneal curvature, because the curvature of both the lens and cornea can change dramatically towards the periphery. In general, a flat-fitting lens will appear to be **loose**. A flat **rigid lens** fit, when examined using **fluorescein**, will display a broad region of central touch and substantial peripheral and **edge lift** off (Figure F.7).

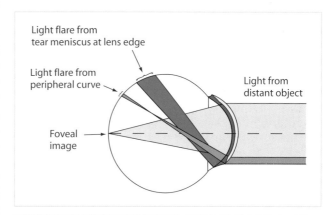

Figure F.6 Causes of rigid lens flare.

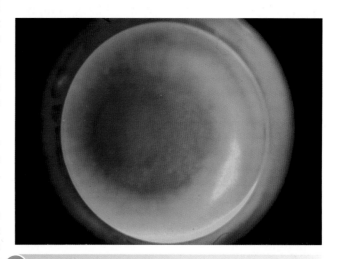

Figure F.7 Flat-fitting rigid lens revealed by fluorescein.

flexure

See dimensional instability, rigid lens.

FLOMs

See fitting scleral lenses.

fluid lens

See tear lens.

fluorescein sodium

Fluorescein sodium is a water-soluble dye. It absorbs most light in the blue part of the spectrum but the majority of its emitted light is in the yellow part of the spectrum, with some in the green. The intensity of light emitted is governed by the concentration and pH of the solution and, critically in **rigid lens** fitting, the thickness of the fluorescein sample. Fluorescein is not visible until a critical thickness of about 15 μm is reached. The intensity of fluorescence increases with increasing thickness until another critical thickness of about 60 μm is reached, beyond which the fluorescein is seen as a uniform bright yellow colour.

This dye has three main uses in contact lens practice:

1. Assessing the adequacy of fit of a **rigid lens**
2. Assessing the ocular surface for evidence of trauma or physiological decompensation
3. Highlighting the **tear film** for the purpose of measuring **tear break-up time**.

In rigid lens fitting, the fluorescein pattern is a simple two-dimensional representation of a complex three-dimensional shape. This provides useful information about the relationship of the lens with the shape of the eye. Areas of tear pooling appear bright yellow. Where the tear layer is absent or extremely thin, there is no visible fluorescence and the area appears dark blue or black. Between these extremes, varying thicknesses of post-lens tear film are seen as varying intensities of yellow/green. Fluorescein therefore provides a contour map of the thickness of the tear film.

Fluorescein will fill spaces on the corneal surface where tissue is missing. It will also enter and stain the cytoplasm of dead or devitalized epithelial cells. Therefore, bright areas of fluorescence on the corneal surface observed following instillation of fluorescein indicate either cell damage or cell loss. A dull glow around a bright area of fluorescence indicates that fluorescein has diffused into surrounding epithelial and/or stromal tissue.

If fluorescein is instilled into an eye and the eye is held open for a few seconds, dark areas will begin to appear among the normal even fluorescent glow across the cornea; these dark areas indicate tear thinning or break-up. This phenomenon forms the basis of the **tear break-up time** test.

fluorescein sodium, instillation of

The preferred method of instilling fluorescein sodium into the eye is to use a filter strip impregnated with this dye (i.e. a 'fluorescein strip'). A drop of non-preserved **saline** is placed on the orange (impregnated) tip of the fluorescein strip. The patient is instructed to look down and the strip is lightly touched on the superior conjunctiva for less than one second. The patient is instructed to execute a couple of blinks in order to spread the fluorescein. Placing a drop of fluorescein on the superior sclera will maximize the length of time the dye remains in the eye.

In **rigid contact lens** wearers, the process can be simplified by touching the fluorescein strip against the front of the lens. A thick fluorescein-stained pre-lens tear film may confound interpretation of the true post-lens fluorescein pattern (the object of interest), so it may be necessary to wait until this has dissipated before assessing the pattern.

fluoro-silicone-acrylates

See rigid contact lens.

fluting

Lifting off of the edge of the lens from the surface of the eyeball. This phenomenon can occur with lenses of relatively high modulus (stiffness), such as thick, low water content **soft lenses**, **silicone elastomer lenses**, and **silicone hydrogel lenses**. Lens fluting should be avoided; if it is observed, a different lens base curve should be chosen (typically steeper).

focimeter

A standard optical focimeter (also known as a lensometer or vertometer) can be used to measure the **back vertex power** (BVP) of a contact lens (Figure F.8). Care must be taken to prevent flexure and damage to the lens. A flat plastic disc with a range of circular apertures is often used to support the lens during focimetry. An automatic **focimeter** can also be used. Any surface droplets, distortions or lens surface depositions (even fingerprints) will decrease the quality of the viewed image, especially with soft lenses, and this increases the likelihood of an error in assessing BVP. The recommended technique, therefore, is to **surfactant-clean** the lens, dab it dry with a lint-free tissue, and place the lens on the focimeter support using rubber-tipped tweezers. It is important to measure the BVP of a **soft lens** as soon as possible following removal from its storage medium to avoid possible effects of lens

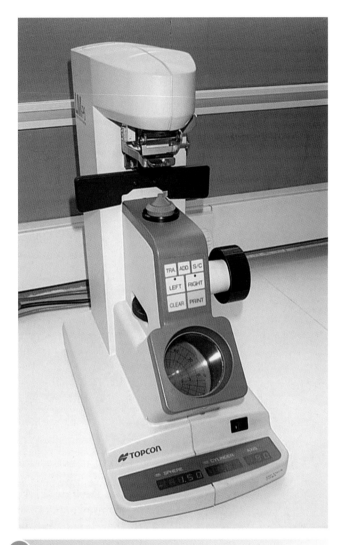

Figure F.8 Focimeter with reduced aperture stop suitable for measuring the power of contact lenses.

dehydration. A graduated rotating device is useful for checking **toric lenses**.

The standard focimeter is calibrated for spectacle lenses placed at a specific location on the instrument measuring stop. The physical limitations of the focimeter combined with the highly curved back surface of the lens cause the lens to rest in a position away from this location. This will result in a systematic error when reading off lens power, and this error is significant especially when checking high-powered lenses. The particular focimeter should be recalibrated for contact lens checking, and ideally a dedicated focimeter should be set aside for the exclusive purpose of checking the powers of contact lenses. The focimeter is also used to measure the magnitude and direction of prismatic power in prism ballast and **scleral lenses**. In addition to the quantitative data obtained using this technique, the clarity of the viewed image formed by transmission through the contact lens can provide an indication of lens optical quality.

The optical configuration of most focimeters is such that lens power is checked by sampling over an aperture of approximately 4 mm diameter. In many advanced **rigid lens** designs (e.g. bifocal, multifocal and aspheric) there can be significant power variations within such a small range, and this will not be detected by standard focimetry. Reducing the aperture can help; however, in advanced optical designs lens power variations are best checked using optical interferometric techniques such as the Twyman–Green interferometer.

folds
See oedema.

Food and Drug Administration
In the United States of America, the control of contact lenses and contact lens care products is governed by the Food and Drug Administration (FDA). The FDA has classified contact lenses as a drug, and therefore demands rigorous testing and evaluation before contact lenses can be released onto the market. This process is controlled by the Centre for Devices and Radiological Health, which has the following mission: 'Protecting the public health by providing reasonable assurance of the safety and effectiveness of medical devices and by eliminating unnecessary human exposure to radiation emitted from electronic products.'

forces acting on a rigid lens
A number of forces that act on a **rigid lens** have to be suitably balanced in order to achieve a satisfactory fit (Figure F.9). The gravitational force of the lens and pre-lens **tear film** causes the lens to drop. The effect will be greater, and the lens less stable, the further forward the centre of gravity lies. The centre of gravity is further forward in plus lenses compared with minus lenses. It is shifted posteriorly by increasing the diameter, steepening the back optic zone radius, or decreasing the thickness of the lens. With both plus and minus lenses, the greatest shift and most effective stabilization is achieved through changing the lens diameter.

The lens is held in place by the capillary forces in the post-lens tear film and the surface tensional force in the tear meniscus at the lens edge. The capillary force increases with increasingly closer alignment of the lens and the **cornea**. The force is therefore greater with spherical corneas compared with **astigmatic** corneas.

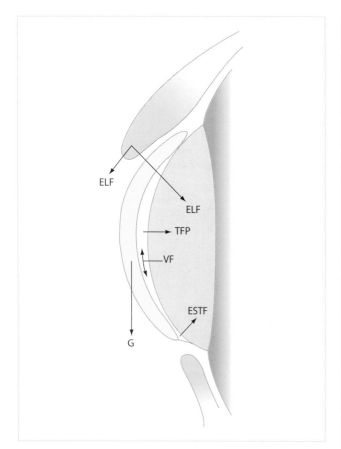

Figure F.9 Forces acting on a lid-attached rigid lens. ELF = eyelid forces; ESTF = edge surface tension force; G = gravity; TPF = tear fluid pressure; VF = viscous forces.

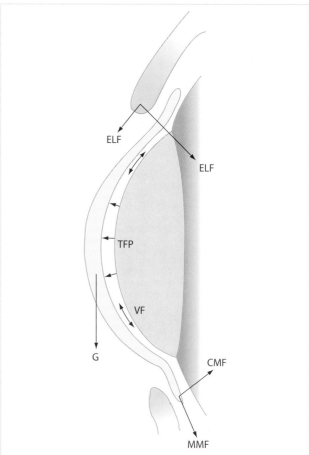

Figure F.10 Forces acting on a soft lens. CMF = circumferential membrane force; ELF = eyelid force; G = gravity; MMF = meridional membrane force; TFP = tear fluid pressure; VF = viscous forces.

Surface tension forces act at the lens edge where the edge meniscus is not covered by the lid. There will be no surface tension where a meniscus is absent due to excessive edge clearance. This force can be increased by reducing edge clearance and edge thickness.

Eyelid forces (primarily the upper lid) act to move the lens in a vertical direction during the blink. Between blinks these forces help to stabilize the lens in the case of an extra-palpebral fit, but have no effect in the case of an intra-palpebral fit.

forces acting on a soft lens

A range of forces act on a **soft lens**, which keeps the lens in place on the eye but allows it to move a small amount between blinks (Figure F.10). Soft lenses are usually required to flex in two directions in order to align to the shape of the **cornea** and sclera. Since soft lenses are generally flatter than the central corneal curvature they steepen in order to align with the cornea, but at the periphery they are required to flatten so as to align with the sclera. The stresses formed in the lens are proportional to the mechanical properties of the material as well as the dimensions of the lens. Due to the viscous nature of the tear fluid, this deformation of the lens to match the shape of the eye results in a 'squeeze pressure' being developed in the post-lens **tear film**. This squeeze pressure is related to the amount of force required to move the lens across the eye, and will therefore influence lens fit. The amount of force required to move the lens is also related to the viscosity of the post-lens tear film. This helps to explain why the movement of a soft lens can vary markedly during a given wearing period. Soft lens retaining forces are relatively large compared with those of **rigid lenses**, and therefore gravitational force has less of an effect.

FOZD
See front optic zone diameter.

FOZR
See front optic zone radius.

front optic zone diameter (FOZD)
This is the diameter of the optic zone of the front surface of the lens as measured through the lens centre (see Figure B.1). The front optic zone diameter (FOZD) of a rigid lens should be at least 0.5 mm larger than the **back optic zone diameter** (BOZD). Except in low powers, most **rigid lenses** are lenticulated to reduce thickness and weight. Lenses occasionally incorporate a negative carrier in order to encourage lid attachment and centre the lens. A negative carrier is a peripheral zone that is thinner at the optic zone junction than the lens periphery. A positive carrier or tapered edge design – where the peripheral zone is thicker at the optic zone junction than the lens periphery – is occasionally used to discourage lid attachment in a high riding lens. *See* high plus power contact lens design.

front optic zone radius (FOZR)
The front optic zone radius (FOZR) is the radius of curvature of the front surface of a contact lens (see Figure B.1). This parameter is varied to achieve the desired optical correction once the **BOZR** has been determined to achieve an optimum fit.

front surface rigid toric lenses
See cylindrical power equivalent rigid toric lenses.

Fuchs's dystrophy
See dystrophies of the corneal epithelium, therapeutic lenses for.

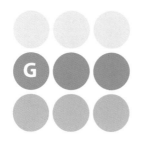

gap junctions
See corneal epithelium.

gas-permeable scleral lenses
See fitting scleral lenses.

General Optical Council (GOC)
The GOC is the regulatory authority in the United Kingdom and Northern Ireland responsible for the regulation of optometrists and dispensing opticians. It does this by providing for statutory registration, the accreditation and monitoring of education, training, and examination. It also enforces proper standards of practice and conduct. The GOC is separate from and independent of any other optical bodies that represent the interests of opticians.

In the UK, optometrists and dispensing opticians must be registered by the GOC in order to practise in the UK according to legal requirements. In order to register, they must have undertaken training at, and passed examinations of, a university or other training institute approved by the GOC. However, European Community Directives provide for the recognition of qualifications awarded in countries of the European Economic Area (EEA), and there are special arrangements, including an examination, for those qualified in countries outside of the EEA.

The law in the UK states that (apart from medical practitioners) only an optometrist can test sight. Optometrists can also fit and supply optical appliances such as spectacles and contact lenses, but may only fit and supply contact lenses if they have gained an appropriate qualification. Dispensing opticians are not permitted to test eyes, but they can fit and supply optical appliances according to a prescription from an optometrist, and can fit and supply contact lenses, again if they have undertaken special training.

By the powers vested in it by the Opticians Act 1985 (section 31), the General Optical Council in the UK has made rules regulating the prescription, supply and fitting of contact lenses by registered optometrists, opticians or companies and their employees. The Rules on the Fitting of Contact Lenses (SI 1985/856) cover the details with respect to the circumstances in which trainee optometrists or opticians may fit contact lenses. The Contact Lens (Qualifications etc) Rules (SI 1988/1305) and The Contact Lens (Qualifications etc) Rules 1989 (SI 1989/375) provide for a minimum level of educa-

tion, training and qualification before a registered optometrist or optician can undertake fitting of contact lenses in the UK. The Contact Lens (Specification) Rules 1989 (SI 1989/791) require that an optometrist or optician who fits contact lenses shall on completion of the fitting give the patient a written specification of the lenses in sufficient detail to enable the lens to be replicated.

ghost vessels
See neovascularization.

glands of Krause
See accessory lacrimal glands.

glands of Moll
These are ciliary glands found in association with eyelash follicles (Figure G.1). Glands of Moll are modified sweat glands consisting of an unbranched spiral tubule. The exact function of these glands is unclear.

glands of Wolfring
See accessory lacrimal glands.

glands of Zeis
These are ciliary glands found in association with eyelash follicles (*see* Figure G.1). The glands of Zeis are unilobular sebaceous glands that open directly into the follicle. The function of their oily secretion is to lubricate the lashes to prevent them from drying out and becoming brittle.

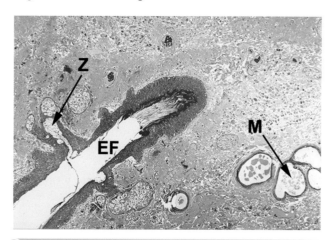

Figure G.1 Histological section through the ciliary zone of the eyelid. Glands of Zeis (Z) discharge their contents into an eyelash follicle (EF), which contains the remnants of an eyelash. M = gland of Moll.

glycocalyx
See corneal epithelium.

GOC
See General Optical Council.

Gothenburg Study
A critically important research study, conducted in Gothenburg, Sweden, during the 1980s, that revealed the long-term adverse effects of extended hydrogel contact lens wear on the **cornea**. Specifically, a contralateral-eye paradigm was employed by examining a cohort of contact lens patients who had worn lenses in one eye only (due to unilateral amblyopia or unilateral **myopia**) for an average of 62 months. Any changes observed were compared with the contralateral non-lens-wearing eye. This methodology afforded an extremely powerful and sensitive assessment of the physiological changes induced by lens wear, as it obviated variability due to intersubject differences. It was discovered that the **extended wear** of hydrogel lenses induces a reduction in epithelial oxygen uptake and thickness, the induction of epithelial **microcysts**, **stromal thinning** (Figure A.2), and increased **endothelial polymegethism**. Although the epithelial changes recovered within 1 month, the principle of ocular compromise *during* lens wear was firmly established.

The Gothenburg Study also revealed four key strategies for alleviating these changes: removing lenses more frequently, regularly replacing lenses, fitting lenses of higher oxygen performance, and improving tear exchange beneath lenses. These strategies formed the blueprint for future contact lens developments, such as the development of mass production manufacturing facilities for disposable lenses and silicone hydrogel lenses. (Holden, B. A., Sweeney, D. F., Vannas, A., Nilsson, K. T. and Efron, N. (1985). Effects of long-term extended contact lens wear on the human cornea. *Invest. Ophthalmol. Vis. Sci.*, **26(11)**, 1489–1501.)

grading contact lens complications
The severity of contact lens complications can be assessed with the aid of **grading scales**. Grading is effected by observing the tissue change of interest directly or with the aid of a **slit-lamp biomicroscope**, under low and/or high magnification as required, and estimating the grading to the nearest 0.1 scale unit. For example, a tissue change that is judged to be considerably more severe than Grade 2 but not quite as severe as Grade 3 may be assigned a grade of 2.8 or 2.9. Although this procedure can sometimes be difficult, grading to the nearest 0.1 scale unit (rather than simply assigning a whole digit grade of 0, 1, 2, 3 or 4) affords much greater precision and increases the sensitivity of the grading scale for detecting real changes or differences in severity.

It is important to designate clearly the grading system used and the specific tissue change being graded. A more expedient approach would be to print or stamp the names of the various complications onto a record card, each with an accompanying box for entering the assigned grade. It may be necessary to make additional annotations to describe the condition more fully – e.g. to indicate the location of the pathology.

The five-stage 0 to 4 grading scale is based on a universally accepted concept whereby a higher numeric grade denotes greater clinical severity. This schema can be applied to any tissue change. The designation and general interpretation of each grading step is shown in Table G.1. It must be recognized that these are only very general guidelines, and are not intended to replace sound professional judgement.

When using grading scales for the first time, a confidence range of about 1.2 is to be expected; however, with experience this confidence range may reduce to 0.7 grading scale units. In general, a change or difference of more than about 1.0 grading scale unit, or a level of severity of more than Grade 2, is considered to be clinically significant.

grading scales
As an aid to accurate record keeping, health care practitioners of all disciplines often resort to the use of standardized grading scales of various conditions. Two grading systems for complications of contact lens wear, each containing a wide range of grading scales, are readily available to practitioners:

Table G.1 Designation and interpretation of the various levels of severity depicted in the Efron Grading Scales

grade	severity	colour band	clinical interpretation
0	normal	green	clinical action not required
1	trace	lime	clinical action rarely required
2	mild	yellow	clinical action possibly required
3	moderate	orange	clinical action usually required
4	severe	red	clinical action certainly required

1. Efron Grading Scales for Contact Lens Complications (supplied by **CooperVision**; also shown in Appendix A)
2. CCLRU Grading Scales (supplied by Vistakon; **Johnson & Johnson**)

These grading scales provide a simple, convenient and accurate means by which clinicians can record and communicate the severity of complications of contact lens wear. The Efron Grading Scales were painted by an ophthalmic artist, and the CCLRU Grading Scales are a mosaic of clinical photographs. The advantage of using painted (versus photographic) grading scales is that greater clarity can be achieved because the precise level of severity can be depicted, all other factors can be kept constant, potentially confounding artefacts can be avoided, and artistic license can be adopted. The grading assigned to a particular condition can serve as a reference against which any future tissue change may be assessed, and can therefore influence clinical decision-making. These grading scales may act as a standard clinical reference for describing the severity of contact lens complications.

The primary design criteria upon which the Efron Grading Scales are based are simplicity, convenience, and ease of use by clinicians. Sixteen sets of grading images are depicted in two panels, each comprising eight complications. These 16 grading scales show the key anterior ocular complications of contact lens wear. Each complication is illustrated in five stages of increasing severity, from 0 to 4, with 'traffic-light' colour banding from green (normal, Grade 0) to red (severe, Grade 4). The severity of the complications is based on an appraisal of accumulated evidence in the literature and clinical experience.

Each complication in the Efron Grading Scales has been painted to an equivalent level of magnification that addresses the compromise between being large enough to depict the key features of the tissue changes, and being low enough to relate to what practitioners can observe with available clinical techniques. The magnification of the complications varies from $\times 1$ (i.e. the whole **cornea**) to $\times 600$. A consequence of these magnification levels is that, although epithelial **microcysts** and **endothelial blebs** can be detected and graded at $\times 40$ magnification on a **slit-lamp biomicroscope**, they will not be viewed at the resolution depicted. Furthermore, **endothelial polymegethism** can only be assessed with the aid of a **specular microscope**. All other complications can be viewed at the resolution depicted and are capable of being graded by direct observation and/or using a slit-lamp biomicroscope up to $\times 40$ magnification. *See* grading contact lens complications.

gravimetry, soft lens

The **water content** of a soft lens can be estimated by weighing the sample in air (W1), completely dehydrating the lens in a suitable oven, and then re-weighing the dried sample (W2). The water content is defined by $(W1 - W2)/W1 \times 100\%$. Alternatively, dehydration can be achieved by placing the lens above an active desiccant such as anhydrous $CaSO_4$. Although the above techniques constitute a useful approach in a research environment, they are destructive and therefore of no value to the clinician.

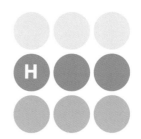

halos

If the optic zone of a **rigid lens** is small and the eye pupil is large, the outer zones of the pupil will be imperfectly corrected, leading to the formation of bright rings or 'halos' when viewing bright light sources under dim lighting conditions (e.g. oncoming headlamps when driving at night). Similar effects may occur with smaller pupils if the lenses are badly decentred.

hand grooming

See hygiene, practitioner and patient.

handling tints

These are also known as 'visibility tints' or 'locator tints', and are incorporated into **soft lenses** so that these lenses can be easily seen in the lens case or on a domestic surface if accidentally dropped (Figure H.1). Such tints are very light and do not alter iris colour; however, they make the lens slightly more visible on the eye by virtue of the handling tint being visible where the lens edge impinges over the sclera. Handling tints do not affect vision or colour perception. *See* tinted lenses.

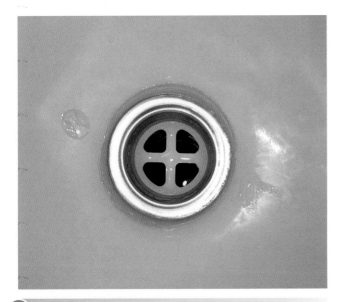

Figure H.1 Lenses 'dropped' in a bathroom sink. The lens with the handling tint can be seen at the half-past 9 o'clock position (relative to the drain hole), whereas the untinted lens is barely visible at the 4 o'clock position.

hardness, rigid lens

The hardness of a **rigid lens** material can be defined as its resistance to penetration. In a hardness test, an indentation device (e.g. a 'nail-like' probe) is pressed on the surface of the material under test, and the extent to which it sinks into the material for a given pressure and time is an inverse measure of the hardness. There are many hardness testing instruments available commercially that are suitable for plastics and rubbers, including the Vickers indenter, the Rockwell hardness tester and the Shore durometer. Other types of hardness testing include resistance to scratching and recovery efficiency (resilience). There is no common method of measurement in these tests; each uses an arbitrary scale and, although the scales can be approximately compared, precise correlation is not possible. The only true form of hardness evaluation is to consider relative data generated using the same instrument at the same time under identical test conditions.

Hartmann–Shack aberrometry

A variety of subjective and objective techniques are available for measuring the wavefront **aberration** of the eye. Probably the most elegant, which is beginning to be commercially available, involves the use of a Hartmann–Shack wavefront. A hexagonal array of identical microlenses allows the slope of the wavefront across a lattice of points in the pupil to be determined. The principle can be understood with reference to Figure H.2. Suppose there is a point source on the retina of a perfect **emmetropic** eye. The light leaving the eye can either be envisaged as a bundle of parallel rays or as a series of plane wavefronts. The array of microlenses is now placed in the path of the emerging light. Each lens will converge the parallel rays to its second focal point, so that an absolutely regular array of image points will form in the common focal plane. If now the eye suffers from aberration, the emergent rays are no longer parallel and the associated wavefronts are no longer flat. Thus the rays no longer come to a focus on the axes of the lenses: the lateral displacement from the focal point of each lens is directly proportional to the local inclination of the ray or the slope of the wavefront. It is, then, easy to calculate the form of the emergent wavefronts and the wavefront aberration from the distorted pattern of image points.

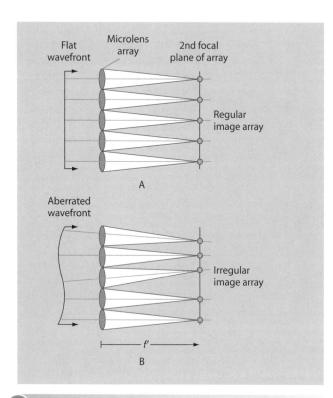

Figure H.2 Principle of the Hartmann–Shack technique. (A) Effects with a perfect emmetropic eye, where the images are formed on the axis of each lens and hence are regularly spaced. (B) Effects with an aberrated eye, where the image ray is irregular since the images are no longer formed on the axes of the lenses.

Departures from a reference sphere of more than a quarter of a wavelength would be expected to degrade image quality. The aberration in the central 2–3 mm of the pupil is usually modest, but much larger amounts may be found in the periphery of dilated pupils. On the basis of wavefront aberration results, it is possible to calculate monochromatic point and line-spread functions, and also the ocular modulation and phase-transfer functions for any pupil diameter.

haze
See oedema.

heat disinfection, soft lens
This physical method of **soft lens** disinfection relies on thermal energy being imparted to micro-organisms to cause lethal cell changes. Heating was the first soft lens disinfection method approved by the USA **Food and Drug Administration** (in 1972). Disinfection using this approach requires a temperature of 80°C to be maintained for at least 10 minutes. A representative example of one of the heating units available at this time was the **Bausch & Lomb** sys-

tem, which reached 96°C for a period of about 20 minutes (Figure H.3). In terms of lens disinfection, the heating systems were recognized as being highly effective, even against the protozoan **Acanthamoeba**. Furthermore, after the initial purchase of the heat unit, the ongoing costs of operation were minimal.

There were a number of disadvantages associated with heat disinfection. In normal circumstances the protein that spoils the surface of a soft contact lens does not denature, but heating the lens tends to denature protein, with adverse clinical consequences such as reduced acuity, the potential for ocular surface reactions such as **papillary conjunctivitis**, and altered physical lens parameters. With the popularity of low water content, non-ionic lenses in the early and mid-1970s, this was not a significant problem. However, heat disinfection is unsuitable with the higher water content materials

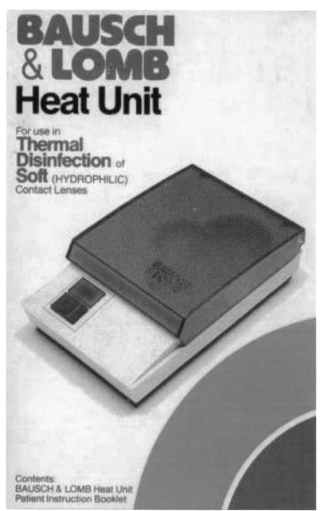

Figure H.3 Early advertisement for the Bausch & Lomb Heat Unit.

that dominate the market today; such lenses, especially if ionic in nature, absorb much greater quantities of proteins, and turn yellow and become deformed when heated.

The heating process is also inconvenient for many wearers. Not only does this method require a nearby source of electricity, but the system also uses unpreserved **saline**, which does not offer any antimicrobial activity. The opportunity for microbial contamination arises if the lenses remain in the cooled saline for a prolonged period, so this disinfection system requires the process to be repeated each day with fresh solution if the lenses are not used. With the advent of **planned replacement** lenses, which are generally of mid-to-high water content and are often manufactured from ionic materials more prone to parameter changes, the popularity of heat disinfection has waned and this technique is rarely used today.

HEMA
See poly (2-hydroxyethyl methacrylate).

hemi-desmosomes
See corneal epithelium.

herpes simplex keratitis
See filamentary keratitis, therapeutic lenses for.

herpes zoster ophthalmicus
See eyelid pathology, therapeutic lenses for.

Herschell, John
In a footnote in his treatise on light in the 1845 edition of the *Encyclopedia Metropolitana*, Sir John Herschel suggested two possible methods of correcting 'very bad cases of irregular **cornea**'. These were '. . . applying to the cornea a spherical capsule of glass filled with animal jelly' (Figure H.4), or '. . . taking a mould of the cornea and impressing it on

some transparent medium'. Although it seems that Herschel did not attempt to conduct such trials, his latter suggestion was ultimately adopted some 40 years later by a number of inventors, working independently and unbeknown to each other, who were all apparently unaware of the writings of Herschel.

high minus power contact lens design
A **rigid contact lens** of −10.00 D would have an unfinished edge thickness of approximately 0.32–0.35 mm if the diameter was 8.8–9.6 mm. Because unfinished edge thickness for best comfort and lens stability should be approximately 0.10 mm, lenticularization of high minus lenses is essential (Figure H.5). A computer-numeric controlled lathe can be used to cut a steeper anterior lenticular radius to obtain the proper edge thickness.

Typical **front optic zone diameters** range from 7.2 mm (in a lens of 8.8 mm total diameter) to 7.8 mm (in a lens of 9.6 mm total diameter) and are about 0.2 mm larger than the back optic zone. The lenticular radius may be cut flatter for a smaller front optic zone or steeper for a larger front optic zone. The latter design will result in higher mid-peripheral thickness. The higher the power (with the same front optic zone), the thicker will be this mid-peripheral area. This may complicate the fit and cause **discomfort** if the lens does not attach to the

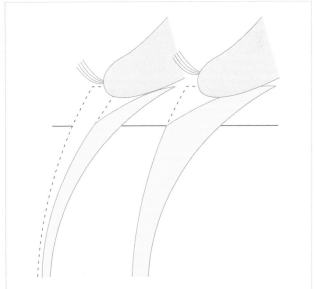

Figure H.5 Low minus power lens (left) with same front optic zone diameter as high minus power lens (right). Junction thickness (horizontal straight line) is greater for the high minus power lens.

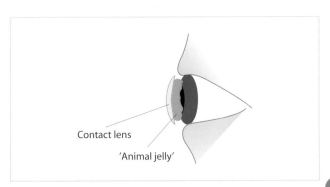

Contact lens

'Animal jelly'

Figure H.4 'Animal jelly' sandwiched between a 'spherical capsule of glass' (contact lens) and cornea, as proposed by Sir John Herschel.

upper **eyelid**. Greater mid-peripheral thickness may also cause a high-riding lens to ride even higher. Mid-peripheral thickness can be reduced with proper polishing or advanced multi-curve computer-controlled anterior surface lathing.

high plus power contact lens design

Silicone lenses of high plus power are typically 11.3–12.5 mm in diameter and are fitted with base curve near (or only slightly flatter than) K. **Silicone hydrogel** high plus lenses are fitted like **soft contact lenses**, and will be beneficial for these patients when they are available.

High plus **rigid lenses**, unless they are of very small diameter (8.5 mm or less) and fit steep, must be made in regular (parallel) carrier form or minus (edge thicker than junction) carrier form (Figure H.6). Lenticular lenses are thinner, have less mass, and centre better than non-lenticular designs. Typically these lenses are 9.0–10.5 mm in diameter. Regular carrier designs are better for lens positioning between the **eyelids**. Minus carrier lenses are better for lid-attachment fitting. The smaller the front optic zone diameter, the thinner the lens. The **front optic zone diameter** may be equal to, larger than or smaller than the **back optic zone diameter**. Typically the front optic zone diameter is 7.0–8.0 mm in diameter, and the back optic zone is designed as needed for fitting. Junction thickness for lenticular rigid plus lenses should be thin enough to minimize **lens thickness** but thick enough to allow adequate lens strength (about 0.15 mm). Regular carrier unfinished edge thickness is typically 0.10–0.12 mm, and minus carrier unfinished edge thickness is typically approximately 0.2 mm. Lenticular (front peripheral) radii range from approximately 0.2 mm flatter than the posterior secondary curve (regular carrier) to 3.0 mm flatter than the posterior secondary curve (minus carrier).

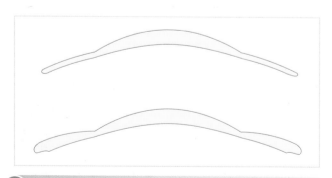

Figure H.6 Lenticular designs for plus powered lenses. Top: regular (parallel) carrier. Bottom: minus carrier.

Hir-Cal grid

See non-invasive tear break-up time.

home delivery plans

See lens supply routes.

hormonal changes

See indications and contraindications for contact lens wear.

hydrogel

It is simplest to regard hydrogels as 'washing line' polymers having a long backbone (the 'washing line') from which a variety of chemical groups may be suspended (the 'washing'). The function of the chemical groups in hydrogels is primarily to attract and bind water within the structure. Greater physical stability is achieved by fastening the washing lines together at intervals by the use of cross-links. Cross-links are introduced by the use of cross-linking agents, which are simply monomers with two active carbon–carbon double bonds. Networks are never perfect, and contain entanglements, chain loops and wasted chain ends. In addition to **hydroxyethyl methacrylate** (HEMA), other important monomers used to achieve an attraction for water include N-vinyl pyrrolidone (used in FDA Group II materials) and methacrylic acid (used in all FDA Group IV materials). In the **silicone hydrogels** the same 'washing line' principle applies, but here groups that contain silicon–oxygen bonds (silicones) are attached, in order to increase oxygen permeability. This is achieved with the monomer commonly referred to as 'TRIS', which is a component of both rigid and silicone hydrogel materials.

Hydrogels are, both historically and potentially, the largest group of contact lens materials in terms of structural variety. PolyHEMA is in many ways typical of other hydrogels, and is still undoubtedly the most important single material of its class across a wide range of biomedical applications.

hydrogen peroxide disinfecting solution

Hydrogen peroxide has been used as an antimicrobial agent for about 200 years. It is widely used medically for disinfection and sterilization, and is generally available in concentrations ranging from 3 to 90%, depending on its purpose. Hydrogen peroxide has a broad-spectrum efficacy against bacteria, viruses and yeast by producing hydroxyl free radicals that attach essential cell components such as lipid and proteins, and is often considered to be the 'gold standard' in terms of soft contact lens disinfection. For example, 3% hydrogen peroxide will kill trophozoites and cysts of **Acanthamoeba** castellanii in 3 min and 9 h of soaking, respectively. Hydrogen peroxide can be chemically broken down into oxygen and water, and is therefore considered to be environmentally friendly. It tends to decompose on standing, and therefore needs to be stabilized, typically with phosphates or phosphorates. The use of stannate as a stabilizer has been associated with hazing of ionic lenses due to an interaction between the stannate ions, methacrylic acid groups in the lens material and tear-derived lysozyme.

Although hydrogen peroxide has a high efficacy in terms of its antimicrobial action it is toxic to the eye, and neutralization is required before a lens that has been placed in hydrogen peroxide can be worn comfortably. Conjunctival hyperaemia is induced by levels of hydrogen peroxide greater than 200 ppm, and concentrations in excess of 100 ppm are associated with subjective stinging; however, concentrations of this order of magnitude do not cause **corneal** or **conjunctival staining**.

Storage in hydrogen peroxide has been reported to alter lens parameters. There is a temporary reduction in lens hydration after prolonged lens storage in hydrogen peroxide. High water ionic lenses (FDA Group IV) appear to be most susceptible to changes in diameter and base curve, although the clinical consequences of these changes are generally not significant because of their temporary nature – for example, a soaking period of 20 minutes in neutralizer returns lens parameters to their original specification within 1 hour of lens wear.

The approaches to neutralization have varied since the introduction of hydrogen peroxide as a contact lens disinfectant. The initial approach was to allow for the storage of the lenses in 3% hydrogen peroxide, with neutralization undertaken as a secondary process before lens insertion. These two-step systems are considered to provide the best antimicrobial action, especially when the lens is exposed to 3% hydrogen peroxide overnight. The two most popular approaches for neutralization in a two-step hydrogen peroxide system are the catalytic and reactive methods. In the Oxysept system (Allergan), a solution containing the enzyme catalase is added to the lens storage case after the hydrogen peroxide has been discarded. This quickly breaks down the remaining hydrogen peroxide into water and oxygen, with the production of the latter requiring a vented storage case. With this system, no hydrogen peroxide is detectable 1 minute after the introduction of the neutralizer. An example of the reactive method is the 10 : 10 product (CIBA Vision). Here, after the hydrogen peroxide storage solution has been discarded, the lens case is filled with a solution containing sodium pyruvate, which completely neutralizes the hydrogen peroxide in about 6 minutes.

Despite the **antimicrobial efficacy** of two-step systems, this approach is probably the most complex of all soft lens disinfection regimens and carries an unacceptably high risk of the patient suffering a severe 'peroxide burn' after accidentally placing a lens directly into the eye from the 3% hydrogen peroxide solution. This led to a reduction of the popularity of two-step systems and the subsequent development of one-step systems. The one-step systems negate the requirement for a separate neutralization process by the contact lens user. After the lens storage case is closed, the disinfection and neutralization steps take place without further intervention from the wearer. Two approaches are common. In the first, such as in the Oxysept 1-Step system (Allergan), the lens case is filled with hydrogen peroxide and a coated tablet containing catalase is added. The coating of the tablet is dissolved, releasing catalase into the solution and leading to neutralization of the hydrogen peroxide within about 2 hours. A number of products use a second method of neutralization – a platinum disc (Figure H.7). In this approach, the disc is either attached as an integral part of the lens holder or is permanently lodged in the base of the storage case. There is a rapid neutralization over the first 2 minutes – from the original 30 000 ppm (or 3% concentration) to about 9000 ppm – followed by a slower phase to 50 ppm after 3 hours and 15 ppm after 6 hours.

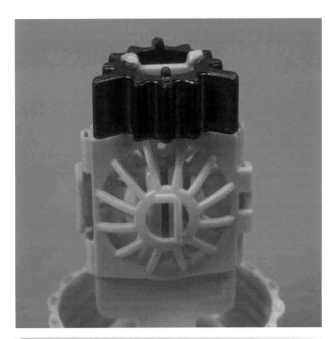

Figure H.7 The neutralizing platinum disc in this one-step hydrogen peroxide system is attached to the lens holder. In other systems, it is fixed in the base of the case.

The trade-off for the increased convenience for the user of a one-step system is two-fold. First, as the lenses are held only in neutralized solution within a few hours of entering the case, long-term storage is not advisable because the residual solution has no antimicrobial capabilities. Secondly, the reduced time in relatively high concentration hydrogen peroxide compared with the two-step systems affords a reduced antimicrobial power to the system. Furthermore, the speed of hydrogen peroxide neutralization differs between the tablet systems and the platinum disc systems. Although activity against bacteria is likely to be adequate with these systems, the storage period is unlikely to be sufficient for efficacy against Acanthamoeba. However, antimicrobial efficacy can be enhanced by appropriate lens cleaning and rinsing.

hydroxyethyl methacrylate
See poly (2-hydroxyethyl methacrylate).

hygiene, practitioner and patient
It is imperative that the importance of hand washing prior to lens handling is reinforced in the course of contact lens patient education. The best way of achieving this without appearing to be patronizing to the patient is for the instructor to wash his or her hands prior to lens handling, in full view of the patient. A very brief explanation as to why this is so important – the prevention of lens contamination and reduction of the risks of infection – can be given to patients before inviting them to wash their hands. At all future instruction or **aftercare** visits, patients should be prompted to wash their hands if they forget to do this before proceeding to handle lenses.

Hand grooming is an important factor related to hygiene. The nails of all fingers that are likely to be involved in lens manipulation should be cut short and filed smooth to avoid both lens damage and the potential for **corneal** insult.

hygienist, contact lens
See patient education.

hypercapnia
This term refers to a level of carbon dioxide in excess of that normally found in a specified condition. For example, the partial pressure of carbon dioxide in the atmosphere is 0.3 mmHg at sea level under conditions of standard temperature and pressure. This is considered to be the baseline reference at the anterior **corneal** surface, where higher levels of carbon dioxide infer hypercapnia.

hypermetropia
Often referred to by the foreshortened term 'hyperopia', this is a refractive defect of the eye in which light from a distant object is focused behind the retina when **accommodation** is relaxed, resulting in blurred distance and near vision. The **hypermetropic** patient can make distance objects appear clear by accommodating the eye, assuming that the accommodation facility equals or exceeds the dioptric degree of the refractive defect; however, constant accommodation to clear distance object can lead to eye strain. Plus powered lenses can be used to obviate the need for constant accommodation and afford comfortable and clear distance vision.

hyperopia
See hypermetropia.

hyperthyroidism
See systemic disease, contact lens wear in.

hypoxia
This term refers to a finite level of oxygen less than that normally found in the atmosphere, which is 155 mmHg at sea level under conditions of standard temperature and pressure, and allowing for a water vapour pressure of 4 mmHg. *Adj*: hypoxic.

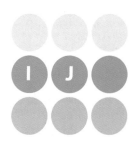

IACLE
See International Association of Contact Lens Educators.

identification tint
Polymer buttons used for **rigid lens** manufacture are often colour-coded with light tints by some manufacturers who supply a wide range of products, so as to facilitate correct product identification at the lens fabrication stage. Such tints are barely visible in the finished lens, and do not affect vision or colour perception. *See* tinted lenses.

impression fitting, scleral lens
See fitting scleral lenses.

indications and contraindications for contact lens wear
As part of an initial assessment as to the suitability of a patient for contact lens wear, any specific indications or contraindications for lens wear must be established. These are best considered in the following categories:

1. *Ocular anatomy.* In elective fitting (i.e. non-therapeutic use) there are few anatomical features that influence the suitability for contact lenses. However, extremely steep or flat **corneas** or extremes of corneal **astigmatism** may present particular fitting difficulties that could increase the time spent on fitting. With **bifocal contact lens** fitting, lower lid tension and position may be critical to the visual outcome and **pupil** size may also influence fitting success. In such cases, the implications for likely success and the increased fitting time and expense should be explained carefully to the patient.
2. *Ocular health.* Since a contact lens will come into intimate contact with the ocular surfaces, it is essential that there are no presenting ocular conditions that might be aggravated by lens wear. Disorders such as recurrent infection, irregular corneal surface, recurrent erosions, **dry eye** or **meibomian gland dysfunction** may be partial contraindications for elective contact lens wear, depending on severity.
3. *General health.* There are numerous health problems that may influence the suitability for contact lenses, including those that have a direct effect on the ocular tissues and those that may cause secondary problems. In addition, several systemic medications may influence the **tear film** and thus the ability to wear lenses comfortably.
4. *Allergies.* Those who are susceptible to allergies may experience problems from two sources. Wearers with atopy may be more intolerant to contact lens wear by a factor of five times compared to non-atopic wearers. Wearing time should be limited during the allergy season. Those with other more specific allergies may be at risk from reactions to the chemicals within preservative-based lens care systems. These chemicals can interact with deposits on the lens surface, creating an allergic-type response. In such cases, preservative-free systems or daily disposable lenses are indicated.
5. *Chronic infection.* Those with chronic sinusitis or catarrh may be more at risk of developing infection secondary to corneal abrasion. The associated **mucus in the tears** may cause visual problems from lens surface wetting anomalies, as well as blocking the nasolacrimal ducts and causing epiphora.
6. *Metabolic disorders.* Disorders of metabolism may have varying effects on the eye and its physiology. Hyperthyroidism, with its associated exophthalmos, may create problems in tear film distribution, while **diabetes** may influence the stability of refractive error, corneal deturgescence and epithelial wound healing.
7. *Pregnancy, lactation and hormonal changes.* Owing to hormonal changes during pregnancy and lactation, female patients may be prone to corneal **oedema** and mucus build-up. Comfort and overall tolerance can be reduced, although the response of a previously-adapted lens wearer during pregnancy may often be good. It is less desirable to commence fitting lenses during pregnancy and lactation. Disruption to the tear film can occur during puberty and the menopause, and while taking oral contraceptives or hormone replacement therapy, giving rise to chronic or transient problems of intolerance and **dryness**.
8. *Systemic medication.* As well as the systemic conditions that can affect tolerance to lenses, medication used in the treatment or control of those conditions can also have undesirable side effects. These generally affect the tear film, either causing symptoms of dryness or in some cases leading to **soft lens** discoloration.

9. *Psychological factors, including motivation.* In addition to anatomical and health-related issues, it is important to judge the motivation to wear contact lenses and the personality type of the potential wearer. Contact lenses are considered to give a more normal cosmetic appearance and may significantly enhance overall appearance, particularly when the refractive error is high. In addition, there are cases where lenses can be used specifically to conceal significant cosmetic defects such as iris anomalies, corneal opacities, inoperable squint or microphthalmos. A particularly exacting personality type may find the adaptation period and the initial learning of handling techniques too intrusive to outweigh the overall benefits of lens wear.

10. *Lifestyle/occupational issues.* In addition to motivational and psychological factors, consideration should be given to lifestyle and occupational issues. Often contact lenses are believed to be inappropriate for certain occupations, and while this may be true for particularly contaminated atmospheres, contact lenses may provide some protection from both foreign bodies and chemicals. In certain vocations, contact lenses may offer no obvious disadvantages and therefore employees should not necessarily be precluded from wearing lenses (e.g. in the fire service). Whatever the situation, hygiene is important, and attention to this factor must be of the highest order. Additionally, lens handling requires some degree of dexterity, and particularly rough or calloused hands may render lens handling and cleaning process difficult, leading to frustration and inadvertent lens damage.

11. *Financial considerations.* It is important that the patient understands the financial implications of the fitting and, perhaps more importantly, the ongoing costs relating to continuing clinical care, lens care solutions and lens replacements. Fitting lenses to a patient without the financial means to care for them will inevitably lead to **non-compliance** and an increased potential for adverse events to occur.

indirect illumination, slit-lamp technique of

This refers to any technique with the **slit-lamp biomicroscope** where the focus of the illuminating beam does not coincide with the focal point of the observation system. Indirect illumination can be achieved by 'uncoupling' the instrument and manually displacing the slit beam to the side. However, it is possible to effect indirect illumination without uncoupling the instrument; this is simply achieved by directing a slit beam on to a section of the **cornea** *adjacent* to that of interest.

The following two specific types of indirect illumination are possible:

1. *Sclerotic scatter.* This technique is used to investigate any subtle changes in corneal clarity occurring over a large area, such as central corneal **oedema**. The slit lamp is set up for a wide-angle parallelepiped (45–60°) and the viewing system is focused centrally. The beam is manually offset ('uncoupled') and focused on the limbus (Figure I.1). The slit beam is totally internally reflected across the cornea, and a bright limbal glow is seen around the entire cornea. Any specific area of abnormality, such as a corneal scar, will interrupt the beam in its passage and produce a light reflection in the otherwise dark cornea.

2. *Retro-illumination.* This refers to any technique in which light is reflected from the iris, anterior crystalline lens surface or retina, and is used to back-illuminate an area more anteriorly positioned. The area may be seen against a light background (direct retro-illumination, Figure I.2) or a dark background (indirect retro-illumination, Figure I.3), depending whether or not the illumination and viewing systems are coincident. Direct retro-illumination is used most often, and here corneal opacities will appear black against a bright field. Retro-illumination is particularly useful for examining epithelial **microcysts**, **neovascularization**, scars, degenerations and dystrophies.

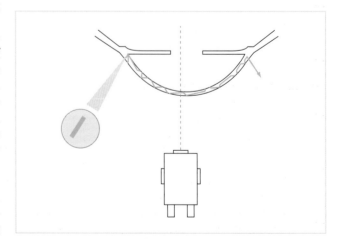

Figure I.1 Sclerotic scatter slit-lamp technique. Adapted from L. W. Jones and D. A. Jones (2001) Slit lamp biomicroscopy. In *The Cornea: its Examination in Contact Lens Practice* (N. Efron, ed.), pp.1–49, Butterworth-Heinemann.

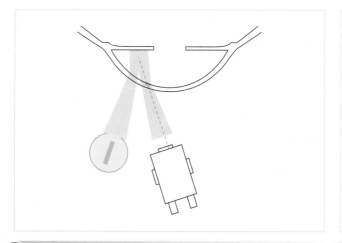

Figure I.2 Direct retro-illumination slit-lamp technique. Adapted from L. W. Jones and D.A. Jones (2001) Slit lamp biomicroscopy. In *The Cornea: its Examination in Contact Lens Practice* (N. Efron, ed.), pp.1–49, Butterworth-Heinemann.

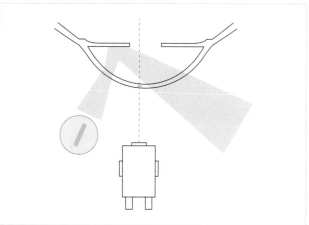

Figure I.3 Indirect retro-illumination slit-lamp technique. Adapted from L. W. Jones and D.A. Jones (2001) Slit lamp biomicroscopy. In *The Cornea: its Examination in Contact Lens Practice* (N. Efron, ed.), pp.1–49, Butterworth-Heinemann.

induced astigmatism with rigid toric lenses

This is the astigmatic effect created in the contact lens/tear lens system by the toroidal back optic zone bounding two surfaces of different **refractive index** – namely the lens (refractive index 1.432 to 1.490 depending on the material) and the tears (refractive index 1.336). *See* compensated rigid bitoric lenses; cylindrical power equivalent rigid toric lenses; residual astigmatism with rigid toric lenses; stabilization of rigid toric lenses; toric lens design, rigid; toric lens, rigid.

infants

See paediatric contact lenses; paediatric contact lens examination; paediatric contact lens fitting.

informed consent

Informed consent means that a patient embarking on contact lens wear should be made aware of both the risks and benefits of contact lens wear, as well as having the opportunity to ask questions. The information provided verbally should be reinforced with written material. As well as providing the patient with information about the recommended lenses and/or solution system of choice, the practitioner must also have discussed the possible alternatives.

A comprehensive list of every possible contact lens complication does not need to be discussed, but a practitioner is required to discuss those that any reasonable member of the profession would expect to be told. A practitioner would be expected to mention the more common non-serious aspects of lens wear, such as the normal adaptation symptoms, in addition to the less common risks that could lead to a serious complication such as visual loss from corneal infection.

Prospective wearers should also be made aware of the consequences of not following the recommended instructions. This may be perceived by some practitioners as a negative approach, as it does not present contact lenses in a positive light. However, discussing such possible scenarios will preclude patients from claiming lack of informed consent should they be non-compliant with advice.

A standard form can be used, which patients sign to acknowledge that they have been given the necessary advice and instructions. They should be given a copy of this, with the other copy retained in their records. In the case of minors, the form should be signed by both the child (where possible) and the parent or guardian.

insertion and removal, rigid lens

Before inserting a **rigid lens** in a new wearer, it is helpful to prepare the patient for some initial discomfort, to advise that this will recede, and to suggest that any discomfort will be minimized by raising the chin and looking downwards (this posture causes the upper lid to stabilize the lens). Anxiety may also be reduced by explaining that any irritation will be to the **eyelid** rather than the eye itself, which will be unaffected. Applying wetting solution to the lens prior to insertion will tend to make the lens more comfortable and transfer more readily to the eye, but care should be taken to avoid applying more than a small drop as too much can make **fluorescein** assessment more difficult. For reasons of **hygiene**, the hands of the practitioner (and the patient, if handling lenses) should be washed and dried immediately prior to lens handling.

The standard technique that a practitioner will use to insert a rigid lens into the eye of a patient is as follows:

1. If you intend inserting the lens with your right hand, stand on the right-hand side of the patient. Lenses can be inserted into both eyes of the patient from the same side using the same hand. The opposite arrangement applies if you intend inserting the lens with your left hand. The following description assumes insertion with the right hand.
2. Ask the patient to fixate a distant object, straight ahead, so as to steady the eyes.
3. Place the lens on the forefinger of your right hand.
4. Hold the top lid using the forefinger or thumb of the left hand. If this proves difficult, have the patient first look down until the lid is securely held.
5. Hold the bottom lid using the middle finger of the right hand, and place the lens directly on to the **cornea**. Instruct the patient to blink (Figure I.4).
6. Release the bottom lid but continue to hold the top lid, and ask the patient to look down.
7. At this point, the lens is often quite comfortable. Warn the patient that once you let go of the lid, he or she will be more aware of the lens.

If the lens locates onto the sclera, the lens will probably not be uncomfortable. Have the patient look in the opposite direction to where the lens is located, e.g. upwards if located on the lower sclera. With two fingers, manipulate the lids to push the lens so that it is manoeuvred back onto the cornea. If this proves difficult, remove the lens by lid manipulation or by using a suction holder (miniature suctions holders are available for in-office lens removal by practitioners only; such devices should not be given to patients).

A practitioner can remove a rigid lens from the eye of a patient as follows:

1. Place the forefinger of one hand on the middle of the bottom lid and the forefinger of the other hand on the middle of the top lid.
2. Gently pull the lids apart, away from the nose and then together so that the tightened lids flick the lens from the cornea (Figure I.5).

The standard technique that a patient can be advised in order to insert a rigid lens into his or her eye is as follows:

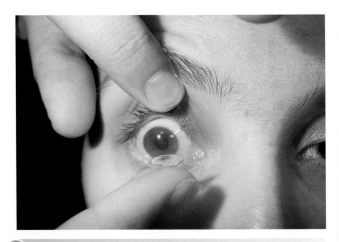

Figure I.4 Lids retracted and rigid lens in position ready for insertion.

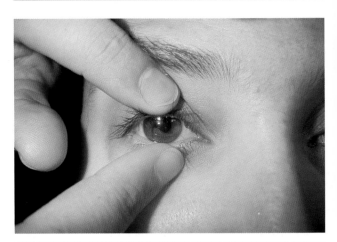

Figure I.5 Preparing to remove a rigid lens by 'flicking' it from the eye.

1. Use the same hand for inserting lenses into either eye. The following description assumes insertion and removal with the right hand.
2. Fixate a distant object, straight ahead, so as to steady the eyes.
3. Place the lens on the forefinger of the right hand.
4. With the forefinger of the left hand (approaching from above the head) hold open the top lid, while with the middle finger of the right hand hold open the bottom lid.
5. Place the lens directly on to the cornea and slowly remove your finger.
6. Release your lids, raise your chin and look down. This will initially stabilize the lens and decrease any discomfort.
7. Let go of the lid and start blinking normally. You will now be more aware of the lens. If the lens

locates onto the sclera, the lens will probably not be uncomfortable. Look in the opposite direction to where the lens is located, e.g. upwards if located on the lower sclera. With two fingers, manipulate the lids to push the lens so that it is manoeuvred back onto the cornea. If this proves difficult, remove the lens by lid squeezing.

A patient can remove a rigid lens from his/her eye as follows:

1. To remove a lens from the right eye, place the forefinger of the right hand towards the outer canthus of the upper lid and place the middle of the right hand towards the outer canthus of the lower lid.
2. Open the eyes wide so that the upper and lower lid margins are above and below the top and bottom lens edge, respectively.
3. Cup the left hand beneath the right eye, resting the edge of the cupped hand against the cheek.
4. Tilt the head slightly downwards, pull the lids taut (away from the nose) and execute a firm blink.
5. The lens will be flipped out of the eye into the cupped hand (or it may end up resting on the lower lid). If the lens remains in the eye, try again.
6. Use the opposite hands to remove a lens from the left eye.

insertion and removal, scleral lens
To insert a **scleral lens** into the eye of a patient, the following procedure is followed:

1. If you intend inserting the lens with your right hand, stand on the right-hand side of the patient. Lenses can be inserted into both eyes of the patient from the same side using the same hand. The opposite arrangement applies if you intend inserting the lens with your left hand. The following description assumes insertion with the right hand.
2. Hold the lens between the thumb and either the index or the middle finger of the right hand.
3. Retract the upper lid and lift it away from the globe, using the thumb and forefinger of the left hand to pull on the lashes.
4. Place the upper edge of the lens under the upper lid and hold it firmly in place with the left hand.
5. Evert the lower lid over the lower lens edge, using the right hand.

Sealed gas-permeable scleral lenses must be inserted filled with saline, so it is necessary to have the patient bend forward and look down to the floor so that the lens is horizontal. This can be difficult to do without letting in bubbles. Manually closing the upper lid over the lens before everting the lower lid often helps.

A scleral lens can be removed from the eye of a patient as follows:

1. Retract the upper lid with the thumb of the left hand and press the lid margin behind the upper edge of the lens.
2. A small movement of the lid over the globe towards the temporal side is usually enough to ease the suction between the lens and eye.
3. Instruct the patient to make a small upwards eye movement to release the lens from the surface of the eye.

A sealed gas-permeable scleral lens may be more difficult to release, in which case a small solid suction holder applied to the front of the lens, as the lid is pressed behind the lens, will help ease the lens off the eye.

The standard technique that a patient can be advised in order to insert a scleral lens into his or her eye is as follows:

1. Use the same hand for inserting lenses into either eye. The following description assumes insertion and removal with the right hand.
2. Hold the lens between the thumb and either the index or the middle finger of the right hand.
3. Retract the upper lid and lift it away from the globe using the thumb and forefinger of the left hand to pull on the lashes.
4. Place the upper edge of the lens under the upper lid and hold it firmly in place with the left hand.
5. Evert the lower lid over the lower lens edge with the right hand.

When instructing patients how to handle lenses, it is often necessary repeatedly to remind them not to let go until the lower lid is fully over the lower edge of the lens. Sealed gas-permeable scleral lenses must be inserted filled with **saline**, so it is necessary for the patient to bend forward and look downwards so that the lens is horizontal. This can be difficult to do without letting in bubbles. Manually closing the upper lid over the lens before everting the lower lid often helps.

The standard technique that a patient can be advised in order to remove a scleral lens from his or her eye is as follows:

1. Retract the upper lid with the forefinger of the left hand and press the lid margin behind the upper edge of the lens.

2. Move the lid a small amount over the globe towards the temporal side; this is usually enough to ease the suction between the lens and eye.
3. Look upwards slightly; this will release the lens from the surface of the eye.

insertion and removal, soft lens

For reasons of hygiene, the hands of the practitioner (and the patient, if handling lenses) should be washed and dried immediately prior to lens handling.

The standard technique that a practitioner will use to insert a **soft lens** into the eye of a patient is as follows:

1. If you intend inserting the lens with your right hand, stand on the right-hand side of the patient. Lenses can be inserted into both eyes of the patient from the same side using the same hand. The opposite arrangement applies if you intend inserting the lens with your left hand. The following description assumes insertion with the right hand.
2. Prior to inserting a soft lens, place it between the forefinger and middle finger of the right hand and rinse with saline to remove any debris.
3. Allow the excess saline to drain before placing the lens on the dry forefinger of the right hand.
4. Use the forefinger or thumb of the left hand to hold the top lid open while, with the middle finger of the right hand, holding the bottom lid open.
5. With the patient looking superiorly and nasally, apply the lens to the exposed bulbar **conjunctiva**. Then press the lens firmly to expel any air bubbles from under it.
6. Slide the lens onto the **cornea** (Figure I.6). Once the soft lens is centred on the cornea, and without air bubbles beneath it, your finger can be

removed. Instruct the patient to look straight ahead. Hold the lids open for a few seconds to allow the lens to settle, and then ask the patient to look down. With thin soft lenses, the lens can be easily folded or dislodged if it has not settled properly.

If the patient finds the lens uncomfortable, debris may have inadvertently become trapped beneath the lens. In such a case, temporarily dislodge the lens onto the sclera and then re-centre the lens.

A practitioner can remove a soft lens from the eye of a patient as follows:

1. Ask the patient to look up or away.
2. Hold open the top lid with the forefinger or thumb of one hand.
3. Hold down the bottom lid with the middle finger of the same hand.
4. Pinch and remove the lens with the thumb and forefinger of the other hand (Figure I.7).

The standard technique that a patient can be advised in order to insert a soft lens into his or her eye is as follows:

1. Use the same hand for inserting and removing lenses into either eye. The following description assumes insertion and removal with the right hand.
2. Prior to inserting a soft lens, place it between the forefinger and middle finger of the right hand and rinse with saline to remove any debris.
3. Allow the excess saline to drain before placing the lens on the dry forefinger of the right hand.
4. With the forefinger of the left hand (approaching from above the head), hold open the top lid while, with the middle finger of the right hand, hold open the bottom lid.

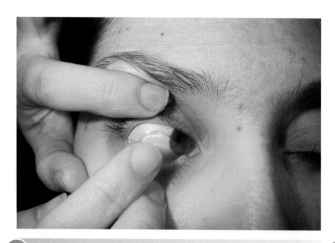

Figure I.6 Insertion of a soft lens.

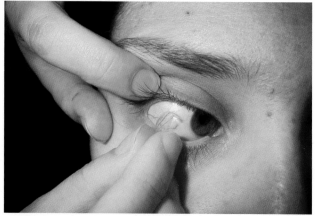

Figure I.7 Removal of a soft lens.

5. Look slightly upwards and apply the lens to the inferior bulbar conjunctiva. Then press the lens firmly to expel any air bubbles from under it.
6. Slide the lens up onto the cornea. Once the soft lens is centred on the cornea, and without air bubbles beneath it, your finger can be removed. Look straight ahead. Hold the lids open for a few seconds to allow the lens to settle and then look down. With thin soft lenses, the lens can be easily folded or dislodged if the lens has not properly settled.
7. The lens will sometimes be uncomfortable immediately after insertion because debris may have inadvertently become trapped beneath it. In such a case, temporarily dislodge the lens onto the sclera and then re-centre the lens.

A patient can remove a soft lens from his or her eye as follows:

1. Look up.
2. Hold open the top lid with the forefinger of the left hand (approaching from above the head).
3. Hold down the bottom lid with the middle finger of the right hand.
4. Place your finger on the bottom of the lens and slide it downwards. Pinch and remove the lens with the thumb and forefinger of the right hand.

inside-out check, soft lens

Before inserting a **soft lens** into the eye, it is necessary to perform an 'inside-out' check. The lens is balanced on the forefinger and the lens profile is examined. If the lens is inside out, its edge will be slightly turned out. The profile will resemble that of a 'dish' rather than a 'bowl' (Figure I.8). A lens that is placed on the eye 'inside-out' may display excessive movement and be slightly uncomfortable.

instructing patients
See patient education.

interferometric measurement of back optic zone radius (BOZR)

There are two types of interferometry, optical and geometric. Optical interferometry is one of the most precise methods for estimating the shape of a reflecting surface relative to a test surface of known parameters. Using Newton's rings, or a similar optical arrangement, the resolution of the technique is of the order $\lambda/2$. A Newton's rings arrangement is cumbersome, time consuming and difficult to use with unstable devices such as **soft lenses**. This has limited its popularity. The technique is eminently suitable for checking non-spherical surfaces, and for any minute imperfections on either the front or back surface of a contact lens.

'Moiré fringes' are geometric interference patterns produced when two gratings overlap. An example of this enigmatic pattern is shown in Figure I.9, where two gratings consisting of parallel dark and clear lines are inclined by an angle θ relative to each other. The angular direction of the resultant pattern (φ) depends on the ratio of the frequency of one grating relative to the other and the angular separation of the two gratings (θ). The ratio of frequencies is the same as the ratio of the apparent sizes of the gratings. If the apparent size of one grating is known for a particular Moiré pattern, as well as the values of θ and φ, then the apparent size of the other grating can be calculated as follows:

$$B/A = \{\sin \theta / \tan \varphi\} + \cos \theta$$

where A is the apparent size of the lines in grating 1, and B is the apparent size of the lines in grating 2 at

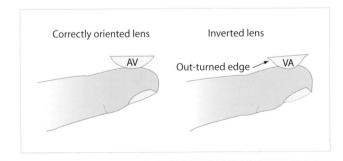

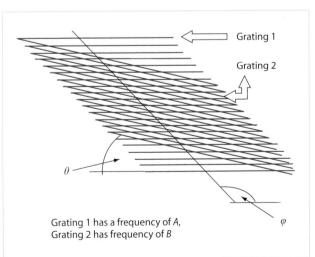

Grating 1

Grating 2

θ

φ

Grating 1 has a frequency of A,
Grating 2 has frequency of B

Figure I.8 A lens can be checked for inversion by examining the lens rim at eye level.

Correctly oriented lens

Inverted lens

AV

Out-turned edge

VA

Figure I.9 Moiré pattern resulting from an overlap of two gratings.

the viewing plane. In Figure I.9, $A = B$. However, keeping θ constant and separating the gratings along the viewing axis (i.e. out of the plane of the paper), the direction of the Moiré pattern φ would change because A would no longer equal B at the plane of observation. A curved reflecting surface has magnifying properties, depending on its radius. If the image of a grating of known frequency is formed by reflection from the back surface of a soft lens, and this image is analysed in a Moiré pattern arrangement, it is possible to create an optical system whereby the radius of the unknown surface is a relatively simple function of φ. Soft lens measuring devices are commercially available which contain a built-in programme that analyses the resulting Moiré pattern and allows an assessment of the form and regularity of aspheric lens surfaces and lens power distribution over a central 5-mm aperture. Moiré pattern systems are valuable for checking non-spherical surfaces in multifocal lenses.

International Association of Contact Lens Educators (IACLE)

This is a global educational organization dedicated to raising the standard of contact lens education world-wide and promoting the widespread, safe use of contact lenses. This is accomplished by: helping to improve the quality of contact lens teaching; providing educational infrastructure; increasing the number of skilled contact lens practitioners throughout the world; and increasing the number of qualified contact lens educators.

The association presently has 462 members in 60 countries; their members include optometrists, ophthalmologists, opticians and 'contactologists'. Membership is open to persons who are significantly involved either full-time or part-time in contact lens education and are members of staff of a recognized teaching institution. Membership applications are approved by the Executive Board.

IACLE operates an accreditation system, publishes a contact lens curriculum, distributes educational resources, sponsors a teacher exchange programme, and hosts numerous courses and workshops around the world. Website: www.iacle.org

International Society for Contact Lens Research (ISCLR)

The ISCLR is a group committed to international communication in the field of contact lens research and related sciences. Established in 1978 by an international group of leading researchers, ISCLR has become a crucial way in which researchers and industry in the field of contact lenses may be brought rapidly up to date with important developments and directions.

The ISCLR is a 'closed' society in that its membership is limited to only about 100 active workers in the contact lens field. There are strict requirements for admission to, and for retaining, membership; members must demonstrate that they are actively engaged in ongoing research in the contact lens field, and are required to attend all biennial meetings. The society is heavily supported by the contact lens industry, whose representatives participate in its meetings. Website: www.isclr.org

internet supply
See lens supply routes.

inventory
See practice logistics.

iron deposition
See deposits, lens.

ISCLR
See International Society for Contact Lens Research.

J

jelly bumps
See deposits, lens.

Johnson & Johnson Vision Care
Formerly known in the UK as Vistakon, Johnson & Johnson Vision Care is the manufacturer of Acuvue™ disposable **soft contact lenses**. It operates in all major international markets, with headquarters in Jacksonville, Florida, USA. Website: www.vistakon.co.uk

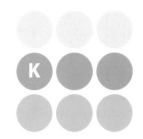
Kalt, Eugène

French ophthalmologist Eugène Kalt (Figure K.1) fitted two keratoconic patients with afocal glass **scleral shells** and obtained a significant improvement in vision. A report of this work, presented to the Paris Academy of Medicine on 20 March 1888 by Kalt's senior medical colleague, Professor Photinos Panas, acknowledges and therefore effectively pre-dates the work of A. E. **Fick**.

keratitis, microbial

Contact lens induced **microbial (infectious) keratitis** (CLMK) can be ulcerative (e.g. *Pseudomonas aeruginosa* keratitis) or non-ulcerative (e.g. epidemic keratoconjunctivitis); the latter form is unrelated to lens wear. A positive culture result for bacteria, virus, fungus or amoeba will provide strong evidence that the keratitis is infectious (microbial), but a negative culture result simply means that microbial agents could not be detected in the tissue. In the latter case, a ker-

atitis may still be classified clinically as 'infectious' based upon the size of the ulcer and associated signs and symptoms. The incidence of CLMK is 4 per 10 000 patients per year for daily hydrogel lens wear and 21 per 10 000 patients per year for **extended hydrogel lens wear**.

An early symptom of CLMK is a foreign body sensation in the eyes associated with an increasing desire to remove the lenses. Continuing or worsening discomfort following lens removal should lead a clinician to suspect CLMK. Associated symptoms include:

- pain
- eye redness
- swollen lids
- increased lacrimation
- photophobia
- discharge
- loss of vision.

Bacterial keratitis (e.g. *Pseudomonas aeruginosa* **keratitis**) can have a rapid and devastating time course. Epithelial and stromal haze, lacrimation and **limbal redness** adjacent to the lesion will be noticed initially, followed by anterior chamber flare, iritis, hypopyon, and a serous or mucopurulent discharge (Figure K.2). If not properly treated, the **stroma** can melt away, leading to corneal perforation in a matter of days. The time course of **Acanthamoeba keratitis** is not as rapid; typical

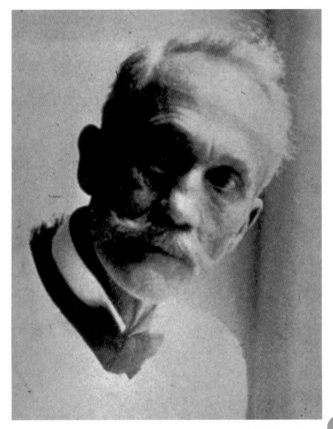

Figure K.1 Eugène Kalt.

Figure K.2 Advanced microbial keratitis (*Pseudomonas aeruginosa*) resulting in a corneal ulcer.

signs include **corneal staining**, pseudodendrites, epithelial and anterior stromal infiltrates (which may be focal or diffuse), and a classic radial keratoneuritis – this being a circular formation of opacification that becomes apparent relatively early in the disease process. A fully developed corneal ulcer may take weeks to form.

The factors leading to the development of CLMK include:

- sleeping in lenses (extended wear)
- patient **non-compliance**
- use of inefficacious lens care systems (especially **chlorine** and unpreserved **saline**)
- **diabetes**
- tobacco use
- travel to warm climates.

A corneal scraping is usually performed to determine if the condition is infectious and possibly to identify the offending micro-organism. Medical therapies may include the use of:

- antibiotics
- mydriatics
- collagenase inhibitors
- non-steroidal anti-inflammatory agents
- analgesics
- tissue adhesives
- debridement
- bandage lenses
- collagen shields.

Steroids may be prescribed with extreme caution in the late healing phase to dampen the host response. Surgical interventions include penetrating graft, which may need to be performed in the case of large perforations or non-healing deep central ulceration, or possibly lamellar graft. The prognosis for recovery from CLMK is variable, ranging from a few weeks in the case of *Pseudomonas aeruginosa* **keratitis** to many months of regression and recurrence in the case of **Acanthamoeba keratitis**.

keratitis, sterile

An inflammation of **corneal** tissue in the absence of infectious agents is considered to be a sterile keratitis. This condition is indicated by the presence of corneal infiltrates. Sterile infiltrates in the **stroma**, in the absence of significant epithelial compromise or associated pathology, are usually benign; however, they can also be a key sign of infectious keratitis, which is potentially sight threatening and must be treated as a medical emergency. It is critical, therefore, to be able to differentially diagnose sterile versus infective keratitis quickly and accurately.

Contact lens associated sterile (non-infectious) keratitis (CLSK) can result from a variety of mechanisms, such as solution toxicity, bacterial endotoxicity (as distinct from infectivity), immunological reaction, trauma, **hypoxia** and metabolic disturbance. Other aetiological factors include breakdown of trapped post-lens **tear film** debris, lens deposits, and poor patient hygiene. The condition may be ulcerative (e.g. **culture-negative peripheral ulcer**) or non-ulcerative (e.g. **contact lens induced acute red eye**).

In CLSK, infiltrates are usually small, forming a multiple or arcuate pattern. A broad band of infiltration may also appear (Figure K.3). There may be slight discomfort, but no pain. Overlying epithelial defects are noted in about 50% of patients who are diagnosed as having CLSK. There may be a mild anterior chamber reaction, but no hypopyon. Histopathological analysis of human tissue from patients suffering from CLSK reveals focal areas of epithelial loss, attenuated epithelium, and stromal infiltration with polymorphonuclear leukocytes; Bowman's layer is unaffected.

Severe ocular **discomfort** is alleviated immediately upon lens removal, although photophobia may persist for some hours. The patient should be examined urgently to determine if the keratitis is infectious, which will be indicated by one or more of the following:

- severe ocular pain that persists following lens removal

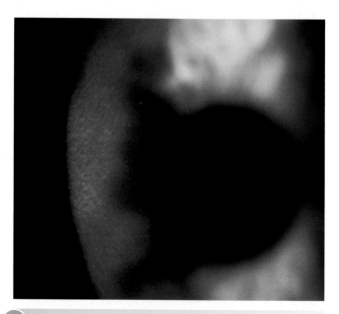

Figure K.3 Broad band of sterile infiltrative keratitis.

- extensive and/or intensive epithelial staining overlying the infiltrates
- significant anterior chamber flare
- extreme **conjunctival redness** that persists following lens removal
- significant loss of vision.

In mild cases of CLSK the patient must cease lens wear and be examined later the same day, and daily thereafter for at least a week, to verify that all signs and symptoms are resolving. Prophylactic topical antibiotics may be prescribed, as well as steroids if strict guidelines are followed (i.e. an active infection is ruled out). If the signs and symptoms do not appear to be resolving after 3–4 days, or if there is a worsening of any aspect of the condition, medical treatment may be required (*see* keratitis, microbial). If there is a progressive recovery, lens wear should not be resumed until there has been a 75% resolution of infiltrates and a complete resolution of all other signs and symptoms.

Discomfort can be alleviated by applying a cold compress to the eye. Treatment strategies to prevent a recurrence of CLSK include replacing lenses more frequently, improving or eliminating lens care solutions, improving overall hygiene, changing from extended wear to daily wear, and fitting lenses of higher oxygen performance. Symptoms and signs generally resolve within 48 hours except for infiltrates, which will slowly resolve over 3–6 months.

keratoconus

Keratoconus is a progressive, asymmetric, non-inflammatory disease of the **cornea** characterized by steepening and distortion, apical thinning, and central scarring of the cornea (see Figure D.9). These corneal changes lead to a mild to marked decrease in vision secondary to high irregular **astigmatism** and, frequently, central corneal scarring. There are several characteristic biomicroscopic corneal signs that become more prevalent as the disease progresses, including:

- an inferiorly displaced, thinned protrusion of the cornea
- corneal thinning over the apex of the cone
- scars in Bowman's layer
- Vogt's striae in the posterior stroma
- Fleischer's ring, consisting of iron in the **corneal epithelium** at the base of the cone.

Although the aetiology of keratoconus is unknown, this condition has been putatively associated with atopic disease, eye rubbing, inheritance, and contact lens wear. Estimates of the prevalence of keratoconus vary from 4–108 per 100 000 population.

Management varies with disease severity. Non-surgical alternatives are the primary method of patient management in keratoconus. Although the visual disturbances in keratoconus may be managed with spectacles or **soft lenses** early in the disease process, **rigid lenses** are the treatment of choice for the irregular astigmatism associated with the condition. Occasionally, in later stages soft lenses are used in conjunction with rigid lenses in a '**piggyback**' combination, or **scleral lenses** are prescribed.

Patients are generally referred for penetrating keratoplasty when they can no longer tolerate contact lenses or when contact lenses provide inadequate vision. Poor vision with contact lenses is often accompanied by apical corneal scarring, but vision can be compromised even with optimal contact lens correction and no corneal scarring. With concerted effort, the vast majority of patients initially referred for corneal transplants can be successfully refitted with contact lenses without surgery, yielding improved visual acuity and contact lens wearing time.

keratoconus, contact lens correction of

The use of **rigid contact lenses** is the mainstay of the optical management of keratoconus. These lenses, which are manufactured in a large variety of unique designs, effectively resurface the irregular **cornea** and allow the intervening fluid lens to correct the corneal **astigmatism** adequately in most cases.

Certainly, a rigid contact lens allows for a far more uniform refracting surface than the irregular astigmatic surface of the keratoconic cornea. The local irregularities of the (often) stained and (sometimes) raised epithelial lesion are filled in by the tears behind the rigid lens. However, the lacrimal lens only eliminates about 90% of the astigmatic error of the cornea due to the index difference between the tears and cornea. Corneal scarring and epithelial staining diffuse light and result in worse low contrast visual acuity. The rigid lens may also further distort the cornea. A flat or steep fit may cause wrinkling of the epithelium, and a very flat fit may decrease axial length.

Although rigid lenses often position over the apex of the displaced ectatic area, they eliminate the difficulties associated with this displacement by also superimposing the visual axis. Rigid lens fitting in keratoconus is, however, by no means simple. Numerous lenses are often required, even for an initial fitting, and achieving an adequate cornea–lens fitting relationship with reasonable vision becomes more difficult as the disease progresses. Although most practitioners who fit a large variety of keratoconus patients have their preferences for lens design, most practising clinicians still find each keratoconus patient a trial-and-error experience.

The major rigid lens fitting techniques are:

- apical bearing, with primary lens support on the apex of the cornea, where the central optic zone of the lens actually touches or bears on the central **corneal epithelium**
- apical clearance, with lens support and bearing directed off the apex and onto the paracentral cornea, with clearance of the apex of the cornea
- divided support or 'three-point touch', with lens support and bearing shared between the corneal apex and the paracentral cornea.

Typically, an apical bearing fit is the easiest to achieve in keratoconus. Almost all rigid contact lenses touch the apex of the cone unless steps are taken to alleviate the bearing or to clear the corneal apex. In three-point touch – although possibly viewed as a variant of apical touch – the objective is to minimize the touch on the corneal apex by steepening the lens centrally and allowing the peripheral cornea to show areas of light touch, thereby minimizing trauma to all areas of the cornea (Figure K.4). The major disadvantage of apical touch is the possibility of epithelial trauma and the inducement of corneal scarring. The advantages of apical touch include the possibility of superior acuity. In lenses fitted with an apical clearance technique, trauma to the central cornea and epithelium is presumably minimized. Lens wearing time may be lessened relative to lenses supported more by the central cornea. *See* fitting scleral lenses.

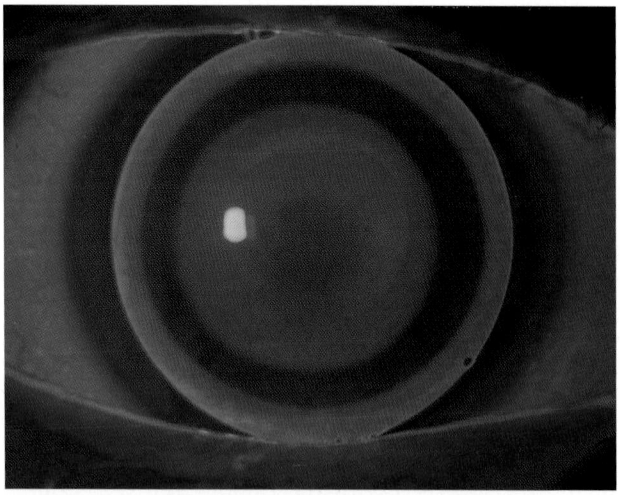

keratocytes
See corneal stroma.

keratoglobus
See distorted corneal shape, therapeutic lenses for.

keratometer, for contact lens curvature measurement
With slight modification, a keratometer can be adapted for measuring any reflective curved surface. In conjunction with a mirror and wet cell, this is a precise although cumbersome method for measuring the **back optic zone radius** (BOZR) (Figure K.5) or **front optic zone radius** (FOZR) of **soft** or **rigid lenses**. Keratometer scales are calibrated for corneal radius and/or corneal surface power, and thus the keratometer scale needs to be re-calibrated when using it for estimating the BOZR of a soft lens. Recalibration can be achieved using rigid contact lenses of known BOZR.

keratometer, for corneal curvature measurement
Knowledge of corneal curvature is primarily of interest as an aid in determining the initial contact lens to be placed on the eye in cases of **rigid contact lens** fitting. The amount of keratometric **astigmatism** can be compared to the ocular astigmatism. This identifies lenticular astigmatism, which may be the cause of residual astigmatism in rigid lens wear. For soft lens fitting, particularly **disposable lenses**, which might, for example, be available in only two **back optic zone radii** (BOZR), keratometry may be used simply to identify steeper **corneas**, which require the lens with the smaller BOZR.

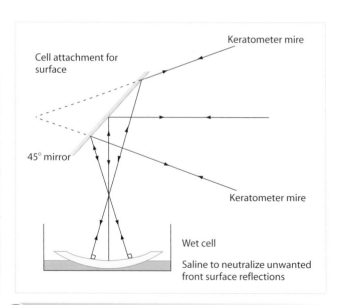

Figure K.4 Three-point-touch technique of fitting a rigid lens to a keratoconic eye.

Figure K.5 Optics of measuring the BOZR of a rigid lens using a keratometer.

For all lens wearers (and indeed non-lens-wearers), keratometry can provide an indication of progressive or rapid changes in curvature, which can be indicative of a compromised cornea. Keratometric assessment can also aid in the diagnosis of keratoconus.

Keratometric measurement of the radius of curvature of the cornea is based on the fact that the front surface of the cornea acts as a convex mirror. The reflection of an object (or mire, from the French for 'target') of known size at a known distance is viewed using a short focus telescope, and a relatively simple equation allows the corneal front surface radius of curvature to be determined directly from the instrument. The corneal power that results from a given radius is often also indicated on the keratometer; alternatively, this can be calculated or determined from tables (Appendix D).

Keratometry is a simple, rapid and non-invasive test (Figure K.6), but it does have some limitations. The actual region over which the standard keratometer measures corneal radius is that of two small areas approximately 1.5 mm on either side of the central fixation point. Different types of keratometers use differing sized mires at differing separations. It is thus of no surprise that different keratometers may give differing radius values on the same eye. The keratometer only measures at one corneal radius, it assumes regular astigmatism (i.e. that the principle axes are orthogonal), and it has a limited range of powers (36.00–53.00 D). The latter problem can be overcome by interposing a −1.00 D lens (for low corneal powers, i.e. very flat corneas) or a +1.25 D lens (for high corneal powers, i.e. very steep corneas) in front of the entrance aperture of the keratometer (on the patient side of the instrument). The doubled mires are aligned in the usual way, and the keratometer reading is converted to the actual corneal power using tables such as those given in Appendix C.

The latest development in automated keratometry involves the use of infrared devices that rapidly and automatically determine central keratometry and refractive error simultaneously.

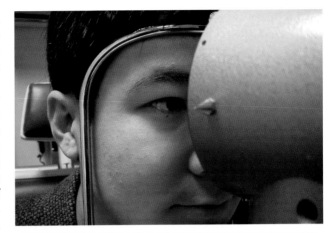

Figure K.6 Alignment of the keratometer with the eye of a patient.

In addition to determining central radius of curvature, it is useful to measure peripheral radius values, particularly in complicated conditions such as post-penetrating keratoplasty and post-refractive surgery. Conventional keratometers have been traditionally adapted by using peripheral fixation points. However, in reality keratometers cannot be used to determine corneal curvature accurately if the surface being measured does not have a constant radius of curvature or is not radially symmetric. For this reason, dedicated instruments using other technologies, such as computer-assisted **corneal topographic analysis**, have been developed to measure the overall corneal topography.

keratoplasty, lens fitting following
See post-keratoplasty, contact lens fitting.

keratoscopy
See corneal topographic analysis.

Krause gland
See accessory lacrimal glands.

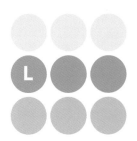

lacrimal drainage system

Tears collect at the medial canthal angle, where they drain into the puncta of the upper and lower lids (Figure L.1). Each punctum is a small oval opening, approximately 0.3 mm in diameter, which is located at the summit of an elevated papilla. From each punctum the canaliculus passes first vertically for about 2 mm and then it turns sharply to run medially for about 8 mm. At the angle, a slight dilation, the ampulla, can be seen. The canaliculi converge towards the lacrimal sac, usually forming a common canaliculus before entry. The lacrimal sac occupies a fossa formed by the maxillary and lacrimal bones. It measures 1.5–2.5 mm in diameter and approximately 12–15 mm in vertical length. From the lacrimal sac tears drain into the nasolacrimal duct, which extends for about 15 mm, passing through a bony canal in the maxillary bone to an opening in the nose beneath the inferior nasal turbinate. A fold of mucosa is often observed at the termination of the duct, which has been termed the 'valve of Hasner', although there is no strong evidence that it functions as a valve.

Tear drainage is an active process mediated by the contraction of the **orbicularis** during blinking. Tears enter the canaliculi principally by capillary action. During the early part of the blink, the puncta are occluded as the orbicularis further contracts. The canaliculi and lacrimal sac are also compressed, forcing fluid into the nose. An alternative hypothesis has been proposed, whereby orbicularis contraction dilates the sac, thus creating a negative pressure that draws in the tears from the canaliculi. A vascular plexus is embedded in the wall of the lacrimal sac and duct, and this may influence tear outflow. It is postulated that opening and closing of the lumen of the lacrimal passages can be achieved by regulating blood flow within this plexus.

lacrimal gland

The main lacrimal gland is the key provider of the aqueous component of the **tears**. The gland is located in a shallow depression of the frontal bone behind the superolateral orbital rim. It is partially split by the aponeurosis of the levator palpebrae into an upper larger orbital lobe and a lower palpebral lobe, which can often be visualized through the **conjunctiva** upon lid eversion. The gland is pinkish in colour, with a lobulated surface. Between 6 and 12 ducts leave the gland through the palpebral lobe and discharge into the conjunctival sac at the upper lateral fornix.

At a microscopic level, the lacrimal gland is tubulo-acinar in form (Figure L.2). Its secretory units (acini) contain secretory cells surrounded by myoepithelial cells. Acinar secretory cells show extensive folding of their plasma membrane and apical microvilli. Adjacent cells are linked by tight junctions, which restrict diffusion between cells. The most prominent feature of these cells is the presence of abundant secretory granules. Two principal secretory cell sub-types have been identified on the basis of their granule content. The majority of cells contain dark granules (dark cells) with a

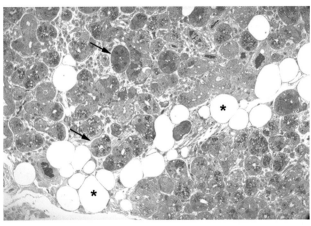

Figure L.2 Low-power light micrograph of the lacrimal gland. Acini are arrowed. Adipose connective tissue (asterisks) extends across the gland.

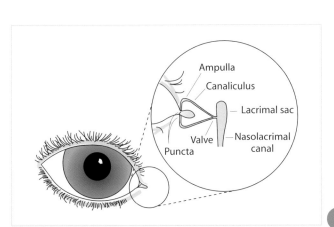

Figure L.1 Lacrimal drainage system.

Ampulla
Canaliculus
Lacrimal sac
Nasolacrimal canal
Valve
Puncta

smaller number of cells containing light granules (light cells). The functional significance of this heterogeneity is uncertain at present. Ducts consist of a single layer of cuboidal cells, which lack secretory granules. Myoepithelial cells are dendritic cells that are closely associated with the perimeter of acini and ducts. It is likely that these contractile cells play a role in the expulsion of tears from the gland. The interstices of the gland contain numerous blood vessels and nerves. A large population of immune cells (particularly IgA-secreting plasma cells) are also found between acini.

The arterial supply to the lacrimal gland is provided by the lacrimal artery, which enters the posterior border of the gland. Venous drainage occurs via the lacrimal vein. A rich autonomic innervation includes secretomotor (parasympathetic) fibres, which issue from the pterygopalatine ganglion, and sympathetic (vasomotor) fibres from the carotid plexus. The lacrimal nerve traverses the gland to provide a sensory innervation to the conjunctiva and lateral aspect of the **eyelid**.

In addition to its role as the principal provider of the aqueous phase of the tear film, the lacrimal gland is also a major component of the ocular sensory immune system, which acts as the first line of defence against microbial infection. The secretory immune system is mediated through secretory IgA. The lacrimal gland is the main source of tear IgA, and the gland contains a large number of IgA-producing plasma cells. The mechanism by which an antigenic challenge of the ocular surface induces a lacrimal antibody response is not fully understood. However, since the administration of an antigen by a gastrointestinal route raises specific IgA levels in tears, one suggested mechanism is that ocular antigens – after drainage through the nasolacrimal duct – stimulate B cells in gut Peyer's patches. These sensitized B cells then populate the lacrimal gland, where they transform into plasma cells.

The lacrimal gland also secretes growth factors into the tears, which are important for the maintenance of the ocular surface and epithelial wound healing. Prominent amongst these growth factors are epidermal growth factor (EGF) and transforming growth factor beta (TGFβ).

lacrimal lens
See tear lens.

lacrimal puncta
See lacrimal drainage system.

lacrimal sac
See lacrimal drainage system.

lacrimal system
The lacrimal apparatus provides for the production and maintenance of the pre-ocular **tear film**. The normal function of this system is essential for the integrity of the ocular surface and the provision of a smooth refractive surface. The lacrimal apparatus comprises a secretory system, which includes the main and accessory **lacrimal glands**, and a drainage system, which consists of the paired puncta and canaliculi, the lacrimal sac and the nasolacrimal duct.

lactate
See oedema.

lactation
See indications and contraindications for contact lens wear.

laminate tint constructions
An opaque tinted iris pattern can be incorporated within a contact lens using a laminate construction. An iris pattern is painted, using opaque dyes and tints, onto the surface of an unhydrated **HEMA** button that has been lathed to the curvature of the intended finished lens. A second pouring of HEMA over the top of this pattern is effected. Once set, the laminate button is lathed to create the finished lens form, which is then hydrated in the usual way. The advantage of this process is that the painted features are encapsulated, and therefore protected, within the lens. The disadvantages are that the lens is thicker, thus reducing **oxygen transmissibility**, and the tensile properties of the lens are altered, which can affect fitting characteristics.

A variation of laminate construction, known as sandwich technology, has been developed. The top and bottom layers of clear HEMA are co-polymerized with a thin middle layer of coloured non-toxic pigments, allowing the composite button to be lathed and then hydrated into an ultra-thin lens design. An alternative approach is to use non-coloured opaquing agents to create an iris pattern in the centre of the two HEMA buttons, and then tinting the top HEMA section to create the desired cosmetic colouration. *See* tinted lenses.

laser-assisted *in situ* keratomileusis (LASIK)
See laser refractive surgery, contact lenses following.

laser refractive surgery, contact lenses following
The contact lens management of the post-photorefractive keratectomy patient poses far fewer problems than those encountered after **radial keratotomy** (RK). Patients may present for contact lens fitting after having laser-assisted *in situ*

keratomileusis (LASIK) surgery performed on both eyes simultaneously. Contact lens fitting differs between the two procedures in that:

- following photorefractive keratectomy (PRK) or LASIK, the mid-peripheral **cornea** remains unchanged from its pre-operative state
- a wider range of **soft contact lens** designs can be used following PRK and LASIK due to the absence of peri-limbal incisions
- the post-PRK and post-LASIK cornea does not have elevated mid-peripheral pivot points secondary to incisional wound healing; these areas are the major cause of rigid lens decentration following RK
- PRK and LASIK offer less diurnal fluctuations in visual acuity due to the stability of the peripheral cornea; this is especially important when soft contact lenses are used post-operatively.

The LASIK flap presents few, if any, problems in the fitting or wearing of contact lenses. In fact, there has been no discernable difference with respect to contact lens fitting or physiologic response between post-PRK and post-LASIK patients.

The amount of corneal tissue removed in a myopic laser procedure will play an important role in the post-surgical management of the patient with contact lenses. Irregular astigmatism is a rare finding in both PRK and LASIK, and therefore it is not a significant issue for the contact lens practitioner.

Three contact lens options are used for post-PRK and post-LASIK patients:

1. *Conventional rigid lens designs.* Many patients who have undergone PRK or LASIK can be successfully fitted with traditional **spherical or aspheric rigid lenses**. With **myopic** ablations, the mid-peripheral cornea (beyond the central 6.0–7.0 mm) remains unchanged. Therefore, the major concern in fitting rigid or **soft contact lenses** is the relative difference between the flatter central cornea and the steeper (normal) mid-peripheral cornea. This difference creates few problems for patients who were low-to-moderate myopes prior to surgery. In such cases, the small amount of tissue ablated does not noticeably affect the contact lens fit or the on-eye lens dynamics. These individuals are often best fitted with a **BOZR** designed to align the mid-peripheral corneal topography 4.0 mm from the centre of the cornea.
2. *Reverse geometry rigid lens designs.* A patient with high pre-operative refractive error (i.e. greater than −10.00 D) might end up with a large difference in thickness between the central and mid-peripheral cornea, such that a traditional rigid lens (designed to align with the mid-peripheral cornea) may exhibit excessive apical clearance. The subsequent large volume of tears centrally can result in unstable optics, and trapped bubbles can form beneath the centre of the lens. In situations such as this, patients may be best managed with **reverse geometry lens** designs. A standard rigid design mimics the prolate shape of the normal, un-operated cornea, which is steeper in the centre than the periphery. The reverse geometry design more closely parallels the post-refractive surgery topography by incorporating a flat central radius of curvature with a steeper mid-peripheral design. This creates a 'plateau' configuration on the posterior lens surface, which dramatically decreases the volume of tear fluid present beneath the central portion of the lens.
3. *Soft lenses.* Most of the currently available daily disposable or frequent replacement soft lenses are viable options for the post-laser correction. However, after surgery a complex relationship exists between visual acuity, defocus (refractive error), diffraction and optical aberrations. The loss of post-operative central corneal asphericity can result in a form of spherical aberration that will be symptomatic, especially in patients with large pupils. Improved optical correction can be achieved with soft lens designs that incorporate aberration-correcting anterior aspheric optics.

With both PRK and LASIK, rigid lens fitting is best delayed until approximately 8–12 weeks after surgery. At this point, the refraction and topography have stabilized. At 3 months post-surgery, the integrity of the flap interface is usually sufficient to withstand the minor trauma associated with lens insertion and removal, as well as the normal on-eye movement that occurs with blinking.

Practitioners need to be aware of the level of **corneal sensitivity** following laser refractive surgery if contact lenses are to be fitted. Following PRK, the decrease in central corneal sensitivity will last for about 1 month. Following LASIK, there is a deep decrease in central corneal sensitivity that takes about 6 months to recover.

Patients frequently experience dry eye symptoms after LASIK; however, the mechanisms that lead to these changes are not well understood. **Tear film** dysfunction has obvious implications if contact lenses are required after surgery.

LASIK

See laser refractive surgery, contact lenses following.

lathe cutting

This technique is used to manufacture both soft and rigid contact lenses. It essentially involves the use of a special contact lens lathe to cut a solid piece of plastic into the required shape. In the case of a **soft lens**, a block of anhydrous plastic material (xerogel) is lathed and then hydrated to form the finished product. In the case of a **rigid lens**, the material is simply cut to the desired final form.

Lathe cutting is labour intensive, which means that the cost of manufacturing soft lenses using lathe-cutting technology is necessarily more expensive than that using **spin casting** or **cast moulding**. Therefore, lathe cutting is generally reserved for the production of rigid lenses and for custom-ordered soft lenses which contain design features that are not amenable to mass production – such as lenses of high spherical power and/or high toric power.

The lens material is supplied to the lens manufacturer in the form of 'rods' or 'buttons'. A rod is a solid cylindrical piece of plastic, about 16 mm in diameter and 40 cm long. The rod is then sliced, tangentially to the long axis, into buttons of about 1 cm thick. More commonly, the materials are fabricated and supplied in button form.

The button is first secured to a back surface lathe in a clamp or 'collet', and this assembly is set spinning at a high rate about its central axis. A diamond-tipped tool cuts the posterior surface lens shape into the button. A second diamond tool advances from the side to reduce the diameter to the required size. The surface is rendered smooth by either fine machining or polishing. The dimensions of these cuts are calculated to allow for eventual expansion when the xerogel is later hydrated.

The button is removed from the collet and the cut posterior surface of the button is mounted onto a support tool of a front surface lathe, using low melting point wax. A diamond-tipped tool cuts the anterior surface down to the required thickness (Figure L.3) and the surface is smoothed. Polishing tools may be used to smooth the lens edge, although some advanced lathes obviate this step. Finally, all relevant lens parameters are inspected and measured.

In the case of soft lenses, the xerogel lens form is hydrated in normal, unpreserved **saline**, re-inspected, sealed in small glass vials, and autoclaved at 120°C for 15 minutes to effect sterilization. Advances in lathing technology and computer-controlled processing have led to the development of semi-automatic systems whereby stacks of buttons are automatically fed into lathes; however, even this technology cannot match the mass-production capabilities of cast moulding.

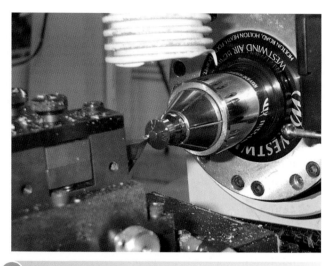

Figure L.3 Front surface curve being lathed onto a rigid lens.

lattice dystrophy

See dystrophies of the corneal epithelium, therapeutic lenses for.

layout, contact lens practice

The layout of a contact lens practice will be governed by the physical limitations of the site and the sequence and order of activities that the patient undergoes during a visit to the practice. The key features are as follows:

1. *Reception area and front desk*. This is the first personal contact position for the visiting patient, and should be a welcoming point as well as a help desk. The reception area will often be the last point of contact before the patient leaves the practice.
2. *Waiting area*. The waiting area needs to be comfortable, with sufficient seating to accommodate potential patients and customers. A 'rule of thumb' worth considering is that this area should be furnished and decorated to a standard similar to that of the sitting rooms of the patients and customers attending the practice.
3. *Consulting room*. Depending on the patient workload of the practice, more than one room may be dedicated to the consultation and examination activity. Increasingly, delegation of data collection tasks (e.g. non-contact tonometry, visual field analysis, auto-refraction etc.) to support staff means that an area or room will be utilized for this pre-examination screening or adjunct data collection. The consulting room will have all the equipment found in a modern contact lens practice, with an emphasis on ante-

rior eye evaluation/recording. In addition to this, it will be necessary to have some contact lens verification equipment. The need for specialist diagnostic fitting sets and materials (e.g. pre-formed rigid **scleral lenses**, **bifocal lenses**, eye impression materials etc.) will be dictated by the profile of patients attending the practice.

4. *Spectacle dispensary.* Every contact lens-wearing patient should be considered to be an optometric patient who happens to be using contact lenses. All contact lens wearers require spectacles. The spectacle dispensary should thus be able to provide for the functional and aesthetic needs of the patient, just as any optometric practice would. In the case of a highly specialized contact lens practice that does not have a spectacle dispensary, there should be the facility to refer patients to a convenient dispensing practice nearby.

5. *Contact lens dispensary.* The contact lens dispensing area is where patients will attend for instruction and for practising insertion and removal of contact lenses (*see* patient education). It is also here that patients will receive their (starter) contact lens care systems, obtain advice on wear, care and hygiene with respect to their contact lenses, and complete the paperwork etc. This area should therefore have the furniture, facilities, materials and equipment to allow this to happen effectively. Employing videos and CD-ROMs in this area to support the education process, along with written materials, is now a common practice.

lens delivery systems

Two main methods for managing the implementation of **planned lens replacement** systems have evolved; manufacturer-driven and practice-driven systems.

Manufacturer-driven systems are common in the UK. The names of new patients are registered with the manufacturer by the practice, along with relevant prescription details. Depending on the lens type, there may also be an option to select a frequency of lens delivery to the practice; for example, monthly replacement lenses may be supplied to the practice in 3- or 6-month quantities. Once the patient is registered, fresh supplies of lenses will be automatically dispatched to the practice until the manufacturer is advised otherwise by the practice.

Manufacturers have, in some cases, branded their systems to promote the service provided. The main benefit to practices is reduced administration. Simple computer programs run the systems (Figure

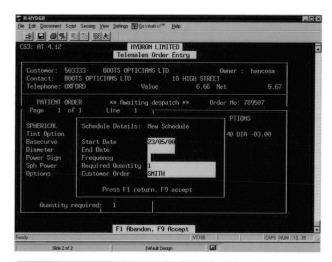

Figure L.4 Order entry screen for planned replacement lenses used by a manufacturer.

L.4), and the arrival of a new supply of lenses for a given patient acts as a trigger for the practice to recall that particular lens wearer.

In the UK, such systems complement the method by which many patients pay for frequent replacement lenses – namely, monthly direct payment from the bank account of the patient to that of the practice. In this way, both payment and regular lens supply is automated, and **compliance** with the designated replacement schedule is encouraged.

Some manufacturers have expanded their service to include direct delivery of lenses and possibly lens care products (so-called 'bundling') to the home address of the patient. The increased convenience afforded by this approach is promoted as a means of retaining the custom of the patient for replacement lenses, given the growth of non-practice sources of supply such as direct mail and the Internet.

If a manufacturer-driven system is not employed, an in-house practice-driven system is required to ensure the timely purchase of replacement lenses and recall of patients. With larger patient bases the amount of stock involved can soon become quite large, and adequate storage space is often an issue. On the other hand, bulk purchasing may allow practices to secure preferential terms from suppliers. A practice operating its own system is also in complete control of the process and less vulnerable to any manufacturer supply problems. *See* lens supply routes.

lens edge fluting
See fluting.

lens insertion
See insertion and removal, rigid lens; insertion and removal, scleral lens; insertion and removal, soft lens.

lens inventory
See practice logistics.

lensometer
See focimeter.

lens modification
A variety of procedures can be adopted to modify or adjust the form of **PMMA** or **rigid contact lenses**. These procedures usually involve the use of paraphernalia such as spinning tools, polishing pads, sponges and suctions caps, and include edge and surface polishing, effecting a small change in lens power, blending peripheral curves, **fenestrating**, **truncating** and engraving. These days most practitioners prefer to return a lens to a specialist rigid lens laboratory for such modifications, although some prefer to undertake such procedures in the practice. Particular care must be exercised to avoid over-polishing (and consequent over-heating) when modifying materials of medium to high **oxygen permeability**, in order to avoid surface damage such as crazing and reducing lens surface wettability.

lens polishing
See lens modification.

lens removal
See insertion and removal, rigid lens; insertion and removal, scleral lens; insertion and removal, soft lens.

lens stock
See practice logistics.

lens supply
See lens delivery systems; lens supply routes.

lens supply routes
The issue of non-optical-practice supply now affects virtually all contact lens types, although **disposable lenses** are particularly susceptible to third party distribution, given the brand awareness that many of these products have with the public. The critical issue here is that it is in the public interest to have a system of lens supply that guarantees the ongoing preservation of the ocular health of lens wearers. A system that provides no disincentives to patients continuing to purchase lenses for many years without having their eyes examined poses a significant public health risk.

Notwithstanding the role of regulatory authorities in discharging their responsibilities of public health and safety, there are strategies that practitioners can employ to retain control of lens supply and to link this to patient care. Fee splitting – where materials are charged at relatively low mark-ups on cost, and these charges are separated from professional fees – helps demonstrate to patients that most of the cost involved in wearing contact lenses is attributed to the professional time involved. Home delivery plans, perhaps operated on behalf of the practice by a supplier, enable practitioners to match the perceived convenience of mail order and Internet supply companies. Many large practices or group practices are able to come to an arrangement with manufacturers so that lenses and solutions supplied by that manufacturers are 're-branded' prior to delivery. The re-branding (or so-called 'own-labelling' or 'private labelling') facilitates an association of the products with the practice, and thereby serves to enhance patient loyalty. *See* lens delivery systems.

lens thickness
The thickness of a contact lens can be specified as the thickness at the geometric centre or edge of the lens. The average thickness over a specified diameter (typically that of the central optical zone) can also be specified. **Soft lens** centre thickness is relevant to ease of lens handling and susceptibility to dehydration. Mid-water lenses (50–59%) are generally manufactured with centre thickness in the range 0.06–0.10 mm, while high water content lenses (> 60%) generally have centre thickness in the range 0.10–0.18 mm. Determination of the average thickness of a soft lens can be useful when considering the physiological impact of a lens on the eye, because the ability of oxygen to permeate through a lens to the eye is inversely related to thickness.

Due to poor measurement repeatability, soft lens peripheral thickness is not the subject of an international standard, and is not always routinely verified during lens manufacture. Nevertheless, variations in peripheral thickness can have a significant effect on lens fit and comfort. Contrary to expectations, lenses with a thicker edge often show a **looser fit** and are less comfortable than lenses of similar basic design with a thinner lens edge.

If rigid lenses are made too thin not only is there greater risk of breakage but the lenses also tend to flex on **astigmatic corneas**, leaving residual astigmatism. Flexure is a function of lens thickness and is therefore more problematic with low minus powered lenses. Fluorosilicone acrylate **polymers** tend to show more flexure than silicone acrylate materials of similar **oxygen permeability** (Dk). Also, for a given material type, flexure tends to increase with increasing *Dk*. It is therefore necessary to increase lens centre thickness with higher *Dk* materials.

lenticulation, lens

The process of altering lens design to minimize edge thickness in a negative-powered lens, or to minimize centre thickness in a positive-powered lens, is referred to as 'lenticulation'. The general strategy is to reduce the optic zone diameter as much as possible without compromising visual function, and form a thin lenticular supporting rim outside the optic zone. *See* high minus power contact lens design; high plus power contact lens design.

levator palpebrae superioris

This muscle is primarily responsible for elevating the upper lid during **blinking**, and for maintaining an open palpebral aperture. The levator palpebrae arises from the lesser wing of the sphenoid, above and anterior to the optic canal, and runs forward along the roof of the orbit above the superior rectus before terminating anteriorly in a fan-shaped tendon known as the aponeurosis. Some fibres are attached to the anterior surface of the tarsal plate, whilst the remainder pass between fascicles of the orbicularis. The superior palpebral sulcus forms at the upper border of the attachment to the orbicularis (Figure L.5).

lice

The louse (*Phthirus pubis*) has two pairs of strong grasping claws on its central and hind legs, allowing it to hold on to eyelashes with considerable tenacity (Figure L.6). Crab louse infestation (phthiriasis) is considered to be a venereal disease because it is passed on by sexual contact, although infestation from contaminated bedding, towels, etc. is another possible mode of transfer.

Signs of phthiriasis include:

- pruritis of the lid margins
- **blepharitis**
- marked conjunctival injection
- madarosis
- presence of lice
- presence of oval, greyish-white nit shells attached to the base of lashes.

Additional signs include preauricular lymphadenopathy and secondary infection along the lid margins at the site of lice bites. The most predominant symptom is intense itching. The initial course of action is to attempt physically to remove as many mites and mite eggs as possible. Patients should be advised to engage in vigorous lid scrubbing twice daily, using commercially available preparations. In general, contact lens wearers presenting with parasitic infestation of the eyelids should be treated in the same way as similarly infested non-lens-wearers.

Syns. Pubic louse; crab louse.

lids

See eyelids.

life expectancy, contact lens

The life expectancy of high water content **soft lenses** is 6 months. In the case of **rigid lenses**, life expectancy

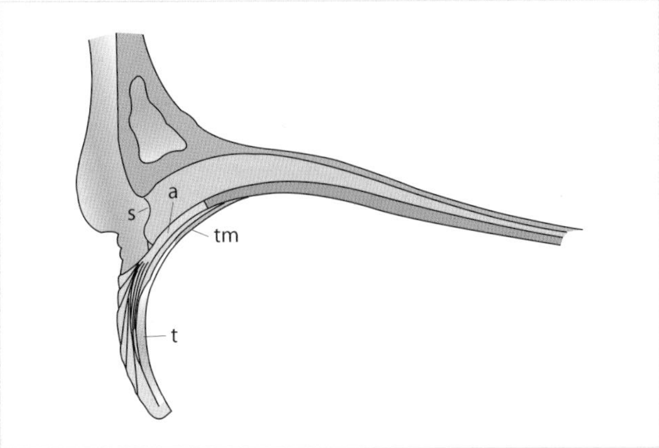

Figure L.5 Relations of the levator palpebrae superioris. a = levator aponeurosis; tm = superior tarsal muscle (of Müller); t = tarsal plate; s = orbital septum. Adapted from H. Gray, L. H. Bannister, M. M. Berry and P.L. Williams (1995) *Gray's Anatomy: The Anatomical Basis of Medicine and Surgery*, 38th edn, Churchill Livingstone.

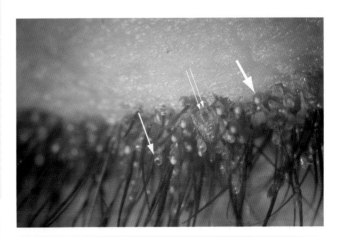

Figure L.6 Lice infestation of the upper eyelashes. A single louse (double arrow) sits at the base of the lashes surrounded by full (thick arrow) and empty (thin arrow) nit shells.

is related to material **oxygen permeability** (*Dk*). The mean life expectancy of rigid lenses is 20 months for low *Dk* materials, 16 months for mid-*Dk* materials, and 9 months for high *Dk* materials.

lifestyle
See indications and contraindications for contact lens wear.

limbal redness
Assuming that a given case of eye redness is lens related, it is necessary to determine whether the source of the problem is the **cornea** or the **conjunctiva**. **Conjunctival redness** associated with a quiet limbus and the absence of pain indicates a primary conjunctival problem. Conjunctival redness associated with an injected limbus and corneal pain indicates corneal involvement, or indeed a problem that is related *exclusively* to the cornea. Careful **slit-lamp** examination of the anterior ocular structures, and inspection of the lens at high magnification, will generally reveal the cause of the problem. It may also be necessary to prescribe different care systems and differentially diagnose the effects of various solutions over time.

In the absence of any clinically observable ocular pathology, corneal **hypoxia** is the likely cause of excessive limbal redness (Figure L.7). Hypoxia stimulates the release of inflammatory mediators from the limbal vessel walls, leading to vasodilatation; this is an automatic reaction designed to facilitate a greater flow of oxygenated blood to the distressed tissue. This mechanism fails in the case of the limbus because limbal blood flow contributes little to corneal oxygenation; the cornea derives virtually all of its oxygen supply from the atmosphere. The result, therefore, is contact lens induced hypoxia maintaining chronic limbal vessel engorgement in a vain attempt to re-oxygenate the cornea.

There is a significant relationship between the **oxygen transmissibility** of the peripheral region of a soft lens and limbal redness. Indeed, one of the key benefits of high-permeability silicone hydrogel lenses is that they induce low levels of limbal redness. Although hypoxia is presumed to be the key determinant of limbal redness, practitioners should be alert to the possibility of other causes, such as poor lens edge design or pathology of the anterior ocular structures – especially the cornea. Recovery from chronic contact lens induced limbal redness after removal of lenses and cessation of wear takes about 7 days.

Syn. limbal hyperaemia, limbal injection.

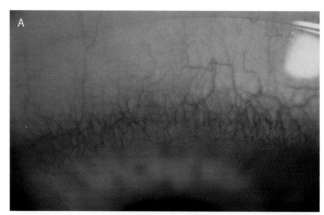

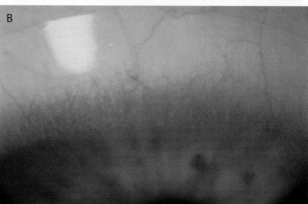

Figure L.7 (A) Hyperaemia is evident at the superior limbus of a patient wearing a low *Dk/t* hydrogel lens in one eye, whereas (B) less hyperaemia is evident at the superior limbus of the contralateral eye wearing a high *Dk/t* silicone hydrogel lens.

lipid deposition
See deposits, lens.

lipids in tears
See tear lipids.

liquid lens
See tear lens.

lissamine green stain
This is a green dye that can reveal the presence of ocular surface damage in patients with keratoconjunctivitis sicca. It is said to be tolerated better than **rose bengal** by patients.

locator tints
See handling tints.

loose lens fit
A lens that moves or lags excessively is deemed to be fitting loosely. Loose-fitting lenses can cause peripheral **corneal staining**, symptoms of **discom-**

fort, and variable vision. Patients may also complain of lenses being displaced from the cornea during wear. The first possibility to consider is whether the lens is inside out. Switching to a similar lens of steeper **back optic zone radius** may not always overcome the problem, particularly with thin lens designs. It may therefore be necessary to change to a lens with a tendency towards tight fitting.

Loveridge grid
See non-invasive tear break-up time.

lubricants
See re-wetting solutions, soft lens; wetting solutions, rigid lens.

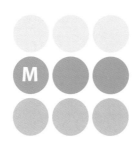

mail order
See lens supply routes.

manufacturing tolerances
See Appendix E; tolerances.

map–dot–fingerprint dystrophy
See recurrent erosion syndrome, therapeutic lenses for.

materials, soft lens
See hydrogel polymers.

McMonnies' dry eye questionnaire
See dry eye questionnaire.

mechanical properties, soft lens
In its dehydrated state, **polyHEMA** is hard and brittle (as are most other hydrogel-forming polymers). In this way it resembles **PMMA**. When swollen in water, however, it becomes soft and rubber-like, with a very low tear and tensile strength. This lack of mechanical strength has a profound effect on the **life expectancy** of the lens, which caused significant problems before the advent of disposability and **planned replacement**. Although water content has a marked effect on mechanical strength within a given family of materials, the chemical structure of the **polymer** also plays a large part. This point is illustrated by comparing the strength of synthetic hydrogels such as polyHEMA with that of natural composite hydrophilic gels, such as articular cartilage, intervertebral discs and the **cornea**. Cartilage has a tensile strength more than 10 times greater than that of polyHEMA, despite having double the water content (around 80%).

The elastic behaviour and rigidity of **hydrogels** is closely governed by monomer structure and effective cross-link density, which includes not only covalent cross-link forces but also ionic, polar and steric interchain forces. By use of modified monomer combinations and cross-linking agents, high **water content** polymers with good stability and elasticity can be prepared. The currently available commercial high water content lenses are vastly superior in strength to the first generation of fragile gels of similar water content based on HEMA-NVP co-polymers. As a general rule, increasing water content reduces durability, particularly resistance to tearing; however, these considerations are of little significance when lenses made from such materials are only intended to last a matter of days or weeks.

Medical Devices Directive
In Europe, the control of contact lenses and contact lens care products is regulated by the European Medical Devices Directive (MDD). This directive sets out requirements to which each device must conform. There are thousands of medical devices covered by the directive. The associated trade must devise appropriate management mechanisms to ensure the conformity of its products. Devices conforming to the directive should carry the European standard CE mark ('CE' stands for the French expression 'Commission Européenne'). Since June 1998, it has been illegal to either sell or buy a contact lens in Europe if it does not have the CE mark affixed to it.

The CE marks are dispensed through what are called Notified Bodies. Companies wishing to affix the CE mark to their products must be registered as an approved manufacturer with a Notified Body, which will provide them with authority to use the mark. In order to get on the approved list of a Notified Body, manufacturers of contact lenses are generally required to have implemented a quality system, typically ISO 9002, and then applied the medical device-specific CE requirements in the form of a further layer of bureaucratic controls set out in EN 46002. This procedure has become the *de facto* approach used by UK contact lens manufacturers who have obtained the CE mark for their products, and looks set to be the normal pathway to complying with the regulations. A principal activity of the Notified Bodies is to audit the device manufacturer to make sure that the procedures in use are such that devices made in the system comply with the directive.

medication with contact lenses
Unpreserved unit-dose eye drops are indicated for concurrent use with **soft lenses**. Preserved eye drops are rarely used in this situation because of concerns that preservatives such as benzalkonium chloride can accumulate in the lens and be toxic to the **corneal epithelium**. This effect is usually of no clinical importance when **disposable lenses** are used for short periods. All topical drugs may be used with **rigid lenses** – both corneal and **scleral**. It is not known whether drugs achieve suitable concentrations in the ocular tissues when sealed **scleral lenses** are being worn. Ointment preparations should not be used concurrently with contact lenses.

Meesmann's dystrophy

See dystrophies of the corneal epithelium, therapeutic lenses for.

meibomian gland

The tarsal plates contain the acini and ducts of the meibomian (tarsal) glands. Ducts are vertically orientated with respect to the lid margins, with multiple secretory acini that open laterally onto each duct. The glands occupy nearly the full length and width of each tarsus, and are fewer and shorter in the lower lid. Histologically, acini are lined by a layer of undifferentiated basal cells that divide, and cells are displaced from the basement membrane. As they progress towards the duct they gradually enlarge and develop lipid droplets in their cytoplasm. Ultimately, cell membranes rupture and cellular debris, together with the lipid product, is discharged into the duct.

The stimulus for meibomian gland secretion is unclear. Although a modest autonomic innervation of the meibomian glands has been demonstrated, there is still some doubt regarding a neuromodulation of glandular secretion, and it is likely that the principal control of the glands is hormonal. Androgens are known to regulate the development, differentiation and secretion of sebaceous glands throughout the body, and are thought also to influence meibomian gland secretion.

meibomian gland dysfunction

The oily secretion from the normal **meibomian gland** is generally clear. The key diagnostic feature of contact lens associated meibomian gland dysfunction (CL-MGD) is a change in the appearance of the clear oil expressed from healthy meibomian glands to a cloudy, creamy-yellow appearance (Figure M.1). Frothing or foaming of the lower tear meniscus is sometimes observed in CL-MGD, especially towards the outer canthus. This appearance is accompanied by symptoms of smeary vision, greasy lenses, **dry eyes**, and reduced tolerance to lens wear. In severe cases where the meibomian orifices are blocked, there may be an absence of gland secretion. Longstanding cases of MGD may be associated with additional signs such as irregularity, distortion and thickening of eyelid margins, slight distension of glands, mild-to-moderate papillary hypertrophy, vascular changes and chronic chalazia. The prevalence of CL-MGD is unrelated to gender but increases with age.

Associated signs of CL-MGD include all those that arise from clinical diagnostic procedures that are designed to indicate the integrity or otherwise of the lipid layer. Specifically, patients suffering from CL-

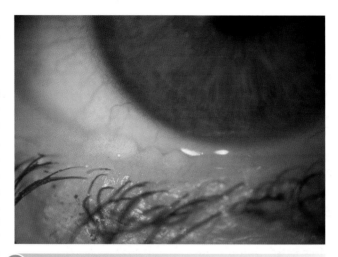

Figure M.1 Inspissated meibomian gland secretion in the lower lid of a female patient wearing rigid lenses.

MGD may display a reduced **tear break-up time** (measured either with **fluorescein** or non-invasively). Examination of the tear layer in specular reflection using a **tearscope** may reveal a contaminated lipid pattern, which is exacerbated by the use of cosmetic eye make-up. Symptoms of blurred or greasy vision can probably be attributed to adhesion of waxy dysfunctional meibomian oils to the surface of the contact lens; this can lead to lens surface drying, lens dehydration and sensations of **dryness**.

Theories for the aetiology of CL-MGD include the following:

1. It is due to excessive eye rubbing causing chronic damage to the meibomian glands
2. It occurs secondary to **papillary conjunctivitis**.

From a tissue pathology standpoint, MGD is characterized by increased keratinization of the epithelial walls of the meibomian gland ducts. As might be expected, therefore, this condition is often observed in combination with seborrhoeic dermatitis and acne rosacea. This leads to the formation of keratinized epithelial plugs that create a physical blockage in meibomian ducts, which in turn restricts or prevents the outflow of meibomian oils.

Although the underlying cause of meibomian gland dysfunction cannot be treated, it is possible to provide symptomatic relief by adopting one or more of the following procedures, all of which should be undertaken with the contact lenses removed:

- application of warm compresses
- lid scrubs
- mechanical expression
- prescription of antibiotics

- use of artificial tears and of **surfactant lens cleaners**.

By adopting these procedures, CL-MGD can be kept under good control and adverse symptoms minimized.

Mengher grid
See non-invasive tear break-up time.

metabolic disorders
See systemic disease, contact lens wear in.

microbial keratitis
See keratitis, microbial.

microcysts
Microcysts appear in the **corneal epithelium** as minute, scattered, opaque grey dots when viewed with the **slit-lamp biomicroscope** using low magnification and focal illumination (Figure M.2), and as transparent refractile inclusions with **indirect retro-illumination**. They are generally of a uniform spherical or ovoid shape and are in the order of 20 µm in diameter. At high magnification (×40) using the observation technique of marginal retro-illumination, microcysts can be observed to display a characteristic optical phenomenon known as 'reversed illumination'; that is, the distribution of light within the microcyst is opposite to the light distribution of the background. This indicates that the microcyst is acting as a converging refractor, and therefore it must consist of material that is of a higher **refractive index** than the surrounding epithelium. Microcysts probably represent apoptotic (dead) cells which either become phagocytosed (ingested) by living neighbouring cells, or remain involuted in the intercellular spaces. In a process similar to that occurring in Cogan's microcystic dystrophy, the epithelial basement membrane duplicates and folds, forming intraepithelial sheets that eventually detach from the basement membrane and encapsulate the cellular material.

Microcysts primarily represent visible evidence of chronic tissue metabolic stress and altered cellular growth patterns. These changes are presumed to be caused by a combination of the direct effects of **hypoxia**, and tissue acidosis created by the indirect effects of hypoxia (producing lactic acid) and **hypercapnia** (producing carbonic acid). They may also have a mechanical aetiology, whereby lens-induced mechanical trauma can induce microcysts.

Whilst the actual presence of microcysts is not thought to be dangerous, their existence in large numbers is worrying, as this is representative of epithelial metabolic distress. Based on the working hypothesis that the severity of the microcyst response is related to the level of hypoxia/hypercapnia induced by lens wear, a variety of strategies can be employed in an attempt to minimize the number of microcysts. Strategies that are likely to be successful include:

- increasing lens **oxygen transmissibility**
- decreasing the frequency of overnight wear
- changing from **extended-wear** to daily-wear lenses
- changing from soft to rigid lenses
- avoiding **defective** lenses.

The prognosis for eliminating microcysts is good, but the time course is peculiar. Following cessation of lens wear there is an initial increase in the number of microcysts over a 7-day period, followed by a subsequent decrease. The initial increase in microcysts is thought to be due to an initial resurgence in epithelial metabolism and growth, resulting in an accelerated removal of cellular debris (formation of microcysts) and a rapid movement of microcysts towards the surface, where they are more readily observed. This is followed by a gradual decrease as the existing microcysts are completely eliminated from the cornea over a period of 3–5 months.

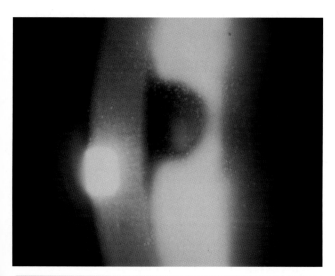

Figure M.2 Extensive microcyst formation in the epithelium of a soft lens wearer.

microdots
Examination of the living human cornea at very high magnification (×680) using a **confocal microscope** will reveal the presence of highly reflective 'microdot deposits' throughout the **corneal stroma** (Figure M.3). Microdots are small, discrete, brightly reflective spots or dots scattered throughout the

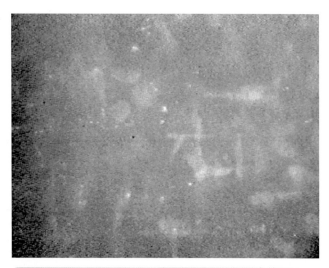

Figure M.3 Microdots in the human corneal stroma of a soft lens wearer.

stroma; they are generally round or oval in shape, and vary in diameter from about 1 to 4 μm. Microdot deposits are observed in all persons, whether contact lenses have been worn or not; however, more microdots are seen in lens wearers, which indicates that contact lens wear is exacerbating otherwise normal corneal morphological features. It should also be recognized that it is not possible at present to determine whether the appearance of microdots is related to the contact lenses, or to solutions used in conjunction with lens wear.

microplicae
See corneal epithelium.

microspherometer
See radiuscope.

microvilli
See corneal epithelium.

microwave disinfection, soft lens
Microwave irradiation has been proposed as a potentially cheap and effective method for soft lens disinfection. Although there are some parameter changes when lenses are repeatedly irradiated with a standard 650-W microwave oven, none of these changes are clinically significant. However, repeated heating (as essentially occurs with microwave radiation) is known rapidly to degrade certain **polymers** and to distort lenses that have absorbed high levels of protein. As patients often need to care for their lenses in locations remote from a microwave oven, this approach is often impractical or inconvenient.

minimum recommended disinfection time (MRDT)
See antimicrobial efficacy.

minus lens carrier
See high plus power contact lens design.

mites
Mite infestation in humans is very common, and infestation of the eyelashes by mites is ubiquitous and generally sub-clinical. If present in excessive numbers, mites can lead to the following signs and symptoms:

- pruritis
- burning
- crusting
- itching
- swelling of the lid margins
- loss and easy removal of lashes.

These symptoms often parallel the 10-day mite reproductive cycle.

Two types of mite can be found in the eyelash region. *Demodex folliculorum* prefers to live in the spaces between the eyelashes and in the outermost region of the eyelash follicles. It shreds the epithelial lining of the follicle, and the shredded material mixes with lipids and sebum to form a clear sleeve around the base of the eyelashes, known as a 'cuff' or 'collarette'. *Demodex brevis* prefers an oily environment, and is found in the **glands of Zeis** (Figure M.4).

Although mites are very difficult to see, their presence is confirmed by the observation of epilated lashes and collarettes under the microscope. Treatment in the first instance is aimed at reducing the level of mites to sub-clinical levels; this can be effected by applying a topical anaesthetic and swabbing the eyelid margins and eyelashes with a cotton-tipped applicator soaked in contact lens cleaning

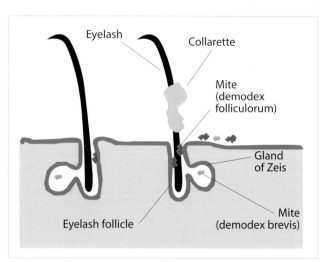

Figure M.4 Mite habitat.

solution. Vigorous twice-daily lid scrubbing and the application of viscous ointments at night (to suffocate the mites) over a 3-week period can cure the condition.

modern orthokeratology
See orthokeratology.

modification of rigid lenses
See lens modification.

Moll gland
See gland of Moll.

monomers
See polymers.

monovision correction for presbyopia
Monovision is an approach for correcting **presbyopia** with contact lenses whereby one eye is given the required distance refractive power and the other eye is given the required near refractive power. This approach is based upon the principle that the visual system can alternate central suppression between the two eyes when viewing is alternating between distance and near targets. The degree of interocular blur suppression, which varies between patients, may be linked to the final success of monovision. Essentially all forms of soft and **rigid contact lenses** can be used for monovision corrections, whether **spherical** or **toric**.

With monovision correction, there is only a slight reduction in performance in distance acuity tests when compared to spectacle correction, and no significant difference in acuity results at near. Distance and near stereopsis is compromised with monovision, but the degree of reduction is patient-specific and may or may not result in failure with this method of fitting. Contrast loss and difficulty in suppressing bright images against dark backgrounds (for example, car headlights) while wearing monovision may also contribute to poor tolerance. Despite such compromises, monovision has high patient acceptance with a success rate of around 75%. Monovision causes minimal compromise in near visual acuity performance in all illumination conditions, and thus this type of fitting option should be considered for presbyopic patients with strong near vision demands. However, when critical or sustained tasks requiring good distance binocularity predominate, it is advisable to avoid monovision or to consider supplementary correction.

No single predictive test exists to identify successful monovision patients, so systematic trial and error is the best approach. However, the initial impression of the patient can be an important indicator of likely success. The more usual fitting approach is to fit the dominant eye (*see* ocular dominance) with the distance vision correcting lens and the non-dominant eye with the near vision correcting lens. It is important to correct any **astigmatism** equal to or greater than 0.75 D in either or both eyes, as uncorrected astigmatism can result in reduced visual performance, asthenopic symptoms, and poor tolerance. Binocular visual acuity similar to that achieved with the spectacle correction – with no significant reduction in stereopsis or contrast sensitivity – is usually a good sign of likely success.

Some patients require spectacles to wear occasionally 'over' their monovision contact lens correction. For example, there may be a requirement for extra minus correction over the near correcting lens/eye and plano over the distance correcting lens to give full binocular vision and optimal distance acuity for night driving, especially when higher reading additions are required.

The following alternative approaches to monovision correction can improve results:

1. *Partial monovision.* In general, the acceptance and therefore success of monovision falls as the reading add increases. As the indicated add exceeds +2.00 D, tolerance can often be improved if a reduced reading addition is given. The patient may need supplementary glasses for small print, a different pair of supplementary glasses for driving, or a secondary distance correcting contact lens. This form of monovision is ideal for social users whose near vision demands will be lower than those of full-time wearers. Partial monovision may also be a useful strategy for patients who have greater intermediate vision needs.

2. *Enhanced monovision.* This approach involves fitting one eye with a **bifocal lens** and the other with a single vision lens. A variety of options exist. The most frequent approach involves fitting the dominant eye with a single vision distance lens (spherical or toric) and the non-dominant eye with a bifocal lens. This improves binocular summation and offers some level of stereo-acuity to the monovision wearer who is experiencing increasing blur with a higher reading add. Alternatively, the same approach can be used when fitting patients who require sharper distance vision than bilateral simultaneous vision can offer with single-vision monovision lenses. The bifocal lens in the non-dominant eye usually needs more bias for near vision. This modification can be achieved effectively by increasing the distance power of the

bifocal lens by +0.50 D to +0.75 D. Other enhanced monovision options include:

- a single-vision near lens in the dominant eye to improve near vision and a distance-bias bifocal lens in the non-dominant eye
- a single-vision lens with slightly excess plus power in the dominant eye and an inter-mediate-bias bifocal lens in the non-dominant eye.

3. *Modified monovision.* This approach involves adjusting the refractive power of the lens or selecting alternative lens designs for each eye to deliberately improve distance vision in one eye, at the expense of near performance in that eye, whilst improving near vision in the other. This can be achieved by increasing minus power/decreasing plus power on the dominant eye to enhance distance vision, while decreasing minus power/increasing plus power in the non-dominant eye. A similar bias can be obtained by using different add powers in each – the lower add power being fitted to the dominant eye to improve distance vision. Similarly, one eye may be fitted with a centre distance simultaneous design and the other with a centre near design.

motivation
See indications and contraindications for contact lens wear.

movement, soft lens
See fitting soft lenses.

mucin balls
Approximately 50% of patients who wear **silicone hydrogel lenses** on an **extended-wear** basis display this phenomenon. Mucin balls can be observed in the post-lens **tear film** as small discrete particles, or 'plugs', and are similar in appearance to tear film debris. In some patients, as many as 200 mucin balls can be seen. At high magnification (×40), mucin balls appear to be of variable size and to take on a characteristic 'flattened doughnut' shape, with a thin circular annulus and broad central depres-sion (Figure M.5). They are observed in greater numbers in patients who sleep in silicone hydrogel lenses. Mucin balls are immovable beneath the lens, and appear to be stuck to the epithelium. A higher number of mucin balls is associated with a **looser lens fit**. Mucin balls generally increase in number over the first months of lens wear and remain constant thereafter.

Mucin balls cause no discomfort or loss of vision, and appear to be of no immediate consequence with respect to ocular health. They are composed prima-

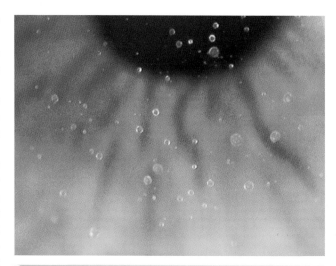

Figure M.5 Mucin balls displaying characteristic 'doughnut' appearance.

rily of collapsed mucin, as well as some lipid and tear proteins. The mechanism by which mucin balls form beneath the lens may in part be related to a physicochemical phenomenon caused by the plasma-treated surface of silicone hydrogel lenses. Specifically, the lipophilic surface of these lenses establishes a complex interfacial relationship with the tear film, which creates a shearing force that has the effect of rolling up tear mucus into small spheres. The mechanical vehicles facilitating such events may be rapid eye movements during sleep and blink-induced lens movement upon awakening. The relatively high modulus of silicone hydrogel lenses may also contribute to the above mechanism. In addition, the more viscous, mucus-rich nature of the closed-eye post-lens tear film is probably of aeti-ological significance in the formation of mucin balls.

Following lens removal, some mucin balls remain 'stuck' to the epithelium and some are washed away with blinking but leave behind pits in the epithelial surface which fill with tear aqueous. Both the remaining mucin balls and surface fluid-filled pits stain with **fluorescein**. When viewed at ×40 magni-fication, the fluid-filled pits give rise to the optical phenomenon of unreversed illumination, which is due to the fact that they are composed of a tear aque-ous which is of lower **refractive index** than the sur-rounding epithelial tissue.

Syn: Mucin plugs, lipid plugs

mucins in tears
See tear mucins.

mucus in tears
See tear mucins.

mulberry deposits

See deposits, lens.

Müller, August

Credit for fitting the first *powered* contact lens must be given to August Müller (Figure M.6), who conducted his work whilst a medical student at Kiel University in Germany. In his inaugural dissertation presented to the Faculty of Medicine in 1889, Müller described the correction of his own high **myopia** with a powered **scleral contact lens**. Paradoxically, Müller lost interest in ophthalmology and went on to practice as an orthopaedic specialist.

multifocal contact lenses

See bifocal and multifocal contact lenses.

multipurpose disinfecting solution

Multipurpose solutions (MPSs) account for about 80% of prescribed care regimens in Europe, Canada and Australia. Most of these products do not require the use of other auxiliary components in the lens care process, especially when used with lenses that are frequently replaced.

Most MPSs contain polyhexanide, which was originally developed as a pre-surgery antimicrobial scrub and then marketed for the sanitization of swimming pools and spas (Figure M.7). Polyhexanide is part of the same pharmaceutical family as **chlorhexidine**, and is active against a wide range of bacteria. The action of polyhexanide is thought to be due to its rapid attraction towards the negatively charged bacterial cell surface, followed by impairment of membrane activity, with the loss of potassium ions and the precipitation of intracellular constituents. Polyhexanide has a larger molecular weight than chlorhexidine, which means that it is not able to enter the matrix of soft lens materials. In turn this reduces the likelihood of the preservative reaching the ocular surface, with the consequent potential for toxic or hypersensitivity reactions.

Various MPSs contain polyhexanide at a range of concentrations from 0.6 ppm to 5 ppm. An increase in concentration of this active ingredient is likely to cause a general increase in its antimicrobial action. For example, a polyhexanide concentration of 5 ppm provides a solution with stand-alone activity against strains of **Acanthamoeba**, but may increase the level of corneal staining seen in wearers of specific lens materials. Excess staining has been observed in some Group II lenses, perhaps because these materials tend to attract lipid to which polyhexanide can bind.

A surfactant component is generally included in MPSs so that they can offer a cleaning action in addition to their disinfection properties. These solutions also contain EDTA as a chelating agent to assist both cleaning and disinfecting, and a buffer to ensure a consistent pH.

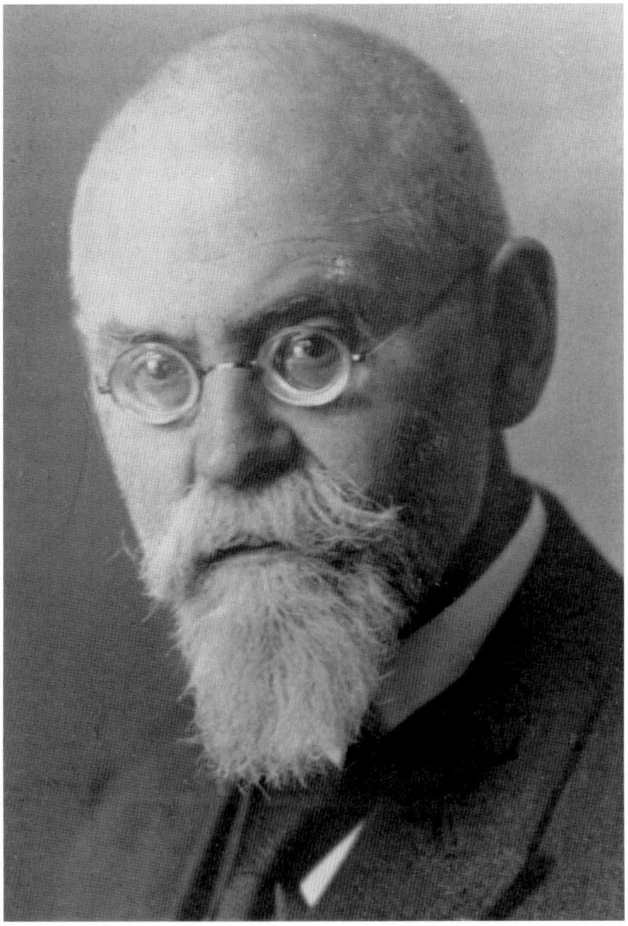

Figure M.6 August Müller.

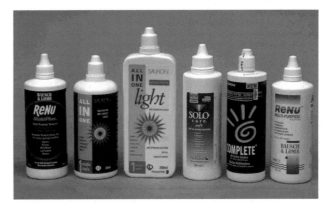

Figure M.7 Polyhexanide-based multipurpose disinfecting solutions.

More recently, 'enhanced' versions of multipurpose solutions have been introduced to the market. In the ReNu MultiPlus (**Bausch & Lomb**) product, hydranate has been incorporated as a sequestering agent to reduce protein deposition. This chemical forms complexes with calcium, which can act as a bridge between the lens surface and proteins. Another example of these newer products is Complete Comfort Plus (**Allergan**), which contains the viscosity agent hydroxypropyl methylcellulose; this ingredient is claimed to improve ocular comfort. Some products are also available in vials, which are more convenient for travelling or for the infrequent wearer.

Some MPSs have polyquaternium-1 (or polyquad) as the preservative. This compound is derived from the same pharmaceutical family as polyhexanide – the polyquats. It is a large molecule, and has a long history of use in the cosmetics industry. A number of **Alcon** disinfectant products have been launched which contain polyquad, such as Opti-Free. This product is usually classified as a 'multipurpose solution'; however, unlike other MPSs it does not contain a **surfactant cleaner**, although the inclusion of a citrate buffer (instead of the phosphate or borate generally found in polyhexanide-based MPSs) provides a cleaning effect. This negatively charged buffer is included in the polyquad products to reduce the adherence of polyquad to the surface of some ionic lens materials; this same property can reduce the protein deposition on **soft lenses** because positively charged proteins, such as lysozyme, can bind with the citrate rather than with the lens surface. However, citrates are not effective against lipid spoilation. Subsequent to the launch of Opti-Free, and its recommended use with a separate cleaner, the identical Opti-1™ was launched as a care product for use with frequently replaced lenses, without the recommended use of a separate cleaner.

More recently, Alcon has introduced a new product which contains polyquad and another antimicrobial agent, myristamidopropyl dimethylamine (MAPD), known as Opti-Free Express. In contrast to original Opti-Free, this product contains a surfactant cleaner in addition to EDTA and a buffer. The antimicrobial performance of this new product is claimed to be similar to disinfection with a one-step hydrogen peroxide system.

Traditionally, rigid lens products were preserved with benzalkonium chloride, thiomersal and chlorhexidine. However, there is some evidence that sufficient levels of chlorhexidine or benzalkonium chloride can bind to the surface of a rigid lens, leading to a toxic reaction at the ocular surface after lens insertion. More recently there has been a move away from these preservative agents or, as in the case of the Boston Advance product, a reduction in chlorhexidine concentration compared with previous care solutions. Also, polyhexanide (more traditionally part of soft lens disinfectant products) has been introduced as a second preservative in rigid lens solutions. For example, Total (Allergan) originally used benzalkonium chloride as its preservative. This was replaced by Total Care, with a new active agent – polixetonium chloride.

myopia

Refractive defect of the eye in which light from a distant object is focused in front of the retina when accommodation is relaxed, resulting in blurred distance vision. Near objects that are closer to the myopic eye than the point conjugate with the retina may appear clear without any optical correction. Minus powered lenses can be used to correct distance vision.

myopia progression, reduction of

It has been suggested that, by prescribing **rigid contact lenses** (instead of **soft contact lenses**) to children displaying a disposition for the development of **myopia**, the rate of progression of myopia can be reduced. The mechanism by which this phenomenon is supposed to occur is unknown, but it is said to be unrelated to any possible lens-induced **corneal** moulding effects. Previous studies that purport to have demonstrated a reduction of myopia regression with rigid lenses have been flawed due to small effects, loss to follow-up, and lack of appropriate controls. Recent carefully controlled studies have failed to demonstrate such an effect, which means that the fitting of rigid lenses as a strategy to arrest myopia progression is unjustified.

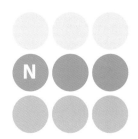

nasolacrimal duct
See lacrimal drainage system.

negative lens carrier
See high plus power contact lens design.

neophyte
See case history, non-lens wearer.

neovascularization
Corneal neovascularization can be defined as the formation and extension of vascular capillaries within and into previously avascular regions of the **cornea**. Superficial neovascularization is the most common of the various forms of contact lens induced vascular response (Figure N.1). Vision loss is rare, and will only occur if vessels encroach on the pupillary axis or if there has been an extensive leakage of lipid into the **stroma** (Grade 4). Deep stromal neovascularization develops insidiously, usually in an already compromised cornea (e.g. keratoconus), and may also progress in the absence of acute symptoms.

In contact lens induced corneal neovascularization, vessel lumina are approximately 15–80 μm in diameter and contain erythrocytes and sometimes leukocytes. Numerous extravascular leukocytes are observed around blood vessels, and the surrounding stromal lamellae are disorganized and separated, with lines of keratocytes lying between them. The overlying **corneal epithelium** is often affected, with general **oedema**, cell loss, and the presence of large, fluid-filled vesicles. The underlying Descemet's layer and **endothelium** are apparently unaffected.

Contact lens induced corneal neovascularization can be explained in terms of a dual aetiology model. Chronic **hypoxia** induces stromal oedema, which 'softens' the stroma and renders this tissue more susceptible to vascular penetration. Some secondary factor must act to stimulate vessel growth – for example, this could be mechanical injury to the epithelium, resulting in a release of enzymes. Inflammatory cells migrate to this site and release vasostimulating agents that cause vessels to grow in that direction.

The limits of 'normal' or 'expected' vascular ingrowth (i.e. less than Grade 1), measured from the limit of visible iris, should be 0.2, 0.4, 0.6 and 1.4 mm for no-wear, daily-wear rigid, daily-wear hydrogel and extended-wear hydrogel regimes, respectively. If corneal neovascularization is a primary concern, the prescription of lenses with design features known to provide minimal interference with corneal physiology are indicated, namely those with:

- high **oxygen transmissibility**, to minimize oedema and metabolic acidosis
- minimal mechanical effect, as judged by patient comfort and good movement, to avoid venous stasis resulting from limbal compression in **soft lenses**.

Other factors to be considered include:

- avoidance of care systems likely to induce toxic or allergic responses
- changing from **extended-wear** to daily-wear lenses
- changing from **hydrogel** to rigid or **silicone hydrogel lenses**
- replacing lenses more frequently
- reducing wearing time
- ceasing lens wear.

Regular aftercare visits are essential. Cessation of lens wear will halt the progression of vessel infiltration into the cornea, but empty 'ghost' vessels may remain in place for months or years. Resumption of lens wear in a previously vascularized cornea will result in immediate refilling of the vessels. Thus, in advanced cases of neovascularization, long-term

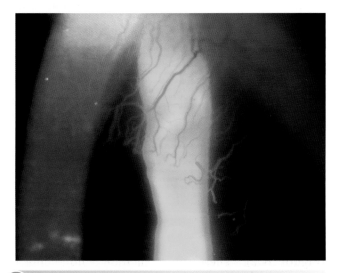

Figure N.1 Contact lens induced corneal neovascularization.

cessation of lens wear is indicated until ghost vessels can no longer be detected.

neutralization of corneal astigmatism

A **rigid lens** of **spherical** power will neutralize virtually all corneal **astigmatism**. In fact the situation is a little more complex than this because of the contribution of the rear surface of the **cornea** to the overall corneal astigmatism, but this is generally a small effect. This neutralization effect does not depend upon the **refractive index** of the correcting lens. Any residual astigmatism due to the crystalline lens will remain uncorrected. Very occasionally a patient may be encountered who has a spherical refractive error but non-zero corneal astigmatism. This therefore implies that the residual (lenticular) astigmatism is of opposite sign to the corneal astigmatism and that correcting the corneal astigmatism with a spherical rigid lens will leave the residual astigmatism manifest. In such cases a spherical **soft lens** will result in better visual acuity, since the failure of the soft lens to correct the corneal astigmatism will allow the balance between the corneal and lenticular astigmatism to be maintained.

Irregular astigmatism and general corneal irregularity will similarly be masked by a spherical rigid lens and its accompanying tear lens. Although nominally a spherical rigid lens will neutralize any value of corneal astigmatism, the fitting relationship is likely to be unsatisfactory for corneal astigmatism greater than about 2.00 DC. Thus for higher levels of astigmatism some form of toroidal correction is required.

NIBUT dome

See non-invasive tear break-up time.

nicotine

See deposits, lens.

non-compliance

'Compliance' can be defined as 'the extent to which a patient's behaviour coincides with the clinical prescription'. This definition highlights the critical importance of the practitioner–patient relationship in avoiding adverse events. Failure of the patient to comply with advice and instructions from an eye care practitioner can compromise the likelihood of success with contact lens wear. In general, non-compliance will result in:

- reduction of treatment efficacy
- secondary problems
- incorrect prescribing
- wasting of practitioner chair time
- wasting of patient time.

Clearly, health care delivery will be enhanced if the above adverse consequences of non-compliance can be minimized or eliminated.

It is not possible simply to characterize the behaviour of a patient as compliant or non-compliant, because there will be variations in the pattern of non-compliance over time, and in the extent of non-compliance at a given instance in time. Such cases are difficult to deal with, because the non-compliant behaviour may continue undetected for some time. There is a greater likelihood of detecting consistent and/or total non-compliant behaviours at an aftercare visit.

About 40–90% of contact lens wearers are non-compliant in at least some aspects of their contact lens care regimens. The types of transgressions that can occur include:

- keeping solutions too long
- failing to clean the lens case
- irregularly cleaning lenses
- failing to disinfect lenses daily
- not washing hands prior to handling lenses
- wearing lenses too long
- failing to rinse lenses after cleaning
- failing to clean lenses
- cleaning lenses in tap water.

The reasons for non-compliance are complex. In some cases patients may be deliberately non-compliant; this intentional non-compliance may be unintelligent (as in a patient adopting a dangerous procedure such as not bothering to clean his or her lenses) or intelligent (as in a patient adding an additional lens rinsing step prior to lens insertion). On the other hand, patients may be unintentionally non-compliant through forgetfulness or misunderstanding. Practitioners detecting non-compliance in a patient should seek to determine which of the reasons outlined above apply. *See* compliance enhancement.

non-contact aesthesiometry

Over the last 10 years a number of devices have been tested and developed to overcome the problems inherent in **contact aesthesiometry**. All of these devices use non-contact means of stimulating the **cornea**. Initially, mechanical stimulation alone was investigated, but more recently aesthesiometers have been produced that stimulate the cornea using a variety of thermal, chemical or mechanical stimuli (Figure N.2). These have included non-contact pneumatic devices, which deliver compressed air as the stimulus, the application of a carbon dioxide laser to determine the threshold for the detection of

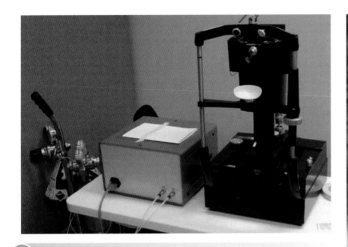

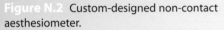
Figure N.2 Custom-designed non-contact aesthesiometer.

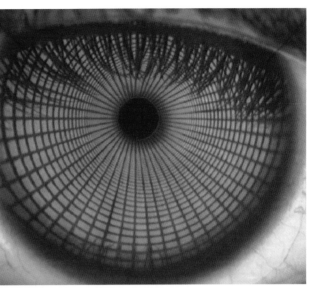

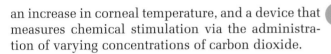
Figure N.3 Reflection of the NIBUT grid attachment of the Tearscope-plus as seen in the pre-corneal tear film.

an increase in corneal temperature, and a device that measures chemical stimulation via the administration of varying concentrations of carbon dioxide.

non-invasive tear break-up time

The non-invasive **tear film** break-up time (NIBUT) can be determined by optically projecting a grid pattern onto the **cornea** and timing how long it takes for the grid to become disrupted. Numerous devices that employ this principle have been produced, including the instrument-stand-mounted 'NIBUT dome' or 'Mengher grid', and hand-held devices such as the **keratometer**-mounted Hir-Cal grid, the Loveridge grid, and the **Tearscope**-plus with NIBUT grid attachment (Figure N.3).

non-planned lens replacement

In certain instances contact lenses can be prescribed to be used for as long as the lenses will last; this is referred to as 'non-planned lens replacement'. Patients for whom non-planned replacement lens use might be indicated include, for example, those who require specially prepared, hand-painted cosmetic lenses; those who wear lenses infrequently and are outside the **daily disposable lens** prescription range; and those who previously have been demonstrated to have few problems with non-planned replacement lenses. However, the main reason for prescribing on a non-planned replacement basis probably relates to a 'traditional' approach

adopted by some practitioners who are perhaps unaware of, or reluctant to embrace, the vast array of planned replacement and disposable lens systems that are available in the marketplace.

The cost of disposable lens systems has come down to such a large extent over the past decade that the current cost to a patient for a monthly lens replacement system would be about the same, or perhaps even less, than the cost of a single pair of lenses for ongoing use (i.e. non-planned replacement) that might last, say, for 12 months. If the more frequent and intensive professional care required for patients wearing lenses on a non-planned replacement basis is factored in, then the cost of this modality of lens wear is prohibitive. Thus, 'cost saving' can no longer be cited as a reason for prescribing lenses on a non-planned replacement basis.

Being outside the available prescription range is also becoming less of a reason for prescribing lenses on a non-planned replacement basis, because planned replacement lenses are now available from many companies in an almost limitless range of parameters in both **spherical** and **toric** designs.

Notified Bodies
See Medical Devices Directive.

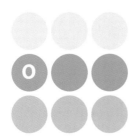

oblique illumination, slit-lamp technique of

The **slit-lamp** technique of oblique illumination is infrequently used in contact lens practice, but is nonetheless a useful technique. Oblique illumination is achieved by setting up a parallelepiped and then moving the illumination system away from the observation system until the angle between them is close to 90°. The illumination arm is adjusted until the light beam is almost tangential to the object of interest. Any raised areas cast a shadow, and this technique is particularly useful for viewing subtle defects within the iris architecture and subtle changes to the epithelial surface.

oblique rigid bitoric lenses

See cylindrical power equivalent rigid toric lenses.

occupation

See indications and contraindications for contact lens wear.

ocular adnexa

The ocular adnexa are those structures that support and protect the eye, and include the **eyelids**, **conjunctiva** and **lacrimal system**. They play an important role in the formation of the pre-ocular **tear film**, and collectively defend the eye against antigenic challenge.

ocular defence mechanisms

The eye has a number of inherent protective mechanisms to resist infection. Potential pathogens are present in the tear film of 5% of a population at any time, yet the prevalence of ocular surface infection falls far short of this value. The **tear film** and the **blinking** process play an important role in the resistance of infection. Basal tear production is of the order of 1–2 μl per minute and the overall tear volume is about 7 μl, which confirms the rapid turnover of tears at the ocular surface with the consequent removal of micro-organisms.

Bacteria in the tear film must also breach the defence provided by proteins in the tear film, such as lysozyme, lactoferrin and transferrin, for an infection to be established. Furthermore, immunoglobulins such as secretory IgA, IgG, IgE and IgM can act to resist infection.

Ocular surface mucus provides a physical barrier to infection because it binds strongly to bacteria, thereby enhancing their removal from the ocular surface (Figure O.1). A bacterium that is able to

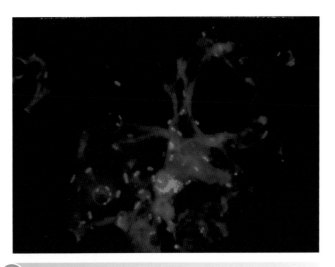

Figure O.1 Pseudomonas bacteria (orange) bound to mucus (green), which is cleared from the eye during blinking. This forms an effective ocular defence mechanism against infection.

defeat all the above systems is still hampered in its quest to invade and infect the **cornea** because of the presence of fibronectin at the epithelial surface, which is known to reduce the bacterial adhesion to epithelial cells in mucosal systems.

Contact lens wear adversely affects a number of these defence mechanisms. Perhaps the most significant effect is the prevention of clearance of debris and micro-organisms from the ocular surface by the blinking mechanism. The level of fibronectin is possibly reduced during contact lens wear, thereby increasing the likelihood of bacterial attachment.

A key reason for the increase in ocular infections amongst contact lens wearers is from the bioburden of micro-organisms introduced to the ocular surface when lenses are inserted. The risk of infection with **Acanthamoeba** is significantly increased when no contact lens disinfection is adopted by the lens wearer, or when weak disinfection systems (e.g. **chlorine**) are employed. The appropriate use of a suitable disinfection system can reduce the incidence of microbial infection of the eye.

ocular dominance

Measurement of the ocular dominance or sighting preference is useful in establishing which eye to correct for distance vision during **monovision** contact lens fitting, or whilst making adjustments during simultaneous contact lens fitting. Ocular dominance can be determined using preferential looking tests, or alternatively by the +2.00 D test. The former is carried out by sitting opposite the patient and asking the patient to look, through a hole in a piece of card, at an open eye of the practitioner. Whichever eye the patient lines up with the open eye of the practitioner is the dominant one. The latter test involves placing the best binocular distance refraction in the trial frame and, while the patient looks at the lowest line that can be read, a +2.00 D lens is placed alternatively in front of each eye. The patient indicates when the vision is clearest. If the +2.00 D lens is in front of the left eye when the image is reported as clearest then the right eye is considered as distance dominant, and *vice versa.* Unsuccessful wearers sometimes become successful after switching near and distance corrections contrary to the dominance as measured by traditional methods, but rarely do so contrary to the +2.00 D test.

Ocular Sciences

Since Ocular Sciences was incorporated in 1985, its strategy has been to market **soft contact lenses** to eye care professionals at competitive prices using a low cost to serve operating structure. The company sells products marketed for reusable and disposable wearing regimens. Ocular Sciences' corporate headquarters are located in Concord, California. The company acquired Lunelle from the French company Essilor International in 2000. Ocular Sciences employs approximately 4000 staff world-wide. Website: www.ocularsciences.com

oedema

Oedema refers to an increase in the fluid content of tissue, and in the contact lens field 'oedema' is usually taken to mean excess fluid in the **corneal stroma**. Since the cornea is only able to swell in the anterior–posterior direction (as a result of the collagen fibre structural network in the stroma), the physical dimensions of the cornea can only increase in that dimension – that is, in thickness. The human **cornea** experiences about 2–4% oedema during sleep. With current generation **hydrogel** and **rigid lenses**, daytime corneal oedema typically varies between 1% and 6%, and the level of overnight oedema measured upon awakening generally falls in the range 5–13%. **Silicone hydrogel lenses** induce about 4% overnight oedema, which is about the same or only slightly more than occurs when sleeping without lenses.

Clinicians can estimate the magnitude of corneal oedema via careful observation with the **slit-lamp biomicroscope**, as a number of structural changes can be identified that correlate with various levels of oedema. Using **direct focal illumination**, striae appear as fine, wispy, white, vertically oriented lines in the posterior stroma when the level of oedema reaches about 5% (Grade 2). Striae are thought to represent fluid separation of the predominantly vertically arranged collagen fibrils in the posterior stroma. Folds can be observed – using specular reflection technique – in the endothelial mosaic as a combination of depressed grooves or raised ridges, or as a general area of apparent buckling, when the level of oedema reaches about 8% (Grade 3). It is thought that folds indicate a physical buckling of the posterior stromal layers in response to high levels of oedema. The stroma takes on a hazy, milky or granular appearance when the level of oedema reaches about 15% (Grade 4); such high levels of oedema are often associated with other signs and symptoms of ocular distress (Figure O.2).

Contact lenses restrict corneal oxygen availability, creating a **hypoxic** environment at the anterior corneal surface. To conserve energy, the corneal epithelium begins to respire anaerobically. Lactate, a by-product of anaerobic metabolism, increases in concentration and moves posteriorly into the corneal stroma. This creates an osmotic load that is balanced by an increased movement of water into the stroma. The sudden influx of water cannot be matched by the removal of water from the stroma by the endothelial pump, resulting in corneal oedema.

The key strategy for reducing the oedema response is to increase corneal oxygen availability during lens wear. Rigid lens oedema can be alleviated by increasing lens **oxygen transmissibility**, or

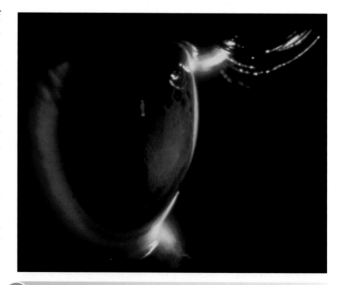

Figure O.2 Severe central corneal oedema, resulting in 'clouding'.

by fitting a lens of flatter base curve, greater edge lift or smaller diameter so as to increase lens-mediated tear exchange. Soft lens oedema can be alleviated by fitting lenses of higher oxygen transmissibility, flattening the base curve or reducing lens diameter. General strategies for reducing oedema include changing from extended to daily wear, changing from soft to rigid lenses, fitting **silicone hydrogel lenses**, or reducing wearing time.

In general, the prognosis for recovery of the cornea from lens-induced oedema is excellent. The oedema induced when a patient wears a contact lens for the first time will resolve within 4 hours of the lens being removed. Chronic lens-induced oedema can take up to 7 days to resolve.

one-day lenses
See daily disposable lenses.

one-step hydrogen peroxide disinfecting solution
See hydrogen peroxide disinfecting solution.

opaque contact lens backing
The matrix of a lens can be tinted with a translucent dye, and an iris pattern and black pupil applied to the back surface of the lens using opaque paints. In this way, the entire back surface of the lens is rendered opaque; light reflects off the opaque layer and the coloured appearance is created from the translucent tint in the lens body. *See* tinted lenses.

optical coherence tomography
Optical coherence tomography (OCT) is a relatively new non-contact optical imaging technique that is capable of high-resolution micrometer-scale cross-sectional imaging of biological tissue. The commercially available OCT used for ophthalmic applications uses 843-nm wavelength near-infrared radiation, which provides a longitudinal resolution of 10–20 μm. The technique uses Michelson interferometry to compare a partially coherent reference beam with one reflected from tissue. The two beams are combined and interference between the two light signals occurs only when their path lengths match to within the coherence length of light. The magnitude and distance within the tissue of the reflected or back-scattered light at a single point are determined using a mirror system. A tomographic image is generated by simultaneously displaying 100 adjacent scans, whose acquisition time takes approximately 1 second.

The technique of OCT is thus analogous to ultrasound B-mode imaging, except that it uses light rather than sound and performs imaging by measuring the back-scattered intensity of light from structures within the tissue. Strong reflections occur at boundaries between materials of differing refractive indices. The OCT two-dimensional scans are subsequently processed by a computer, which corrects for any axial eye movement artefacts that have occurred during the acquisition time. The scans are displayed using a false colour representation scale in which warm colours (red to white) represent areas of high optical reflectivity and cool colours (blue to black) represent areas of minimal optical reflectivity. The image obtained represents a cross-sectional view of the structure under investigation, similar in appearance to a histological section (Figure O.3).

This technique can be used to examine the **cornea**, and has proven useful in determining epithelial and total corneal thickness changes following refractive surgery procedures, in cases of corneal **oedema**, and in evaluating contact lens positioning on the ocular surface. Because OCT enables the non-excisional, *in situ*, real-time imaging of tissue microstructure, it is a powerful and promising technique for corneal imaging purposes.

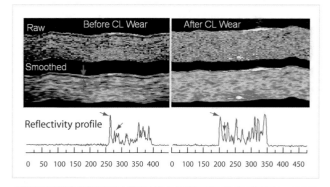

Figure O.3 Optical coherence tomography (OCT) image, before and after closed-eye wear of a thick polyHEMA contact lens. The upper two-dimensional false-colour image indicates the plot obtained from the OCT, the smoothed image being that obtained once background noise is eliminated from the raw image. The lower plot indicates the reflectivity values obtained through the cornea. The data obtained indicate that the cornea has swollen substantially and that the water absorbed has resulted in an increase in the thickness and reflectivity of the corneal tissue. By determining the distance between two peaks from the reflectivity profile, corneal and epithelial thickness can be obtained. Adapted from L. W. Jones (2002) Clinical instruments. In *Contact Lens Practice* (N. Efron, ed.), pp. 52–67, Butterworth-Heinemann.

optical transmittance

Transparency is an essential requisite of a **hydrogel** for contact lens use, but not all hydrogels are optically transparent. Translucence and opacity in hydrogels is associated with microphase separation of water, which produces regions of differing refractive index within the gel. Hydrogels that show this type of behaviour (typically synthesized by making co-polymers with large blocks or segments of hydrophobic and hydrophilic monomers rather then randomly dispersing them) do have advantages in terms of enhanced strength and permeability performance. Phase-separated hydrogels in which the domain sizes are small enough to retain optical transparency are of interest in applications in which strength and/or permeability are particularly important (e.g. **extended-wear** contact lenses and synthetic **cornea**). The lack of optical clarity in simple co-polymers of hydrophilic monomers such as HEMA and TRIS has been a major technical obstacle in the development of **silicone hydrogel lenses**.

optic section, slit-lamp technique of

Once an area or object of interest is located when using the **slit-lamp biomicroscope**, the beam width can be narrowed to approximately 0.2 mm to 'cross-section' the **corneal** tissue (Figure O.4). This provides the ability to assess accurately the depth of an object within the corneal layers. Typical uses include assessment of the depth of a foreign body, location of a corneal scar, and determining whether tissue within an area of staining is excavated, flat or raised.

optics of the eye

The general structure and optical layout of the eye is shown in Figure O.5. About three-quarters of the optical power comes from the anterior **cornea**, with the crystalline lens providing supplementary power which, in the pre-**presbyope**, can be varied to focus objects sharply at different distances. The actual optical design is, however, subtle, in that all the optical surfaces are aspheric, while the lens (and probably also the cornea) displays a complex gradient of **refractive index**. There is little doubt that such refinements play an important role in controlling **aberration**.

Refractive indices of the media vary little between eyes, apart from the refractive index distribution across the lens, which changes with age as the lens grows throughout life. Each dimensional parameter is approximately normally distributed amongst different individuals. The values of the different parameters in the individual eye are, however, correlated so that the resultant distribution of refractive error is strongly peaked near **emmetropia**, rather than being normal. This correlation is thought to be due to a combination of genetic and environmental factors, visual experience helping to actively 'emmetropize' the eyes. The apparently greater incidence of **myopia** in recent times may be attributed to the greater prevalence of near tasks biasing this active process towards myopia rather than emmetropia.

orbicularis oculi

The orbicularis oculi is the sphincter muscle of the **eyelids**, and can be divided anatomically into two main divisions – palpebral and orbital. Fibres of the palpebral division arise from the medial palpebral ligament and arc across the eyelids in a series of half-ellipses, meeting at the lateral canthus to form a lateral raphe. The lateral palpebral ligament also

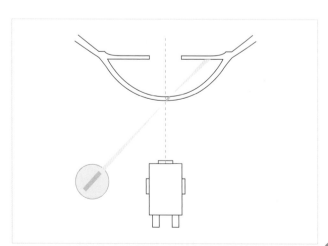

Figure O.4 Optic section slit-lamp technique.

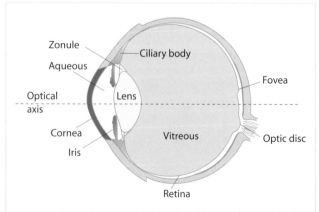

Figure O.5 Schematic horizontal section of the human eye.

acts as an anchor point. The palpebral division can be further subdivided into marginal, pre-tarsal and pre-septal parts (Figure O.6). The marginal part (pars ciliaris), which is also known as Riolans muscle, is responsible for maintaining the apposition of the lid to the cornea during lid closure. A third part of the muscle (pars lacrimalis) is closely associated with the lacrimal outflow pathway. The pars lacrimalis (also known as Horner's muscle) encloses the canaliculus and provides attachments to the lacrimal sac and its associated fascia.

The orbital part of the **orbicularis oculi** lies outside the palpebral division and extends for some distance beyond the orbital margins. Muscle fibres arise predominantly from bone at the medial orbital rim, and appear to sweep around the lids without interruption as a series of complete ellipses. The muscle fibres of the orbital and palpebral divisions of the orbicularis are relatively short (0.4–2.1 mm) and overlapping. The regional divisions of the orbicularis also show a functional distinction. The action of the palpebral part of the muscle is to produce the reflex or voluntary closure of the lids during blinking. Contraction of the orbital division produces the forcible closure of the lids that occurs in sneezing or in response to a painful stimulus.

orientation of toric lenses , soft
See toric lens rotation, soft.

orthokeratology
This refers to a technique of fitting **rigid contact lenses** in such a way as to alter **corneal** morphology

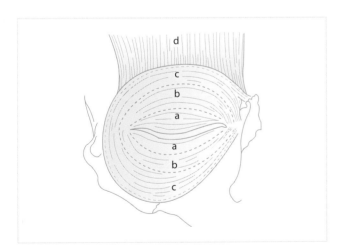

Figure O.6 Schematic representation of the divisions of the orbicularis oculi and the frontalis. a = pre-tarsal; b = pre-septal; c = orbital; d = frontalis. Adapted from A. J. Bron, R. C. Tripathi and B. Tripathi (1997) *Wolff's Anatomy of the Eye and Orbit*, 8th edn, Chapman & Hall.

and thereby reduce the level of **myopia**. It is a technique that has been evolving since the 1960s, and the term 'modern orthokeratology' has been coined to distinguish previous approaches from current methods. More specifically, 'modern orthokeratology' refers to the practice of orthokeratology using **reverse geometry lenses**. Orthokeratology lenses can be made of highly **oxygen-permeable** materials, permitting the wearing of orthokeratology lenses on an overnight basis (i.e. overnight orthokeratology).

The advent and acceptance of keratorefractive surgery for the correction of refractive errors has ensured that interest in other non-surgical approaches, such as orthokeratology, has remained relevant. The resurgence of orthokeratology as a viable alternative to refractive surgery, or indeed traditional contact lens or spectacle corrections, is a consequence of three developments:

1. The availability of new lens designs, particularly reverse geometry lenses, and the ability to design and manufacture lenses to produce a specific tear layer thickness profile
2. The availability of **videokeratoscopes** to assist with contact lens design and evaluate corneal shape changes
3. The availability of new highly oxygen-permeable materials, allowing overnight lens wear.

The average magnitude of the refractive change using orthokeratology lenses is about 1.75 D, and is subject to significant individual variability (Figure O.7). The issue of predictability of those changes is still an important and unresolved one. The corneal changes are not permanent, with significant regression occurring over a few hours. Ongoing use of contact lenses (sometimes referred to as 'retainer lenses'), whether for overnight or daily wear, is still needed to sustain the refractive changes.

The corneal curvature changes in orthokeratology appear to result from a combination of short-term corneal moulding and a longer-term redistribution of anterior corneal tissue. It has also been suggested that the tear reservoir generated by the steeper secondary curves leads to pressure changes, which are responsible for the corneal tissue redistribution.

overnight orthokeratology
See orthokeratology.

overnight wear
See extended wear.

over-refraction
This is the standard technique for determining the power of the contact lens to be ordered for a

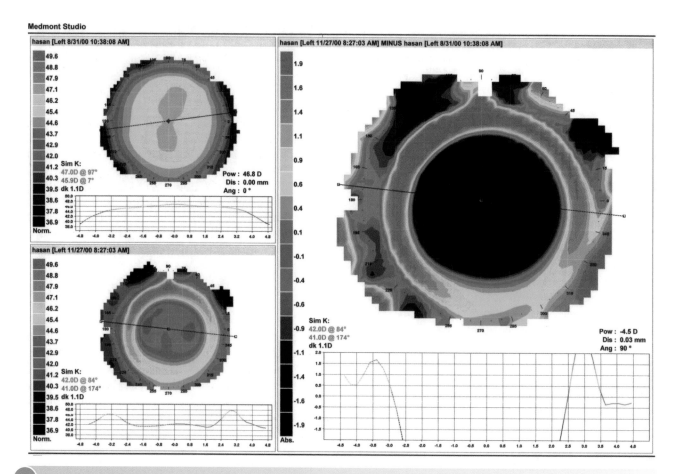

Figure O.7 Corneal topography before (upper left) and after (lower left) wear of reverse geometry lenses in this example of a dramatic change of about 4.00 D (difference plot, right) in corneal power.

patient. The over-refraction is conducted with the best fitting trial lens in place. The procedure is best performed using a trial frame and trial lens set. The technique of conducting the over-refraction is essentially the same as that conducted on a non-lens-wearing patient. A full sphero-cylindrical over-refraction is conducted first, and if the patient is to be fitted with a spherical lens, the best sphere refraction is determined. The result of the over-refraction is simply added to the power of the trial lens to determine the power of the lens to be ordered, after making any corrections for effectivity (*see* Appendix B). In **toric soft lens** fitting, the over-refraction can be used as an indication of the direction of cylinder axis mislocation.

Measuring the over-refraction during a **rigid lens** trial fitting not only helps to determine the final lens power but also gives an indication of whether the optimum fit has been obtained. An unexpected over-refraction suggests that either the lens is wrongly labelled or the fit is not perfect. The steeper the lens fit, the more minus power will be required in order

to compensate for a relatively plus powered tear lens. Variable vision may indicate a decentred or flat fitting and relatively mobile lens fit.

own-labelling
See lens supply routes.

oxygen permeability (*Dk*)
The term 'oxygen permeability' describes the ease with which oxygen may pass through a particular material under standard conditions. It is thus a property of a material, and not of a finished contact lens. Oxygen permeability of a material is a function of the diffusivity (*D*) and solubility (*k*) of oxygen in that material, and is represented by the term *Dk*. The diffusivity (*D*) refers to the speed at which oxygen molecules can pass through the material, and the solubility (*k*) refers to the number of oxygen molecules that can be absorbed into a given volume of material (Figure O.8).

In order to determine the oxygen permeability of a material at a given temperature, it is necessary to measure the rate (volume per unit time) at which oxygen passes through a sample of material of given dimensions (area and thickness) for a given gas pressure. The units of *Dk* take these variables into account, and are quite complex. It is common therefore to quote the value in 'Fatt units' (after Irving Fatt, who pioneered contact lens oxygen permeability measurement) or, more formally, 'Barrer', whereby:

$$Dk \text{ in Barrer (or 'Fatt units')} = 10^{-11}$$
$$(cm^2 \cdot mlO_2)/(s \cdot ml \cdot mmHg)$$

The international standard unit for pressure is the 'pascal' (Pa). Because the term mmHg is now becoming obsolete internationally, it is being advocated that the closest accepted metric unit of pressure – 100 Pa, or 'hectopascal' (hPa) – should replace the term mmHg. Indeed, this approach is specified in the international standard ISO 8321-2 (2000). When hPa is used, *Dk* is quoted as:

$$Dk = 10^{-11} (cm^2 \cdot mlO_2)/(s \cdot ml \cdot hPa)$$

The difficulty here is that converting from the traditional Barrer or Fatt units to ISO units involves multiplying *Dk* by the constant 0.75. For example, a lens quoted with a traditional *Dk* of 40 units will have revised ISO *Dk* of 30 units.

For **soft contact lenses**, there is a well-defined relationship between water content (W, %) and *Dk*; this is given by the Morgan–Efron equation, where:

$$Dk = 1.67 \times 10^{-11} e^{0.0397W} \text{ (at 35°C)}$$

Silicone rubber has an oxygen permeability several times greater than that of water and over 100 times greater than that of either PMMA or dehydrated polyHEMA. Its incorporation into a **hydrogel** therefore produces a marked gain in oxygen permeability. In such materials, as the proportion of silicone-based **polymer** is increased and water content consequently decreases, the *Dk* value rises to values well in excess of 100 Barrer.

oxygen transmissibility (*Dk/t*)

The term 'oxygen transmissibility' describes the ease with which oxygen may pass through a particular material of given thickness. The oxygen transmissibility of a lens is a function of the **oxygen permeability** (*Dk*) of the material from which the lens is made, divided by the thickness of the lens (*t*) (Figure O.9). Thus, 'oxygen transmissibility' is represented by the term *Dk/t*, and describes the passage of oxygen through a finished contact lens.

The units of *Dk/t* are as follows:

$$Dk/t \text{ in Barrer/cm} = 10^{-9} (cm \cdot mlO_2)/(s \cdot ml \cdot mmHg)$$

When hPa is used, *Dk/t* is quoted as:

$$Dk/t \text{ in Barrer/cm} = 10^{-9} (cm \cdot mlO_2)/(s \cdot hPa)$$

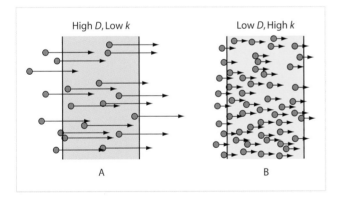

Figure O.8 Schematic representation of the passage of oxygen through two infinitely thin sections of contact lens materials. Each circle represents an oxygen molecule. The length of the arrow indicates the distance moved per unit time. Compared with lens A, more oxygen molecules are observed in lens B (high oxygen solubility, *k*), but each molecule in lens B is moving at a slower speed (low diffusivity, *D*). It can be seen that both materials have the same permeability, since the same number of molecules pass through each section of material per unit time.

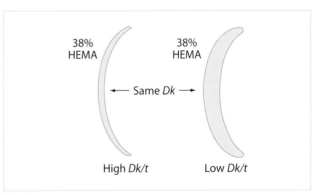

Figure O.9 Illustration of the concept of oxygen permeability (*Dk*) and oxygen transmissibility (*Dk/t*). The *Dk* is an intrinsic property of the lens material. In this example, both lenses are made of the same material (38% HEMA); thus, they have the same *Dk*. However, the thicker lens will offer greater resistance to oxygen flow, and therefore has a lower *Dk/t* than the thinner lens.

To convert from the traditional Barrer or Fatt units to ISO units, *Dk/t* must be multiplied by the constant 0.75.

Contact lens oxygen transmissibility can be expressed as either the central or the average value. The central lens *Dk/t* is derived by dividing *Dk* by the centre thickness of the lens. The average lens *Dk/t* is derived by dividing *Dk* by the average thickness of the lens over a defined lens radius. The average *Dk/t* is always less than the central *Dk/t* for minus powered lenses (which become progressively thicker from the centre to the edge of the lens), and the converse is true for plus powered lenses.

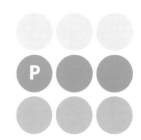

pachometry, optical

Optical pachometry is based on the measurement of the apparent thickness of an optical section of the **cornea**, and its popularity is largely based on the commercial availability of a pachometer attachment for the Haag–Streit **slit lamp**. First, a split image device is inserted into one eyepiece of the slit-lamp biomicroscope. The method depends upon the relative rotation of two glass plates, which are placed on top of each other. Rotation of the upper plate moves the upper half of the image of the cornea with respect to the fixed lower half. When the **corneal endothelium** of the upper field is aligned with the **epithelium** of the lower field, the angle of rotation of the upper plate is read off an externally positioned scale. This measurement is proportional to the apparent thickness of the cornea, with true corneal thickness being determined by means of a conversion table.

Whilst perfectly acceptable for clinical purposes, the arrangement described above is too inaccurate for research purposes. A number of modifications to the technique have resulted in an accuracy of approximately 5 μm being reported. Two such modifications include the use of two or four small light sources to ensure that the incident beam is normal to the corneal surface, and an arrangement whereby the rotation of the glass plate is coupled to a potentiometer such that the angle of rotation is directly converted into an electrical signal, allowing immediate input into a computer program. This enables more rapid data collection, efficient file management, and more accurate, repeatable data collection (Figure P.1).

The Orbscan™ (Orbtek Inc., Salt Lake City) corneal topographer and pachometer is an advanced optical technique that operates by analyzing the anterior and posterior boundaries of a corneal optical section as the incident slit scans over the cornea. The dedicated software quickly generates a two-dimensional pattern of **corneal surface topography** and thickness distribution. The Orbscan can also be used to measure thickness variations within a contact lens.

pachometry, ultrasonic

The ultrasonic pachometer is based on traditional A-scan ultrasonography, where the recording is in one dimension only, as compared with B-scan instru-

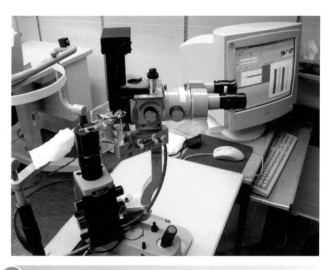

Figure P.1 A computerized optical pachometer. The pachometer is connected to a potentiometer that is directly linked to a computer software program.

ments, which provide a two-dimensional view of the eye. Ultrasound is transmitted to the eye from a transducer. Sound is reflected back to the transducer from tissue interfaces, which possess different acoustic impedances, enabling the distance from the ultrasound probe at the anterior epithelial interface to determine the distance between itself and the endothelium–aqueous interface. The transducer determines the time difference between the pulse signals obtained at the two interfaces, and computes the corneal thickness based on this time delay and the velocity of sound in corneal tissue, which is approximately 1580 ms^{-1} at body temperature. A direct measurement of corneal thickness is then displayed on a digital readout.

Prior to undertaking ultrasonic pachometry, the **cornea** is anaesthetized and the patient slightly reclined (Figure P.2). Potential sources of error in measuring corneal thickness include holding the probe at an oblique angle to the cornea and measuring away from the central corneal apex, both of which would result in elevated readings of central corneal thickness (because corneal thickness increases from the centre to the periphery). The majority of modern instruments include a mechanism whereby a reading is not displayed if the probe is positioned such that there is excessive deviation from the perpendicular. The operator can use the pupil as a centring target,

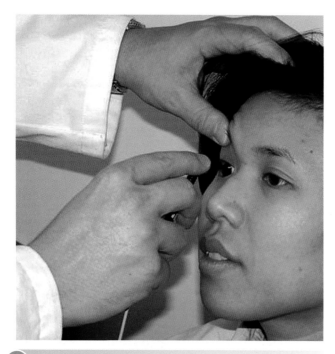

Figure P.2 An ultrasonic pachometer evaluation. The eye is anaesthetized and the probe touched to the cornea. Readings are digitally recorded once the angle of inclination of the probe is correct.

and using these adaptations the measurements obtained are valid for clinical use.

paediatric contact lenses

The key lens choice in paediatric contact lens fitting is between **soft hydrogel lenses**, **silicone elastomer lenses** and **rigid lenses**. Silicone hydrogel lenses may have useful paediatric applications when they become available in high plus and high minus power ranges, and in appropriate paediatric parameters (for small eyes). **Scleral lenses** are rarely required, but may be used, for example, for prosthetic purposes.

Soft lenses are the most frequently used lens types in paediatric contact lens fitting. High **water content** soft lenses – or preferably silicone hydrogel lenses if available in the required parameters – are usually selected, as they can be worn for continuous or daily wear. Daily wear should be considered where possible to reduce the risk of infection, as **oxygen transmission** can be reduced through all forms of high powered lenses, such as those used to correct **aphakia**. However, as babies and young children sleep during the daytime, the lenses can remain in the eye during these periods. Lenses are usually fitted according to age, or based on keratometry readings and corneal diameter.

Advantages of soft lenses:

- they can be custom made in a range of radii, overall size, power and water content
- they are initially comfortable for the child
- parents/carers tend to be less apprehensive about inserting a soft lens into the eye of a baby or young child.

Disadvantages of soft lenses:

- they do not correct significant corneal **astigmatism**
- insertion can be difficult, especially for minus lenses, where there is considerable lid squeezing, or if there is a very small palpebral aperture
- they are prone to dehydration, which can be problematic in babies, who tend to have relatively **dry eyes** due to low **blink** rate
- there is frequent lens loss due to eye rubbing and dehydration.

Silicone rubber lenses are often used in the correction of refractive errors in babies and young children, and are particularly useful where there is frequent lens loss or a dry ocular surface (Figure P.3). The lens fit can be checked using **fluorescein** and UV light after a period of 30 minutes or so of settling.

Advantages of silicone rubber lenses:

- they have a very high **oxygen permeability**
- they are not susceptible to dehydration on the eye
- they are less susceptible to damage
- they are not easily rubbed out due to the negative pressure (eye suction) effect
- they are easier to insert than soft lenses due to their increased rigidity.

Disadvantages of silicone rubber lenses:

- the range of parameters and availability is limited
- they need to be fitted precisely, and require more chair time due to longer settling periods
- negative pressure effects can cause adhesion to the cornea if the lens is too tight
- the surface coating can degenerate, resulting in an uncomfortable hydrophobic surface, so lenses have a relatively short lifespan
- they are more expensive than soft or rigid lenses.

The development of automated hand-held **keratometry** and improvements in rigid lens design have led to the increased use of rigid lenses for paediatric fitting. Rigid lenses have been successfully used for the management of aphakia in infants, and can be fitted without the need for general anaesthesia.

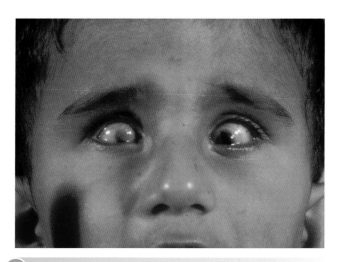

Figure P.3   A silicone rubber lens fitted to the left aphakic eye of an infant with microcornea.

Advantages of rigid lenses:

● they are available in a large range of materials and parameters
● they correct corneal astigmatism
● durability
● their rigidity can help to ease insertion and removal.

Disadvantages of rigid lenses:

● they are not suitable for **continuous wear**
● parents/carers can be more apprehensive about inserting rigid lenses
● there is the risk of abrasion if **insertion** is difficult
● initial **discomfort** may be a problem in older children
● they are easily to dislodge.

See paediatric contact lens examination; paediatric contact lens fitting.

paediatric contact lens examination

All the examination techniques that would normally be conducted on adult contact lens wearers also need to be conducted on the very young, but with an almost exclusive reliance on objective techniques of refraction. The logistics of examination often need to be adjusted to obtain the necessary clinical data. The key aspects of the paediatric contact lens examination are:

1. *Anterior segment examination.* As with the adult patient, examination of the anterior segment in an infant is an important aspect of contact lens fitting and **aftercare**. A very simple method of determining the presence, location and severity of **corneal staining** or ulceration is to use an ultraviolet lamp with **fluorescein**. In babies, a major **slit lamp** can be used with the baby being held horizontally, belly down, and head facing towards the instrument (the 'flying baby' technique, Figure P.4). In the case of infants and young children, a hand-held slit lamp may be preferable for examining the anterior segment in more detail. Older children, from about 3 years upwards, are usually happy to position themselves at a slit-lamp biomicroscope by kneeling on a chair and grasping the headrest support bars.

2. *Keratometry.* A hand-held automated **keratometer** can be used to determine the corneal radius of curvature in young infants and in children who are too young to sit at a conventional keratometer.

3. *Refraction.* Determination of the refractive error or a contact lens **over-refraction** can usually only be performed objectively using retinoscopy and hand-held lenses; a paediatric trial frame may be more convenient in an older child. The use of a cycloplegic drug is recommended in those children with normal **accommodative** function. It is useful sometimes to dilate the pupil in aphakes or pseudophakes where there is a small or displaced pupil, or where significant media opacity is apparent (e.g. posterior capsular thickening).

4. *Biometry.* Prior to cataract surgery, the axial length of the eye can be measured with ultrasound and the corneal radius of curvature determined by keratometry. These measurements can be used to determine the power of the contact lens required post-operatively by using an IOL calculation formula, which can determine the ocular power at the corneal plane post-surgery. This is particularly useful as it allows a lens of more or less correct specifications to be ordered, which alleviates

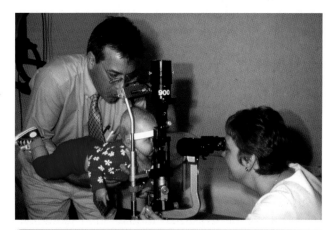

Figure P.4   The 'flying baby' technique of child support for examining an infant at the slit-lamp biomicroscope.

the need for many lenses to be used at the initial fitting and allows fewer lenses to be kept in stock.

See paediatric contact lenses; paediatric contact lens fitting.

paediatric contact lens fitting

Contact lenses play an important role in the correction of complex refractive errors in the paediatric population, and in the management of deprivational amblyopia. Contact lenses also play an important role in prosthetic fitting.

Children over the age of about 12 years are generally capable of being examined, counselled and fitted like adults, albeit with parental guidance. However, there generally needs to be a specific indication for fitting children younger than this. The indications for fitting the very young are as follows:

1. *Aphakia.* Surgical removal of the crystalline lens results in **aphakia**. The most common reason for performing this procedure is congenital cataract, the incidence of which is about 2.1 per 10 000 live births and 7.7 per 10 000 children at 4 years of age. Of theses cases, around 40% and 50%, respectively, have unilateral cataracts. Aphakia can also result from lens subluxation, as seen in Marfan's syndrome, or ectopia lentis. Trauma to the eye may result in the immediate loss of the crystalline lens or subsequent development of traumatic cataract, which may require surgical intervention. Refractive management of bilateral aphakia can be achieved with spectacles. However, the drawbacks of aphakic spectacles include the weight of the lenses and difficulty in achieving good frame fit in babies and young infants. In addition, the maximum power of lenses is restricted, even in lenticulated form, to around +26.00 D. Since infants in the early stages of visual development require a focal length of around 30–50 cm to see a face, the power of the selected contact is usually 2.00–3.00 D greater than the ocular refraction. This over-correction should be reduced at 18 months to 2 years of age, when the toddler becomes more aware of distant objects. A reading correction or bifocal spectacles can be prescribed from around 3–4 years of age, when the child starts pre-school education.

2. *Pseudophakia.* The use of intra-ocular lenses (IOLs) in the management of congenital cataract is increasing, with IOL implantation being carried out in infants as young as 2 weeks of age. The aim of IOL implantation at this early age is to alleviate the need for contact lenses or aphakic glasses when the eye is fully grown. Typically, the young eye will be left 6.00–10.00 D under-corrected with the implant so as to compensate for the expected ongoing 'myopic shift' during childhood. The resultant refractive error can then be corrected with a contact lens in the early months, with a 2.00 D over-correction, gradually reducing lens power until the eye reaches an **emmetropic** state.

3. *Myopia.* **Myopia** is not uncommon in infants and young children, and correction with spectacles is the accepted practice. However, in high myopia, spectacles have the disadvantage of reducing the retinal image size, inducing peripheral distortion and reducing the effective visual field (especially with lenticulated lenses). Contact lens correction is warranted where spectacle correction is problematic or normal visual development is threatened. High myopia (> 10.00 D) may be present from birth, and may be related to a number of ocular and systemic conditions. Also, high myopia may be associated with craniofacial anomalies, which can make the wearing of spectacles difficult. The myopic eye is larger overall, and tends to have a flatter-than-average **corneal** radius and a larger corneal diameter than the emmetropic eye. Adult-sized lenses can often be used in young infants and children. Myopia can also result from buphthalmos, where the corneal diameter is much larger than normal (> 12.5 mm), and so requires a lens that is flatter and larger than an adult equivalent. Contact lenses in unilateral high myopia have been shown to be more satisfactory than spectacle lenses in the management of amblyopia, in regard to cosmesis, comfort and treatment.

4. *Ocular motility disorders.* Contact lenses can be useful in the management of ocular motility disorders. Applications include **aniseikonia** induced by **anisometropia** exceeding 6.00 D, **accommodative** esotropia in older children, nystagmus, and occlusion.

5. *Irregular astigmatism.* This is derived from primary corneal ectasia, and is extremely rare in childhood. Most causes of corneal irregularity are secondary in nature – for example, following corneal infection or laceration. Neutralization of irregular **astigmatism** is important during the visual development period to prevent deprivational amblyopia. The optimum form of contact lens correction here is a **rigid lens**, although sometimes, if the irregularity is less severe, a **toric soft lens** may suffice.

6. *Tinted prosthetic and therapeutic lenses.* **Tinted therapeutic lenses** may be used in children to enhance visual performance by reducing the effect of photophobia. **Tinted prosthetic lenses** may be used for improving the cosmesis of the child by camouflaging a disfigured eye. The most common reasons for fitting prosthetic lenses in childhood are:

- albinism
- aniridia
- achromatopsia
- iris defects (e.g. coloboma)
- nanophthalmus or microphthalmus
- corneal anomalies (e.g. sclerocornea or Peter's anomaly).

A modified technique for insertion and removal is required in the young eye in view of the small palpebral aperture size of an infant (Figure P.5). Some general points to consider when handling contact lenses in babies and young children are as follows:

1. Lenses are easier to insert and remove with the child lying down on a firm, flat surface, e.g. an examination couch.
2. Babies can be 'swaddled' in a blanket to make handling easier.
3. It is far easier to learn how to handle lenses on a young infant than on a more active baby or toddler. It is therefore important to encourage parents/carers to undertake lens handling from the outset of lens fitting.
4. Parents/carers should be advised to keep to regular times for handling, so that this becomes ritualized and accepted as part of daily routine.

5. If handling is difficult in young infants, lenses can be **inserted** or **removed** during sleep.
6. Handling often becomes more difficult from 18 months onward. Bilateral aphakes can start to use spectacles at this point, and **anisometropes** can use a spectacle correction when occluded.
7. Co-operation may be extremely limited in children aged between 2 and 5 years having lenses fitted for the first time. Spectacles may have to suffice at this age if the benefits of contact lenses are outweighed by the distress caused to the child by handling.

See paediatric contact lenses; paediatric contact lens examination.

pain
See discomfort, contact lens induced; discomfort, investigation of.

pannus
This is a particular type of corneal **neovascularization** characterized by a thick plexus of vessels typically observed at the superior limbus. Two forms of pannus may be observed in contact lens wearers; active (inflammatory) and fibrovascular (degenerative) (Figure P.6). An active pannus is initially avascular, and is composed of sub-epithelial inflammatory cells. In the later stages it may be associated with secondary scarring of the **stroma**.

papillary conjunctivitis
This condition refers to the appearance of localized swellings, or 'papillae', on the tarsal **conjunctiva**. Papillae are primarily observed in the upper **eyelid**, and can only be viewed by everting the lid (Figure

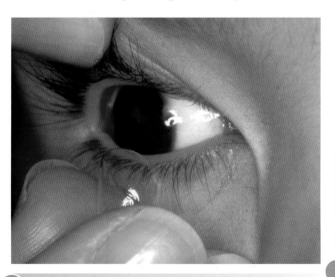

Figure P.5 The small palpebral aperture of a child poses problems for lens insertion.

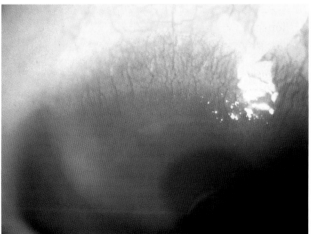

Figure P.6 Contact lens induced fibrovascular pannus with a degenerative leading edge revealed by rose bengal staining.

P.7). Rarely, papillae can be observed on the lower tarsus by pulling the lower lid firmly down. In soft lens wearers, papillae are more numerous; they are located more towards the upper tarsal plate (that is, closer to the fold of the everted lid), and the apex of the papillae take on a more rounded form (Figure P.7). In rigid lens wearers, papillae are flatter and are located more towards the lash margin, with few papillae being present on the upper tarsal plate. Papillae often appear as round light reflexes, giving an irregular specular reflection.

In the early stages (< Grade 1) of contact lens induced papillary conjunctivitis (CLPC), the tarsal conjunctiva may be indistinguishable from the normal tarsal conjunctiva apart from increased redness. In advanced cases (> Grade 2), papillae can exceed 1 mm in diameter and often take on a bright red/orange hue. The distribution of papillae can be more readily appreciated with the aid of **fluorescein**. The hexagonal/pentagonal shape is lost in favour of a more rounded appearance, with a flattened or even slightly depressed apex or tip. A tuft of convoluted capillary vessels is often observed at the apex of papillae; this vascular tuft will typically stain with fluorescein. Other signs in severe CLPC (> Grade 3) include conjunctival oedema, excessive mucus and mild ptosis. The **cornea** may display punctate staining and superior infiltrates. Injection of the superior limbus may also be apparent.

There is general concordance between the severity of signs and symptoms. In the early stages of CLPC, patients may complain of:

- **discomfort** towards the end of the wearing period
- slight itching
- excess mucus upon awakening

- intermittent blurring
- a slight but non-variable vision loss while wearing lenses.

As the condition progresses, patients report itching, discomfort and excessive lens movement.

Key factors implicated in the aetiology of CLPC include lens-induced mechanical irritation, and immediate and delayed hypersensitivity. There is often a link with **meibomian gland dysfunction**, and atopic patients may be more susceptible to developing the condition. Treatment options include:

- altering the lens material
- replacing lenses more frequently
- altering or eliminating the care system
- improving ocular hygiene
- treating any associated meibomian gland dysfunction
- prescribing soft steroids (e.g. loteprednol etabonate)
- prescribing mast cell stabilizers (e.g. 4% cromolyn sodium)
- dispensing ocular lubricants for symptomatic relief
- reducing wearing time
- suspending or ceasing lens wear.

The prognosis for recovery from CLPC after removal of lenses and cessation of wear is good, with symptoms disappearing within 5 days to 2 weeks of lens removal, and redness and excess mucus resolving over a similar time course. Resolution of papillae takes place over a much longer time course – typically many weeks, sometimes as long as 6 months. The more severe the condition, the longer the recovery period. In the longer term, however, the prognosis is less good. The condition can recur, especially in atopic patients who appear to have a propensity for developing CLPC.

parallelepiped, slit-lamp technique of

Using the same **slit lamp** set-up as for **direct focal illumination**, a 0.5–2.0 mm wide illuminating beam is scanned over the ocular surface. This permits assessment of the location, width and height of any object within the **cornea** or adjacent structures (Figure P.8). The parallelepiped is the most commonly used direct illumination technique, and is employed, for example, to assess corneal scarring, infiltrates, and **corneal staining**.

party lenses

See theatric tinted lenses.

patient discharge

A useful strategy to instil confidence in patients who have never worn lenses previously is to have the

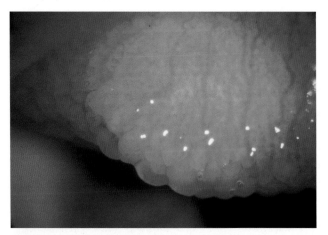

Figure P.7 Papillary conjunctivitis induced by rigid lens wear.

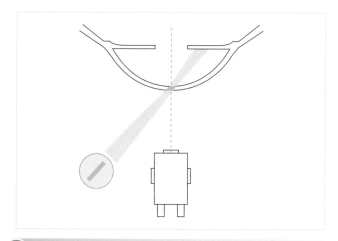

Figure P.8 Parallelepiped slit-lamp technique. Adapted from L. W. Jones and D. A. Jones (2001) Slit lamp biomicroscopy. In *The Cornea: its Examination in Contact Lens Practice* (N. Efron, ed.), pp. 1–49, Butterworth-Heinemann.

patient **insert** his or her lenses at the conclusion of the training session, and to discharge the patient from the practice wearing the lenses. The patient will then be forced to 'confront' the challenge of lens handling (at least lens **removal** in the first instance) rather than, as might occur, putting the lenses aside until enough courage can be mustered to wear lenses at a later date.

An appointment for the next aftercare visit should be made before the patient leaves the practice with the new contact lenses. The patient must appreciate that ongoing success with contact lenses is dependent upon several factors, such as adaptation to the lenses, **compliance** with the instructions given, and attending for regular **aftercare** visits. It should be impressed upon the patient that whilst good vision and comfort are indicators of success, they do not automatically prove there are no adverse ocular effects. All wearers must be made aware of the importance of regular biomicroscopic examination. The standard strategy for encouraging **compliance** with the requirement to return for regular aftercare visits is to restrict the supply of lenses issued to the patient to correspond with the desired time period between aftercare appointments.

Prior to being discharged, patients should be advised how to identify an emergency situation when wearing lenses. At the same time, new wearers need to be aware of normal adaptation symptoms, such as mild foreign body sensation and intermittent blurring of vision. If concerned that there is a problem, contact lens wearers can be advised to check that their eyes 'look good, feel good and see good'. This easy-to-remember adage refers to the following:

- 'look good' – there is no more ocular redness than normal
- 'feel good' – there is no discomfort prior to and after lens insertion
- 'see good' – there is no disturbance to vision (each eye checked monocularly).

Patients should be advised that:

- any significant redness when accompanied by pain needs urgent practitioner attention, especially if the redness and pain do not ease following lens removal
- visual losses should not automatically be put down to contact lens wear, as there may be some form of ocular pathology present that is unrelated to lens wear.

patient education

The quality of instruction and advice given to a patient contributes to the success or failure of the new wearer. Proper and careful tuition of a patient at a dispensing visit will facilitate confident lens handling by the patient, and will help nurture a sound appreciation of how lenses should perform and how to manage various situations that can arise in contact lens wear. Certainly, poor patient education can result in premature discontinuation from lens wear and increase the likelihood of unscheduled visits to the practice.

The dispensing visit seeks to:

- teach the patient the correct methods of lens **insertion** and **removal**
- explain the methods that optimize lens comfort, such as understanding when a lens is **inside-out**, or how to remove post-lens debris
- inform the patient about the likely adaptation issues that may be encountered
- outline the correct use of the prescribed care regimen.

The use of diagnostic lens banks facilitates undertaking both the fitting and dispensing appointment on the same day. Some patients are so motivated following their first experience of contact lens wear that the dispensing can take place immediately after the initial trial fitting. On the other hand, rescheduling the dispensing visit for another day has the benefits of giving patients a break after the fitting visit, and allows them to read through some preliminary literature about their contact lenses.

A trained member of support staff (as opposed to the practitioner) commonly adopts the teaching role, and this person is sometimes referred to as the 'contact lens hygienist'. Having a trained member of the support staff undertaking this task can have several advantages. Some patients feel pressured to have to 'perform' in front of the practitioner, whereas they may feel more relaxed with a member of support staff. The delegation of this role requires careful selection of personnel who can be relied upon to provide accurate information to the patient and refer back to the practitioner when necessary.

Patients who have elected to wear contact lenses are often apprehensive about the process of lens insertion and removal. For this reason, the teaching room should be of a comfortable temperature and well ventilated, as many patients become quite anxious in their frustration if they do not insert the lens on the first attempt. The area should be reasonably private – perhaps screened off from the rest of the practice – and it is essential that the instructor and the patient are free from incidental interruptions. Patients require careful attention when they first handle lenses, and the instructor must not be taken away or distracted from this supervisory task.

Good lighting is important, along with suitable seating for both the patient and the instructor, as flexibility to be able to sit on each side of the patient is needed (Figure P.9). The patient's chair should be set at a desk such that the knees of the patient can fit comfortably under the desk. This is helpful if the patient accidentally drops the lens during handling. An illuminated, double-sided mirror (with one side that magnifies) that is height-adjustable and can be tilted is ideal. The teaching area must be prepared in advance of the lesson, so that all necessary items are to hand, including:

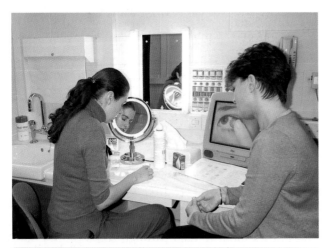

- contact lenses, cross-checked with the record card and spectacle prescription
- a lens case, which may be supplied with the solutions
- a trial pack of solutions, sufficient for the needs of the patient until the first scheduled **aftercare** visit
- additional **saline**, for rinsing during the lesson
- comfort drops (wetting solution), especially for **rigid lens** fitting
- a full box of tissues, with a spare box available
- hand washing facilities (soap in a pump dispenser and lint-free paper towels)
- a mirror, as described above, cleaned and free from fingerprints
- an appropriately-sized plastic bag, for the patient to carry away lenses, solutions and accompanying literature.

The full care regimen should be demonstrated from start to finish, explaining why each step is necessary as well as what could happen if the routine is not strictly adhered to. The patient should be handed written information about the care products being dispensed; this may be information that is supplied by the manufacturer and/or material prepared by the practitioner.

Contact lens handling can be a very frustrating experience for novice lens wearers. Accordingly, patience is the most critical personality trait of the member of staff chosen to instruct contact lens patients. The instruction session should not be rushed, and the patient should feel comfortable asking questions. *See* hygiene, practitioner and patient; informed consent; patient discharge; wearing schedules.

patient instruction
See patient education.

patient scheduling in contact lens practice
Effective practice resource management without compromising clinical care is often dependent on the use of appropriate appointment scheduling methods. In contact lens practice a variety of appointment types are scheduled, such as general eye examinations, preliminary examination and initial **fitting**, evaluation after diagnostic lens wear (return), collection/education, routine **aftercare**, and unscheduled visits (urgent, emergency etc.). Three main approaches to patient scheduling can be employed to accommodate the various appointment types:

1. *Individual appointments.* Here, patients are booked in at regular intervals with equal times set aside for each consultation. For example,

patients are booked in every 20–30 minutes starting and ending at a given time. This approach is simple, which is why it is used so often. However, it does not allow for patients who require longer consultations or patients who require less time, which is an issue that especially relates to contact lens practice. It is thus possible to end up with 'unproductive' portions of time when less time with a patient is needed, and long waiting queues should a patient require a longer consultation.

2. *Block booking*. This is not often used in optometry, but is found in hospitals and general medical practice. This method involves scheduling multiple patients in the same time slot – e.g. three patients may be booked at 9.00 am and then none until 10.00 am, when three more patients are booked, and so on. Individuals who have experienced this approach are often disgruntled to find that they have the same appointment slot as others.

3. *A mixed system*. Some practices find a mixture of traditional and block booking to be a workable combination, using the block system for scheduling shorter 15-minute visits for contact lens follow-up visits, and 20–30 minute individual scheduling for prescribing and fitting contact lenses.

The challenge is to schedule patients so that the 'downtime' and the time taken to 'settle in' in the consulting room does not curb the consultation time of the practitioner.

pemphigoid
See cicatricial conjunctivitis, therapeutic lenses for.

penetrating keratoplasty, lens fitting following
See post-keratoplasty, contact lens fitting.

'per case' lens supply
See fitting rigid lenses.

peri-ballast
See stabilization of soft toric lenses.

peripheral fit, soft lens
See fitting soft lenses.

personnel, contact lens practice
Optometric practices rely on individuals to deliver their professional services and products to patients and customers. Thus, at a minimum level of practice activity, it will be necessary to employ someone to provide reception and general administrative support with respect to the day-to-day activities of the practice. At the other end of the spectrum, a large, busy practice may employ additional optometrists, dispensing staff, contact lens hygienists, technicians, optical receptionists/advisors, secretaries and cleaners. It is important to remember that as part-time employment increases, many more individuals will need to be employed to cover the practice requirements in terms of hours per day etc. The issues of managing the practice staff take more prominence as the size and the activity of the practice increase.

Once a vacancy has been identified and additional hours of staff time justified, it is essential to establish the duties of the new member of staff. Having decided on the qualifications, training needs and skills required to do the job, it is useful to prepare a job description and then to decide on the type of person who would ideally be recruited to fill this vacancy – i.e. a 'person specification' (Table P.1). A 'person specification' should take account of:

- physical make-up
- attainments
- general intelligence
- special aptitudes
- interests
- disposition and circumstances
- impact on others
- qualifications or acquired knowledge
- innate abilities
- motivation and adjustment or emotional balance.

Staff selection involves choosing the right person by interviewing short-listed candidates with a view to selecting the applicant who has the skills, abilities, aptitude and personal qualities to do the job. The job description and the person specification will decide the major selection criteria normally considered during the interview process.

A contract of employment needs to be issued to the staff member; this is simply the legal agreement between the employer and the employee, clarifying their mutual obligations. The law in the UK provides the employee with a number of employment rights and imposes some statutory obligations on the employer. Contracts do not have to be in writing. Employment law in the UK has gone a little further, and even with a verbal contract there is a requirement for employers to give any employee taken on for 1 month or more a written statement setting out the main employment particulars. This statement must be issued within 2 months of the starting date of employment. Covered by common and contract law, contracts of employment in the UK are governed by the Employment Rights Act (1996).

A practice handbook that sets out basic information about the policies and facilities of the practice

Table P.1 Example of the job specification for a person whose primary role would be to provide contact lens patient education

essential qualities	desirable qualities
1. Impact on other people (appearance, speech and manner) clean and tidy presentation good writing and speech	smart presentation gets on well with young adults
2. Qualifications and experience (education, training and work experience) GCSE English and mathematics able to work with a computer	experience in medical reception, nursing assistance or pharmacy experience of data input and output
3. Innate abilities (aptitude for learning) quick to grasp ideas and views	able to prioritize and decide on action
4. Motivation (consistency, determination and success in achieving goals) interested in health care and general cosmesis	interested in a potential career in optics
5. Adjustment (emotional stability, ability to handle stress and ability to get on with people) friendly and able to work as part of a team	comfortable with the pressures of day-to-day practice and the demands of patients and practitioners

can act as a clear guide for all staff to providing optometric and contact lens services. It should be an easily accessible set of ground rules that promote a good working environment in the practice. Should a case of misconduct (breach of rules that merit disciplinary action) arise, the rules in the handbook regarding expected conduct will be invaluable.

philosophy of fitting
See fitting philosophy.

photorefractive keratectomy
See laser refractive surgery, contact lenses following.

piggyback lens fitting
This is when a **soft lens** is fitted to the eye and a **rigid lens** is fitted over the top of the soft lens (Figure P.10). An annular recess, slightly larger than the diameter of the overlying rigid lens, can be incorporated into the front surface of the soft lens to help the rigid lens locate centrally. Indications for piggyback lens fitting include the requirement for full corneal coverage of a distorted **cornea**, and as an aid to counteracting intolerance to rigid lens wear where a rigid lens is required due to corneal distortion.

placido disc
This is the most basic reflective device for assessing **corneal topography**. It is simply a series of concentric black and white rings on a flat circular disc with a central sight hole. The disc is positioned in front of the **cornea**, and the reflections are observed (Fig-

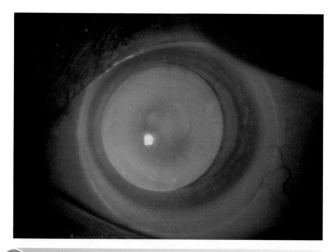

Figure P.10 Piggyback fitting of a rigid lens sitting on top of a soft lens in a patient with keratoconus.

ure P.11). Using this method, only gross irregularities in the corneal surface and very high **astigmatism** can be detected. Improved versions of the Placido disc include the internally-illuminated Klein keratoscope, the Loveridge grid, and the **Tearscope**-plus with corneal topography grid attachment.

planned rigid lens replacement
Rigid lenses, irrespective of **oxygen permeability** (**Dk**) or material type, show a gradual deterioration in wettability and visual performance and an

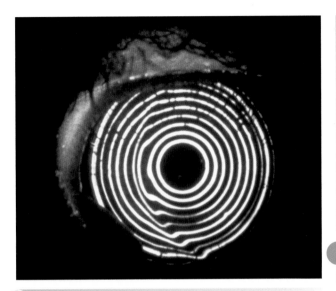

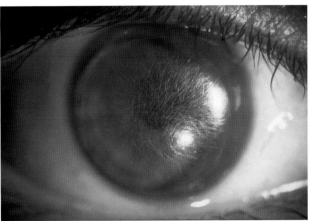

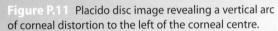

Figure P.12 Heavy scratching on a rigid lens that had been used for 4 years.

Figure P.11 Placido disc image revealing a vertical arc of corneal distortion to the left of the corneal centre.

increase in surface scratching and deposition over time (Figure P.12). Some clinicians believe that re-polishing techniques can be applied to prolong the life of rigid lenses; however, caution should always be exercised with this procedure, as over-polishing can lead to reduced **surface wettability** and ultimately result in reduced comfort and visual performance. An alternative strategy is to replace rigid lenses more frequently; however, this is problematic because rigid lenses are manufactured using the **lathe cutting** method, which makes their unit cost significantly greater than that of **soft lenses**.

If it is accepted that higher Dk materials should be fitted for clinical reasons, that such lenses have a reduced **life-expectancy** and that all lenses show a deterioration in performance with age, then the planned replacement of high Dk rigid lenses would appear to be a logical modality to adopt.

Planned replacement of rigid lenses worn on a daily-wear basis results in significantly less **corneal staining**, limbal hyperaemia and tarsal conjunctival changes compared with identical lenses worn on a non-replacement basis. There is also less surface drying, surface scratching, mucus coating and surface deposition.

In **extended-wear** patients, planned rigid lens replacement results in less **corneal and conjunctival staining** and less corneal binding; however, this modality does not prevent the occurrence of tarsal conjunctival changes.

It is recommended that rigid lenses be replaced every 6 months, based on the argument that lenses should be replaced *before* any adverse ocular or lens surface changes would be expected to occur, and that this is an easy-to-remember calendar-based frequency – which would facilitate patient **compliance**.

planned soft lens replacement

The term 'planned replacement' refers to lens replacement intervals from 1 day to 12 months, and therefore includes all 'disposable lenses', which are defined as lenses replaced at least monthly.

Products replaced at least monthly have invariably been designed, packaged and promoted for replacement at specific intervals. However, the same is less true for lenses replaced 3-monthly, and is almost never true for lenses offered for biannual and annual replacement; such lenses are usually conventional lenses packaged in vials, and many of these lenses were developed prior to widespread use of planned replacement. This does not detract from the benefit of prescribing conventional soft lenses in this way, especially in view of the strong evidence supporting more frequent replacement intervals.

The rationale for the planned replacement of **soft contact lenses** is simple: cleaner lenses should produce fewer adverse ocular effects and afford better vision and comfort. All soft contact lenses suffer gradual spoliation from the environment and **tear film** components over time. Daily cleaning and periodic **protein removal** can slow this rate of deposition but not prevent its occurrence. By ensuring that soft lenses are replaced at a suitable pre-determined interval, one of the most enduring medical management axioms – that of prevention being better than cure – is brought to bear. In practice, patients who replace lenses regularly report fewer symptoms and exhibit less physiological changes, in most instances, compared with patients who do not replace lenses regularly.

The principal benefits of planned replacement soft lenses are as follows:

1. *Use of higher water content materials.* Higher **water content** lenses (i.e. > 50% water) generally offer superior oxygen performance. However, such lenses are generally less durable than lower water content lenses. Planned soft lens replacement provides a rationale for the use of physiologically superior high water content materials; the increased fragility of such lenses is clinically inconsequential as long as the lenses will survive intact for the intended replacement period.
2. *Simple lens care.* Disposability obviates the need for prolonging the life of lenses with elaborate lens care systems. In cases where lens surface spoilation is a problem with monthly replacement, shortening the replacement interval to 2 weeks or even 1 day is likely to be a superior option.
3. *Ready availability of replacement lenses.* Lenses replaced weekly, fortnightly or monthly are normally supplied in three- or six-packs. **Daily disposable lenses** are usually provided in packs of 30 or 90 lenses. It follows that the loss or damage of a lens should not, in most cases, be an inconvenience to a patient wearing disposable lenses.
4. *Enhanced **compliance** with aftercare schedules.* Planned replacement protocols require patients to return at regular intervals for fresh lenses. **Aftercare** visits can be scheduled to coincide with lens collection.
5. *Single use trial lenses.* In the case of **disposable lenses**, new diagnostic or trial lenses are used with each patient and disposed of thereafter (Figure P.13). This eliminates the risk of cross-infection from a previous wearer of the lens. It also has the advantage of eliminating the time-consuming chore of trial lens cleaning, disinfection and storage.
6. *Trial lens fitting with accurate prescription.* With the ready availability of a comprehensive stock of trial lenses, it is nearly always possible to undertake a lens-wearing trial on a prospective disposable lens patient with the required lens parameters, especially with respect to lens power.
7. *Lens parameters are easy to change.* By the very nature of planned replacement, it is straightforward to modify the prescription of a patient, particularly with respect to changes in refractive error.

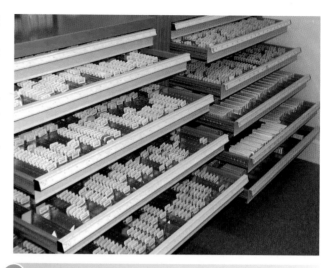

Figure P.13 Single-use diagnostic lenses allow for convenient and accurate fitting assessment.

8. *Superior comfort.* Numerous factors can lead to lenses becoming less comfortable over time; these include the existence of microscopic lens **defects**, physical trauma and/or immunological reaction due to lens deposition, and progressive **hypoxic** effects due to lens **ageing**. Regular lens replacement avoids these problems.
9. *Superior vision.* Deposit accumulation on lenses is associated with vision loss; this is avoided if lenses are regularly replaced.
10. *Superior ocular response.* Lens deposits can facilitate immunological, toxic and traumatic damage to the eye. Therefore, deposit-related problems such as **corneal staining**, corneal infiltrates and conjunctival injection will occur less if lenses are replaced more regularly.

See daily disposable lenses.

PMMA
See poly(methyl methacrylate).

polishing rigid lenses
See lens modification.

poly (2-hydroxyethyl methacrylate)
This hydrophilic material can be fabricated by the incorporation of hydroxyl groups into **poly(methyl methacrylate)** (PMMA), because hydroxyl groups have an affinity for water. That is, poly (2-hydroxyethyl methacrylate), or polyHEMA, is obtained by polymerizing the 2-hydroxyethyl methacrylate (HEMA) monomer (Figure P.14). In the absence of water polyHEMA is a hard glassy material, which upon hydration is transformed into the familiar contact lens material.

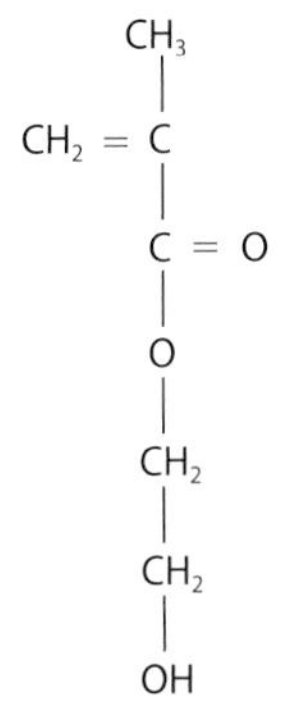

CH₃
|
CH₂ = C
|
C = O
|
O
|
CH₂
|
CH₂
|
OH

Figure P.14 Chemical structure of 2-hydroxyethyl methacrylate monomer (HEMA).

polyHEMA
See poly(2-hydroxyethyl methacrylate).

polymegethism
See endothelial polymegethism.

polymers
The unique properties that polymers possess arise from the ability of certain atoms to link together to form stable bonds. Foremost among the atoms that can do this is carbon (C), which can link together with four other atoms of its own kind or alternatively with atoms of, for example, hydrogen (H), oxygen (O), nitrogen (N), sulphur (S) or chlorine (Cl). Silicon (Si) resembles carbon in this way, especially in its ability to link to carbon, hydrogen and oxygen. It is this property of carbon that forms the basis of what is called organic chemistry, or the chemistry of carbon compounds.

Most of the polymers that are encountered fall within the realm of organic chemistry as defined in this way. These polymers may be purely natural (such as cellulose), modified natural (such as cellulose acetate) or completely synthetic (such as **PMMA**). There is a much smaller family of polymers based on silicon rather than carbon. Their properties differ somewhat from those of the carbon-based polymers and they are best known in the form of siloxane polymers, in which silicon and oxygen alternate in the backbone. These materials are important in relation to contact lenses because both rigid lenses and **silicone hydrogel lenses** incorporate such units, which have the principal benefit of conferring enhanced **oxygen permeability**.

The single characteristic that unites silicon-based and carbon-based polymers is the fact that, as the name (poly-mer) suggests, they are composed of many units linked together in long chains. Thus if we can imagine a molecule of oxygen and a molecule of water enlarged to the size of a tennis ball (the molecular size of water is very similar to that of oxygen), a molecule of polyethylene or poly(methyl methacrylate) on the same scale would be of similar cross-sectional diameter but something like 60 m in length. It is the vast length of polymers (sometimes called macromolecules) in relation to their cross-sectional diameter that gives them their unique properties, such as toughness and elasticity. The links between individual atoms are inclined to each other at an angle (the bond angle), which means that chains are not rod-like but 'kinked'.

The individual building blocks from which polymers are formed are termed 'monomers'. To indicate that a polymer contains more than one type of repeating monomer unit, for example when two different monomers are polymerized together, the description 'co-polymer' is used. 'Co-polymer' is a general term, and can be used to describe polymers obtained from mixtures of more than two monomers. Because most contact lens polymers are formed from monomers that are characterized by the presence of a carbon-to-carbon double bond that opens to form a linked chain, the process can be generalized. It is the way in which the structural and functional groups interact with each other and with their surrounding environment that governs the interaction of polymer chains and the resultant properties of the polymer itself.

Perhaps the best way of visualizing the way in which polymer chains arrange themselves is by taking several pieces of string to represent individual molecules. The most usual arrangement will be a random one in which the pieces of string are loosely entangled rather than being extended. It is the interaction and entanglement of the individual molecules in this way that gives polymers their characteristic physical properties. By changing the chemical nature of the polymer chain and their arrangement together, it is possible to change the physical properties and thus obtain either hard glassy behaviour or, at the other extreme, flexible, elastomeric behaviour. The best example of a hard glassy material is **poly(methyl methacrylate)**, which is formed from methyl methacrylate monomer units. A widely known elastomeric material in the biomedical field is silicone rubber, which is based on the flexible silicon–oxygen backbone.

There is an important way in which a hard glassy polymer can be converted into a flexible material, and that is by the incorporation of a 'plasticizer'. This is a mobile component, often an organic liquid with a high boiling point, that will act as an 'internal lubricant'. Its presence separates the polymer chains and allows them to move more freely. A good example is poly(vinyl chloride), or PVC, which in its unmodified state is a rigid glassy material and will be familiar as the clear corrugated roofing material used on car ports, conservatories and similar domestic extensions. When a plasticizer is incorporated the material is converted into the flexible material used, for example, as 'vinyl' seat coverings in cars and general domestic applications. In these cases, pigments and various processing aids will also have been added in order to enable the polymer to be produced in a variety of colours and textures. An almost identical principle is involved in the formation of **hydrogel** polymers.

poly(methyl methacrylate) (PMMA) lenses

The development of PMMA lenses (also referred to as corneal lenses or hard lenses) began as the result of an error in the laboratory of optical technician Kevin Tuohy. During the lathing of a PMMA **scleral lens**, the haptic and corneal portions separated. Tuohy became curious as to whether the corneal portion could be worn, so he polished the edge, placed it in his own eye and found that the lens could be tolerated. Further trials were conducted, leading to the development of the corneal lens or, in today's terminology, a **rigid lens**. Tuohy filed a patent for his invention in February 1948.

Lenses are made from PMMA by polymerization of methyl methacrylate with a free radical initiation system to form rods or buttons, from which lenses are fabricated by lathing and polishing. PMMA has a number of desirable properties, including optical clarity, ease of fabrication, acceptable surface wettability and excellent durability; however, it is impermeable to oxygen and is thus only used today for the fabrication of trial contact lens fitting sets.

poor vision, investigation of

The causes of vision loss during contact lens wear are not always obvious, and a definitive diagnosis may be difficult due to the transient or inconsistent nature of the problem. In addition to measuring vision with and without contact lenses, additional descriptive information relating to symptoms of poor vision should be obtained from the patient (*see* Table P.2).

Other techniques for assessing vision may help to characterize the problem. These include:

Table P.2 Descriptive information relating to symptoms of poor vision

characteristic	description
severity	mild or severe
consistency	constant or fluctuating
onset	immediate or delayed
proximity	distance or near
persistence	whether the problem persists throughout the period of lens wear and/or following lens removal
type	whether the problem is best described as blur, haze, glare, or some other descriptor

- contrast sensitivity function – this may be suppressed during adaptation, but otherwise should be no different from that obtained with the best corrected spectacle prescription
- high- and low-contrast acuity charts – reduced acuity with a high-contrast chart suggests a refractive problem, and reduced acuity with a low-contrast chart indicates a 'non-refractive' problem (such as poor lens fit, ocular pathology or excess lens deposition)
- glare sensitivity test – a bright light is positioned next to a low-contrast eye chart facing the patient; reduced vision under this condition indicates 'glare sensitivity', which can be due to conditions that scatter light, such as epithelial oedema, epithelial microcysts and anterior chamber flare.

After the symptoms of poor vision with contact lenses have been fully characterized, the following general strategies can be employed to help resolve the problem:

- restoration of vision immediately after lens removal (with a corrective trial lens before the eye) suggests a lens-related problem
- sustained vision loss after lens removal (with a corrective trial lens before the eye) suggests an ocular problem (which may or may not be related to lens wear)
- unilateral vision loss may be due to the lens or uniocular pathology
- bilateral vision loss may be due to a refractive cause or general ocular pathology (e.g. a toxic or allergic solution reaction), or to systemic disease (e.g. **diabetes**)
- worse vision immediately after a blink may signal excessive lens movement and either a flat fit (corrected by fitting the lens more steep) or inap-

propriate lens rotation in the case of a **soft toric lens** (corrected by employing better lens stabilization techniques); this indicator correlates with the appearance of **keratometer** mires before and after the blink

- improved vision immediately after a blink may signal a **tight fit** (corrected by fitting the lens more loosely).

The following causes of vision loss with contact lenses relate to spherical refractive error, and can be identified by the suggested strategies:

- patients may be unaware that the lens has become displaced from the **cornea** on to the sclera, or even lost from the eye, leaving vision uncorrected – inspect the eye
- shifts in refractive error can reduce vision – check the refraction
- lens power may have been ordered (and therefore supplied) incorrectly – check the record card against the power specified on the lens box
- lens power may have been ordered correctly but supplied incorrectly – check the record card against the power specified on the lens box
- lens power may be incorrect (manufacturing/packaging error) – measure the power of the lens and check this against the power specified on the lens box
- the tear layer beneath a rigid lens can have significant optical power – reconcile ocular refraction, **over-refraction**, keratometry readings, lens parameters and observed **fluorescein** pattern
- flexure of thick soft lenses can induce power shifts – fit lenses that are thinner and/or made of a material of lower modulus.

An uncorrected astigmatic component of a refraction with contact lenses can be due to:

- an astigmatic shift in refraction
- residual uncorrected **astigmatism**
- mislocation of toric lens cylinder axis
- the lens power may have been ordered (and therefore supplied) incorrectly – check the record card against the power specified on the lens box
- the lens power may have been ordered correctly but supplied incorrectly – check the record card against the power specified on the lens box
- the lens power may be incorrect (manufacturing/packaging error) – measure the power of the lens and check this against the power specified on the lens box
- **corneal warpage**.

Contact lens correction of **presbyopia** entails a variety of visual compromises, such as:

- **monovision** correction – degrades stereopsis at near
- **alternating vision bifocal lenses** – incomplete or improper lens translation will compromise vision
- **simultaneous vision bifocal lenses** – the visual system may have difficulty in processing clear and blurred images on the same region of retina; non-optimal **pupil** size will degrade vision.

Most non-optical causes of vision loss relate to problems of poor lens fitting, as follows:

- **flat fitting lenses** will decentre away from the pupil
- excessive post-lens movement can degrade vision
- **steep fitting lenses** may buckle in the centre and degrade vision
- hyper-thin **soft lenses** can dehydrate the epithelium, leading to vision loss
- lenses of low **oxygen transmissibility** can induce gross **oedema**, leading to vision loss
- poor lens surface quality (due to manufacturing problems, lens deposits or excessive surface drying) can degrade vision.

A variety of pathological and non-pathological ocular problems relating to lens wear can cause vision loss; these include:

- corneal infection
- corneal epithelial oedema
- corneal stromal oedema
- corneal stromal infiltrates
- corneal epithelial desiccation
- corneal **neovascularization**
- **tear film** dysfunction
- **corneal warpage**
- binocular vision problems.

posterior limiting lamina of the cornea

The posterior limiting lamina of the **cornea** (Descemet's membrane) is the basement membrane of the **corneal endothelium**. It lies between the endothelium and the overlying stroma. At birth it is 3–4 μm thick, and it increases to a thickness of 10–12 μm in the adult. In the periphery of aged corneas the posterior limiting lamina displays periodic sections of thickening, which are known as Hassall–Henle warts. The anterior one-third of the posterior limiting lamina represents that part produced in foetal life and, under the electron microscope, is characterized by a periodic banded pattern. The posterior two-thirds, which is formed postnatally, has a more homogenous granular appearance. The posterior limiting lamina has a unique biochemical composition by contrast with other basement membranes. The major basement membrane collagen is type IV, whereas in the posterior limiting lamina type VIII collagen predominates.

post-keratoplasty, contact lens fitting for

Corneal transplantation, also referred to as 'corneal graft' or 'penetrating keratoplasty' (PKP), is a surgical procedure by which diseased corneal tissue is removed and replaced by donor material. Corneal grafts are performed for the following reasons:

- optical – to restore visual function (e.g. in **keratoconus**)
- therapeutic – to treat disease (e.g. to treat an infection by debulking)
- tectonic – to restore, or preclude loss of, globe integrity
- cosmetic – to improve appearance (e.g. eliminate an unsightly scar in a non-seeing eye).

The main optical challenge following corneal transplantation is irregular surface **astigmatism**, which relates to the way in which the graft sits in the host **cornea**. It can be described as follows: 'nipple', or steep; 'proud', whereby the graft is totally or partially elevated above the host corneal surface; 'sunken', whereby the graft is depressed below the host surface; tilted; or 'eccentric'.

The indications for contact lens use following corneal grafts are post-operative irregular or high astigmatism, and **anisometropia** (e.g. as will occur in **aphakia**). Between 20% and 60% of post-PKP patients will benefit optically from wearing contact lenses. Contact lenses can be fitted when the graft is considered to have healed sufficiently to tolerate lens wear, which may begin as early as 3–6 months post-surgery, and often with one or more sutures remaining *in situ*.

Rigid lenses remain the overwhelming device of choice for the majority of PKP patients because they efficiently and effectively form an optical mask that neutralizes most regular and irregular astigmatism. Large-diameter lenses (9.0–11.0 mm) that over-ride the entire graft without causing hypoxic difficulties allow enhanced stability and centration and often give good results; however, achieving a good fit may still be difficult, especially on sunken or tilted PKPs, as rigid lenses tend to 'ride' over the highest corneal point (Figure P.15). The **back optic zone radius** of a rigid lens should be selected, with initial assis-

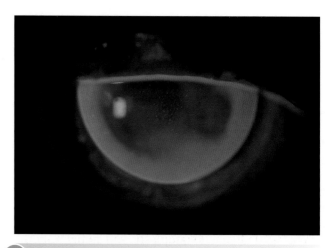

Figure P.15 Fluorescein revealing points of corneal contact in respect of a 'plateau' rigid lens fit on a proud graft.

tance of **keratometry** or **videokeratography** measurements, so as to achieve some form of irregular corneal surface alignment with neither excessive touch nor pooling of tears.

Consideration needs to be given to edge design in fitting rigid lenses to graft corneas. Some corneal surfaces can be fitted with standard edge parameters. Many abnormal corneal shapes require flatter than standard, steeper than standard or even **'reverse geometry'** peripheral lens designs to achieve mechanically acceptable corneal surface alignment and appropriate lens positioning. **Toric and bitoric rigid designs** can be helpful in fitting PKP corneas exhibiting relatively regular astigmatism, and occasionally in tilted and eccentric grafts.

Hydrogel contact lenses, both standard and in custom parameters, may sometimes be helpful, especially for patients who exhibit the following:

- high refractive errors with lesser degrees of astigmatism
- rigid lens intolerance
- acceptance of a less than optimal visual result.

Hybrid lens designs can be beneficial in post-PKP fitting; these include the following:

- **'piggyback'**, where a rigid lens is fitted upon a hydrogel lens
- Sofperm™ (former Saturn II), a lens with a rigid centre and hydrophilic periphery ('skirt')
- over-sized (scleral-like) rigid lenses.

The above hybrid designs will allow optimal vision, similar to rigid lenses, but such lenses are expensive to fit and may induce **hypoxia**, which in turn can increase the prevalence and severity of many complications (e.g. **neovascularization**).

post-refractive surgery, contact lenses for

Fifty years of evolution in refractive surgery procedures has left in its wake a large group of patients with sub-optimal visual results. Today, these patients are faced with three corrective options – glasses, contact lenses or further refractive surgery. For some of these individuals, contact lenses may provide the only option for visual rehabilitation and restoration of binocular vision. Past attempts with refractive surgery have included such procedures as keratophakia, keratomileusis, epi-keratophakia, thermokeratoplasty, automated lamellar keratoplasty and radial keratotomy (RK), and, more recently, photorefractive keratectomy (PRK) and laser assisted *in situ* keratomileusis (LASIK). Each of these procedures modifies the corneal surface in a unique way, necessitating a rethinking of traditional lens designs and fitting techniques for optimal contact lens performance. *See* laser refractive surgery, contact lenses following; radial keratotomy, contact lenses following.

post-surgery

See post-trauma, therapeutic lenses for.

post-trauma, therapeutic lenses for

Persistent or recurrent epithelial defects following trauma or surgery may heal more rapidly following the application of a soft bandage lens. A small aqueous leak following surgery or trauma can often be sealed with such a lens; if the anterior chamber is shallow or absent, a slightly **flat lens** will be needed, and this will have to be changed for a **steeper lens** as the chamber reforms. Custom-made lenses of over 20 mm in diameter and with greater than 70% **water content** have been successfully used as bandage lenses to arrest leakage from trabeculectomy filtration blebs or traumatic wounds (Figure P.16). Corneal transplant problems such as loosening sutures or slippage of the donor disc are usually best dealt with by further surgery – for example, by suture removal and/or re-suturing.

power changes

See soft lens on-eye power changes.

practice accommodation

See practice location, contact lens.

practice location, contact lens

In a contact lens practice, the patient participates, in person, in the buying process. It is therefore important to locate the practice as conveniently for the patient as possible. The decision regarding the location of the practice is crucial, not only in terms of

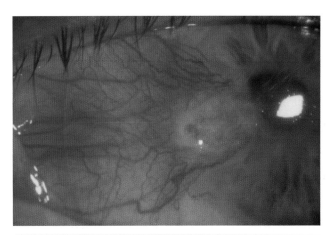

Figure P.16 A 20.5 mm diameter, high water content (77%) soft bandage lens covering a traumatic corneal wound sealed with histo-acryl tissue glue.

the ease of access for potential patients and customers, but also because a wrong or a poor decision cannot easily be reversed – unlike decisions on pricing or product choice. The costs of a mistake include the financial losses involved in acquiring and running a practice (e.g. fixtures and fittings, launch costs etc.) and, just as importantly to many businesses, the indirect cost of not keeping a competitor out of a better location. The suitability of a particular practice location is based on the estimated potential for attracting patients and customers in a given catchment area, and on the location of competitors.

Sophisticated models using a variety of information, including census data, family expenditure surveys, geodemographic characteristics etc., have been developed to help quantify catchment areas and the desirability of differing sites. Checklists with key considerations itemized may also be used to help in the decision-making process, with or without the computer modelling. Other good sources of information about an area include local authorities (e.g. planning department, electoral office, rating office, clerks office), estate agents, and the local and national press. Having decided on the location, it is important to ensure that the physical site will be able to accommodate a contact lens practice, including a waiting area, consulting and data collection rooms, spectacle and contact lens dispensaries, staff room, storage/stock room and washrooms.

practice logistics

There is no doubt that **planned replacement**, particularly when practised with **disposable lenses**, can generate a considerable extra workload in a practice. A critical issue is the maintenance of adequate stock levels.

As an example, a practice with 500 patients using 2-weekly disposable lenses will handle over 4000 six-packs of lenses per annum (ignoring new fits), or over 80 lens packs per week on average. Five hundred patients will also require 500–1000 **aftercare** appointments, depending on the preference of the practitioner. This takes perhaps as much as 30% of annual available chair time. If patients collect their supplies quarterly, practice staff will deal with nearly 40 collections per week.

Assuming the above level of activity, a reasonable stock or inventory of lenses will need to be kept in the practice to ensure good service to patients; however, such stocks can be expensive and can consume a considerable amount of space (Figure P.17). There are several approaches to deciding what levels of stock to maintain. The simplest involves keeping a few boxes of each parameter or 'stock kept unit' (SKU). As next-day delivery is usually available to UK practices it is not necessary to stock large numbers of lenses, although several spherical disposable lens brands now host parameter ranges of over 100 SKUs. Practices may wish to weight their stock towards the more commonly occurring prescriptions, such as the range from −1.00 D to −5.00 D. With very large patient bases it may be helpful to consult with suppliers, who can advise on an appropriate in-practice stock holding based on statistical stock models used to manage their own inventory.

Practices that are computerized may wish to model their stock on the actual prescriptions of their patient base. This approach can be tied in with the aftercare recall system. Due allowance needs to be made for unpredictable purchasing patterns, which can arise, for example, ahead of holiday periods. As well as holding sufficient stock for purchase, an adequate number of trial or diagnostic lenses are needed for ongoing fitting.

practice management, contact lens

Contact lens practice by definition resides within an optometric practice embracing, amongst other products and services, the prescribing, fitting and dispensing of contact lenses and associated products, and services. Thus practice management issues that impact on contact lens practice are, first, all those that impact on an optometric practice, and secondly (if it is possible to separate them), those issues that are regarded as more the domain of contact lens practice.

Practice management may be defined as that activity concerned with planning, organizing and controlling the non-clinical activities of an optometric enterprise to ensure pre-defined outcomes and goals, through the effective use of the available physical, financial, and human resources. The supply of optometric goods and services ranges from very tangible goods (e.g. the supply of a contact lens case) to entirely intangible services such as a contact lens consultation (e.g. aftercare).

The key elements that determine the management issues in a primarily service-orientated enterprise such as a contact lens practice can be categorized as per the following 'six Ps':

- practice location and the accommodation
- personnel at the practice
- products and services provided
- proper fees and charges
- promotional issues
- processes.

These issues have to be considered within the framework of the wider legal, political, economic and institutional environment within which optometry has to operate. Although contact lenses practice can be effected in a variety of settings, such as medical practices, hospitals, dispensing outlets etc.,

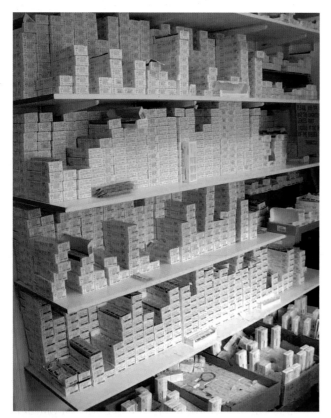

Figure P.17 A considerable amount of storage space is required to carry extensive stocks of planned replacement lenses.

the principles of efficient management can be applied to all of these situations. *See* fees and charges, contact lens; financial management in contact lens practice; layout, contact lens practice; patient scheduling in contact lens practice; personnel, contact lens practice; practice location, contact lens; products and services, contact lens; promotional issues in contact lens practice; staff training in contact lens practice.

pre-formed scleral lens
See fitting scleral lenses.

pregnancy
See indications and contraindications for contact lens wear.

preliminary contact lens examination
This is the initial examination conducted on a prospective contact lens patient. It can be considered to be an extension of a general eye examination, with additional procedures and questioning introduced to allow the practitioner to evaluate suitability for lens wear, and to consider the most suitable options. If the preliminary examination is straightforward – which is often the case – a contact lens fitting can be conducted at the same time.

The procedures conducted at a preliminary consultation may include the following:

- general introductory discussion with patient
- **history taking** – general health, past ocular history and family ocular history
- vision testing
- general external ocular examination
- measurement of ocular dimensions
- **refraction** – objective (**retinoscopy** or automated refractometry) and subjective, at distance and near
- **keratometry** or **videokeratoscopy**
- **slit-lamp biomicroscopy** – with and without **fluorescein**
- binocular vision assessment
- supplementary tests as required – binocular indirect ophthalmoscopy, tonometry, visual fields, gonioscopy, cycloplegic refraction, colour vision analysis, low vision evaluation etc.
- contact lens fitting – if time allows.

pre-ocular tear film
See tear film.

presbyopia
Refractive defect of the eye whereby there is insufficient **accommodative** capacity to focus on near objects. This is a condition that is progressive throughout life, and usually begins to become problematic during the fifth decade of life. Presbyopia is thought to be caused by a progressive sclerosing and hardening of the crystalline lens with age, rendering the lens unable to change shape to create more plus power. This condition is alleviated by introducing plus powered lenses before the eyes.

presbyopic correction
One of the more challenging areas within contact lens practice is fitting **presbyopic** patients with contact lenses so as to allow them to fulfil the majority of their visual requirements. The number of newer designs available in recent years, as well as the availability of single-use disposable trial lenses, has resulted in an increased rate of prescribing of contact lenses for presbyopic patients by practitioners. With the presbyopic population growing in size at an ever increasing rate, practitioners can expect to see an increase in the number of presbyopic patients attending for this form of lens fittings, which should now be considered as an integral, routine part of contact lens practice.

The options for the correction of presbyopia for both existing and new contact lens wearers include:

- distance powered contact lenses and near reading spectacles
- **monovision**
- **bifocal contact lenses** – simultaneous vision or alternating vision.

Each option has different advantages and disadvantages, which vary with the lens type, the fitting approach used and the degree of presbyopia present. Distance powered contact lenses combined with near reading spectacles may be the simplest and least expensive option. However, this does not address the problem for the patient who does not wish to wear spectacles, and may even de-motivate an existing lens wearer. Nevertheless, the quality and stability of vision in this mode of correction is such that it may give the best optical correction when compared to bifocal or monovision contact lenses.

Patient motivation plays an important role in any form of contact lens fitting. However, it is often restricted to those patients who are aware of the contact lens options, which they are then keen to explore further. Perhaps more important is informed choice based on the advantages and disadvantages of the various options available, as the majority of patients are not aware that contact lenses are a possibility for the correction of presbyopia. This more 'proactive' approach may result in lower success rates but, inevitably, in a larger contact lens patient base.

Caution should prevail when considering patients with compromised binocular vision, amblyopia, distance acuity of less than 6/12, or exacting critical vision needs for either distance or near vision. High- and low-contrast visual acuity charts give more information about acuity. In particular, the difference in low-contrast acuity between spectacles and contact lenses may give some indication of possible success. It is important to have access to trial lenses to obtain an idea of potential success for any particular type of bifocal lens or fitting technique based on both patient subjective feedback and objective measurement.

Patients must be given realistic expectations about the likely level of vision, as is the case with any type of vision correction for presbyopia. It is necessary to ensure that they fully understand the basis of presbyopia, and their expectations should be set out in a positive but informative manner. This involves discussing the benefits of combined distance/near correction without the need for spectacles, as well as likely differences between the visual performance of monovision, **simultaneous vision** or **alternating vision lenses**. When compared to spectacles or single vision contact lenses, visual decrements may be noticed, such as reductions in visual acuity (especially in low luminance) and stereopsis, and reduced intermediate vision, depending on the type of lens fitted. It should also be explained that it is quite normal for fitting to require more than one appointment in order to try out alternative lens powers and fitting approaches. *See* alternating vision lenses for presbyopia; bifocal and multifocal contact lenses; monovision correction for presbyopia; ocular dominance; simultaneous vision lenses for presbyopia.

pricing

A 'cost per wear' (CPW) model can be used to assist practitioners and patients when considering the cost implications of various lens replacement frequencies, tailored to the wearing habits of individual patients. The CPW is a simple calculation of the total cost of lenses (and solutions for non-daily lens replacement) and professional fees over a 12-month period divided by an estimate of the number of days lenses will be worn over 12 months (Figure P.18). This model demonstrates that unplanned replacement lenses provide the cheapest option for the full-time wearer, although the difference in CPW between **unplanned replacement** and monthly replacement lenses is small. For part-time wearers, **daily disposable lenses** are usually cheaper than monthly replacement lenses.

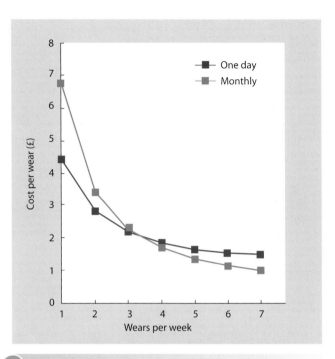

Figure P.18 'Cost per wear' of daily-disposable versus monthly-disposable lenses based on the average number of days lenses are worn each week over a 12-month period. This model assumes an annual professional fee of £60 and solution costs.

print tinting

Dye can be placed on the surface of a **soft lens** in a controlled manner using a printing process similar to that used for ink printing on paper. In this way, realistic iris patterns containing many colour elements can be applied, and the pupil region can be kept clear. *See* tinted lenses.

prism ballast

See stabilization of rigid toric lenses; stabilization of soft toric lenses.

prismatic effects

When ordinary spectacles are worn and the visual axes do not pass through the optical centres, prismatic effects are introduced of the magnitude given by Prentice's rule $P = cF$, where P is the induced prism power, c the decentration in cm and F the lens power. If the corrections are the same for both eyes, these prismatic effects cause no problems for the spectacle wearer. In **anisometropia**, however, the prismatic effects will be different for each eye. For example, in reading, the visual axes of a young anisometrope would normally intercept the lenses of the distance correction at some distance below the optical centres. Assuming this distance to be 8 mm and the corrections to be RE -3.00 D, LE -6.00 D, the prismatic effects would be RE $2.4\,\Delta$ and LE $4.8\,\Delta$, both base-down. In this example, the difference in vertical prism power ($2.4\,\Delta$) exceeds normal vertical fusional reserves, so that to avoid the problem the spectacle-corrected anisometrope would have to execute head turns during reading rather than simply depress the visual axes. This problem is absent with well-centred contact lenses.

Prismatic effects may arise as a result of a rigid lens either decentring or tilting, the latter often being due to pressure from the upper lid. To a reasonable approximation, the contact lens and the associated tear lens will both become decentred by the same amount with respect to the pupil centre; these effects can again be calculated using the Prentice rule. If, for example, $F = \pm10.00$ D and a there is 1 mm of lens decentration, a $1\,\Delta$ prism can be induced, which will be of little importance if similar effects occur in both eyes – that is, if the correcting powers are similar and fitting has ensured that similar amounts of movement occur in the two eyes. *See* accommodation demand; convergence demand.

private labelling
See lens supply routes.

PRK
See laser refractive surgery, contact lenses following.

products and services, contact lens
Income generated in an optometric practice is derived from provision and sales of:

1. *Eye examinations.* The vast majority of patients attend for eye examinations, which is the key value driver in optometric practice. It is only after a complete eye examination has been conducted that contact lenses are prescribed and dispensed.
2. *Spectacle dispensing.* Regardless of how much contact lens activity a practice has, the supply of complete spectacles will almost always be a necessary part of contact lens practice.
3. *Contact lenses.* Apart from a stock of 'off-the-shelf' designs, the practice may need to have to hand specialist contact designs and products.
4. *Accessories.* A range of appropriate contact lens care systems and other accessories must be available, such as sunglasses, spectacle chains, contact lens and spectacle cases, etc.
5. *Subscription schemes.* Both contact lens and spectacle wearing patients benefit from 'service agreement' schemes, which enable them to obtain replacement products and specific professional services at preferential terms. Such

schemes are now common, and maintain a degree of continuity to the practice.

The tangible products supplied by contact lens practices include all those products normally supplied in general optometric practice and, additionally, contact lenses, contact lens care systems and associated products. In view of concerns about contamination and cross-infection, the use of empirically fitted **rigid lenses** is now the preferred option, and the use of stock disposable **soft lenses** a practical alternative. It is thus necessary for contact lens practices to stock a variety of lens types for fitting and, possibly, initial supply. However it must be borne in mind that this stock, if paid for by the practice, is only creating value if sold. Similarly, the stocking of a variety of contact lens care systems and accessories is essential in providing a complete service. Like contact lenses, stock that is held in the practice only creates value if it is sold or supplied to patients and customers. Bar-coding of contact lenses and care systems will help manage the inventory of both contact lenses and solutions; however, the value of this process in the absence of a standardized bar-coding scheme is somewhat limited.

professional regulation
See General Optical Council.

profile matching, soft lens
The **back optic zone radius** (BOZR) of a soft lens can be estimated by placing the lens in a wet cell with its circular edge in contact with an optical flat. The lens is then illuminated from the side using a cold light projector, and a magnified profile of the lens back surface is projected onto a series of curves of varying radii. After correcting for magnification, the radius of the curve best fitting the profile is an indication of lens BOZR. Another similar technique (but one requiring contact with the lens) involves placing the lens on a series of perspex domes of known and varying curvature. This has been termed the 'template method' (Figure P.19). If the lens is steeper than the dome, an air bubble will appear between the lens and dome and/or central lens warpage will be observed. The lens is placed on progressively steeper domes until an air bubble no longer forms and the lens surface is smooth. If the lens is flatter than the dome, a section of the lens edge will be seen to lift off the periphery of the dome. This is a very crude although rapid method of radius assessment.

projection magnifier
The **total diameter** of **soft** and **rigid lenses** can be measured using a projection magnifier and a graduated scale (Figure P.20). Such devices typically have a

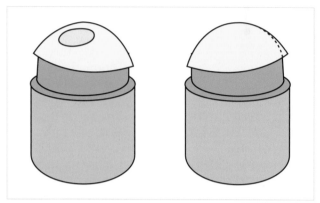

Figure P.19 Estimation of soft lens BOZR using the template method. Left: the lens has a bubble beneath it, indicating that the lens BOZR is steeper than the curvature of the template. Right: the lens edge is lifting off the surface of the template, indicating that the lens BOZR is flatter than the curvature of the template.

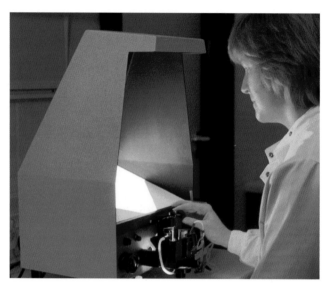

Figure P.20 Projection magnifier in use.

magnification of between ×10 and ×20. The lens is placed in **saline** and illuminated with a cold light source, and the projected image is focused on to a fixed scale. The projected image can be checked for any optical defects and regularity of the circumference.

The same device can be used to check the optic zones, and the body of the lens and the lens periphery for physical **defects**. For **toric**, truncated lenses, the smoothness of edge transition can also be checked. The measuring device should be calibrated regularly.

promotional issues in contact lens practice

Communicating the availability of products and services that have been identified as 'needs and wants' by patients and customers, at a price that creates sustained value for the practice, is what promotions are about. A variety of options are open to the owner/manager of a contact lens practice regarding communication with existing and potential patients and customers. The mix of these will often be determined by the stage at which the practice is in its life cycle. For example, a new practice with mostly new patients will rely more on external promotions, whilst an existing mature practice will rely more on internal communications and promotions.

Internal promotions embrace all aspects of communication to existing patients and include the spectrum from personal contact at the practice – which embraces the practice ambience and point-of-sale literature – through to special mailings. Personal communication is by far the most significant mode of internal contact with the patient, and can adopt the following guises:

- the recall letter – with careful database management, it is possible not only to send out recall letters for routine optometric review visits, but also to tailor promotions of specific products and services to patients by criteria other than clinical need
- special mailings – some practitioners will send patients thank-you cards for referrals, cards on the arrival of a new family member etc.
- practice newsletters, via both conventional mail and e-mail – these are increasingly used, and are indeed a good way of educating and maintaining contact with patients, and keeping them aware about the practice, its personnel, and its activities.

The use of a website as an internal communication tool merits some mention. Practice web sites and electronic mail will increasingly play a role in the following functions: facilitating patient education; e-mail recall letters; e-promotions and opportunities for patients to contact the practice to order sun wear, accessories and replacement products; to book an appointment; and even to submit medical history. Similarly, it makes sense to consider an appointment reminder communication via e-mail.

External promotions include all activities whereby potential patients might be exposed to the activities, personnel or products at the practice. These include national and regional newspapers, trade and professional magazines, radio and television broadcasts, telephone directories, exhibitions and health fairs, direct mail, public relations, speaking engagements and the Internet (world-wide web). This last method enables practices to broaden their catchment area, and to offer sun wear, accessories, frames and spectacles along with practice information and opportunities to book appointments on-line.

prophylactic tints

The purpose of a prophylactic tint is to *prevent* the eye from injury or disease. The primary prophylactic application of tinted lenses is protection from excess ultraviolet (UV) light. Lenses with UV-protection tints may be beneficial to lens wearers who are frequently exposed to UV radiation, such as those who:

- have an active outdoor lifestyle, especially near snow, sand and sea
- work outdoors (such as professional tennis players)
- use photosensitizing drugs
- are often exposed to artificial UV sources during work or recreation
- are **aphakic**.

Some argue that everyone can benefit from UV tints to prevent chronic ocular damage, such as lens yellowing with age – although, paradoxically, an aged crystalline lens that has become yellow will intrinsically absorb UV light, obviating the need for UV protection later in life. Non-tinted lenses and lenses with standard cosmetic tints transmit light of wavelengths down to 230 nm and thus do not provide UV protection. Lenses with special UV tints block light with wavelengths lower than about 350 nm from entering the eye, thus affording the desired protective effect.

Patients must be warned of the limitations of UV-tinted contact lenses. For example, solar keratitis can occur in exposed regions of the **cornea** and **conjunctiva** in UV-tinted **rigid lens** wearers, and areas of the conjunctiva not covered by the lens are susceptible to solar damage in **soft lens** wearers. Accordingly, patients should be advised to wear UV-protecting sunglasses or goggles during prolonged periods of UV exposure, and to protect exposed regions of skin in extreme conditions. *See* tinted lenses.

prosthetic tinted lenses

A prosthetic tinted lens can be defined as a lens that is designed to normalize an otherwise abnormal appearance. Typical cases for which such lenses are indicated include the aftermath of trauma, ocular disease and congenital abnormalities. Visible deformities of the anterior ocular structures – in particular the **cornea**, iris and crystalline lens – can be effectively masked using opaque tints (Figure P.21). Specific tinting configurations can be tailored for different circumstances – for example, a painted iris

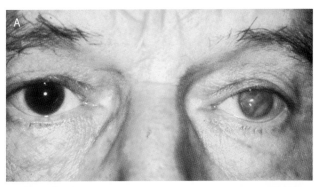

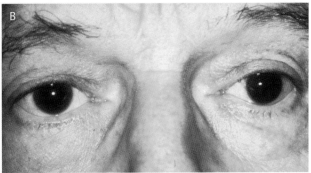

Figure P.21 (A) Patient with severe opaque scarring of the cornea of the left eye. (B) Vastly improved cosmetic appearance with a prosthetic lens in the left eye that has a painted iris and black pupil.

and clear pupil for a sighted eye with a disfigured iris; a painted iris and opaque pupil for a non-sighted eye; or a clear iris and opaque pupil for a non-sighted eye with a dense cataract. *See* tinted lenses.

protein deposition
See deposits, lens.

proteins in tears
See tear proteins.

protein removal systems

Although **surfactant cleaning** may remove loose protein from the surface of **soft** and **rigid lenses**, it is less capable of removing denatured or bound tear proteins. The build-up of protein deposition has been linked to discomfort, visual compromise, and adverse reactions such as **papillary conjunctivitis**. Protein removal can be undertaken with enzymatic treatment, generally with products containing papain, pancreatin or subtilisin-A. When prescribed, they are used typically on a weekly basis. Traditionally, enzymatic cleaners were developed in tablet form and treatment was a distinctly separate part of the lens care process. More recently, **Alcon** has introduced the SupraClens product, which is a liquid formulation of purified pancreatin that is added to the overnight disinfectant on a daily basis. Other manufacturers also make protein removal tablets, which can be dissolved in either **multipurpose** or **hydrogen peroxide solutions**. Clinical benefits have been shown with regular enzymatic treatment, but the use of these products has declined with the use of more frequently replaced soft lenses, as the issue of protein spoilation is seen as less of a clinical problem.

Protein removal is arguably more important with rigid lenses than with soft lenses, in view of the fact that most soft lenses prescribed today are replaced more regularly than rigid lenses. With few exceptions, protein removal systems that were originally designed for use with soft lenses can also be used with rigid lenses. The frequency with which patients should be advised to use **protein removal systems**, and the way in which such systems should be applied to the lenses, will vary depending on the lens material and the strength of the active ingredient in the protein removal system. Advice on these issues should be obtained from the manufacturer.

Individual patient factors will also impact upon the way protein removal systems should be applied. Patients who display a propensity for depositing protein on lenses, and who wear their lenses more frequently and for longer periods of time, may need to treat their lenses more regularly. Typical frequencies of usage of protein removal systems vary from weekly to monthly.

Pseudomonas aeruginosa keratitis

Pseudomonas aeruginosa infection of the **cornea** can have a rapid and devastating time course, and be associated with anterior chamber flare, iritis and hypopyon. A mucopurulent discharge will be evident, although the discharge can sometimes be serous. If not properly treated, the **corneal stroma** can melt away, leading to corneal perforation in a matter of days.

Extended wear of **hydrogel** lenses increases Pseudomonas adherence to human corneal epithelial cells (Figure P.22). This bacterium does *not* adhere to the healthy cornea, because of the natural protective layers of the corneal surface; specifically, the mucus layer of the **tear film** and the epithelial cell surface glycocalyx (which also contains mucin molecules). The basolateral epithelial cell surfaces (the sides and the bottoms of cells) are much more susceptible to infection than the apical cell membrane (the top surface of cells). Notwithstanding these defence mechanisms, it is now known that some strains of Pseudomonas invade **corneal epithe-**

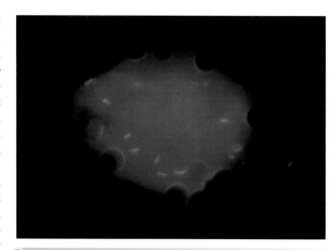

Figure P.22 Pseudomonas bacteria adherent to a human corneal epithelial cell taken from a patient wearing extended wear hydrogel lenses.

lial cells during corneal infection. Once the bacterium is inside a cell it then has the potential to alter host cell function internally. Meanwhile, it is protected from factors of the host immune system and from most forms of antibiotic therapy – neither of which can enter epithelial cells.

Another important recent discovery is that there are two types of Pseudomonas that cause clinical disease, and that the pathogenesis of the two types is entirely different. One type, an invasive strain, invades corneal epithelial cells without killing the host cell, and probably causes disease largely via the host immune response. The other type, a cytotoxic strain, is cytotoxic for corneal and other epithelial cells; that is, these bacteria kill the host cell.

Pseudomonas infections may appear to worsen slightly during the first 24 hours after medication has commenced (*see* **microbial keratitis**). The condition will gradually improve thereafter, with the micro-organism persisting for 14 days or longer.

psoriasis

See systemic disease, contact lens wear in.

psychological factors

See indications and contraindications for contact lens wear.

ptosis

The classical appearance of ptosis is of a narrowing of the palpebral fissure and a relatively large gap between the upper lid margin and the skin fold at the top of the **eyelid** (Figure P.23). **Rigid lenses** can cause narrowing of the palpebral fissue by about 0.4 mm, whereas **soft lenses** do not affect palpebral

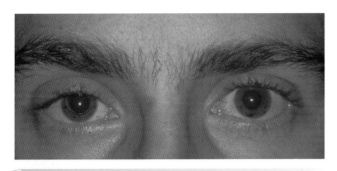

Figure P.23 Unilateral ptosis of the right eye in a patient who had been wearing a rigid lens in that eye, and a soft lens in the contralateral eye, for 4 weeks.

aperture size. Clinically significant ptosis occurs when the distance between the centre of the pupil and the lower margin of the upper lid is less than 2.8 mm. Using this criterion, contact lens induced ptosis (CLIP) occurs in about 10% of rigid lens wearers. The ptosis takes 4–6 weeks to develop fully, and is generally noticed by patients in advanced cases. There are no associated signs or symptoms.

A number of mechanisms have been advanced as possible causes of CLIP. Those involving some form of dysfunction of the aponeurosis (*see* levator palpebrae superioris) include forced repeated lid squeezing and lateral eyelid stretching during lens removal, rigid lens displacement of the tarsus, and blink-induced eye rubbing. Non-aponeurogenic causes of CLIP include lens-induced lid oedema, blepharospasm and **papillary conjunctivitis**.

To differentiate between these possible causes, patients demonstrating CLIP should be required to cease lens wear for at least 1 month (to detect any trends towards recovery) and perhaps as long as 3 months (to demonstrate complete resolution). If the CLIP partially or completely resolves after ceasing lens wear for 1 month, then the cause is lid oedema and/or involuntary blepharospasm, and the patient may need to be refitted with soft lenses (which do not induce ptosis). The eyelids should also be everted to determine if papillary conjunctivitis is involved, and if so, appropriate action should be taken to alleviate the condition. If the ptosis persists after resolution of the papillary conjunctivitis, or after ceasing lens wear for 1 month, then the cause is most likely damage to the aponeurosis, whereby surgical correction is the preferred option. Management strategies available to patients with severe CLIP who do not wish to undergo lid surgery include being fitted with a 'ptosis crutch'.

The prognosis for recovery from aponeurogenic CLIP is poor; the condition can only be reversed by

surgical correction or other management options as described above. The prognosis for recovery from non-aponeurogenic CLIP is good. If the cause of ptosis is papillary conjunctivitis, the time course of resolution of the ptosis will parallel the time course of recovery of the papillary conjunctivitis. If a contact lens wearer presents with ptosis, the numerous other possible causes of this condition must be considered so that the appropriate course of management can be adopted.

pupil diameter

While the retinal image is always blurred by both aberration and diffraction, in **ametropia** and **presbyopia** it is often defocus blur that is the major source of visual degradation. Defocus will occur whenever the object point lies outside the range of object distances embraced by the far and near points of the individual. Even within this range small errors of focus will normally occur, due to the steady-state errors that are characteristic of the **accommodation** system. Such blur depends on the dioptric error of focus and the pupil diameter. For any object point and assuming that the eye pupil is circular, spherical defocus produces a 'blur circle' on the retina. It is easy to show that the diameter, d mm, of this blur circle is:

$$d = \Delta F{\cdot}D/K'$$

where ΔF is the dioptric error of focus with respect to the object point, D is the pupil diameter in mm, and K' is the dioptric length of the eye. If astigmatism is present, the blur patch is an ellipse, with major and minor axes corresponding to the focus errors in the two principal meridians.

The blur circle diameter can be expressed in angular terms as:

$$\alpha = \Delta F{\cdot}D{\cdot}10^{-3} \text{ rads} = 3.44{\cdot}\Delta F{\cdot}D \text{ min arc}$$

Thus, for a 3 mm diameter pupil, the blur circle diameter increases by roughly 10 min arc per dioptre of defocus. The impact of blur on visual acuity depends somewhat on the acuity target chosen and the criteria and observation conditions used. The minimum angle of resolution (MAR) would be expected to be somewhat smaller than the blur circle diameter. For errors of focus above about a dioptre, letter targets, a 50% recognition rate, and normal chart luminances of about 150 cd/m² (giving pupil diameters of about 4 mm),

$$\text{MAR} = 0.65{\cdot}\Delta F{\cdot}D \text{ min arc}$$

With errors of focus smaller than about 1 dioptre, diffraction, **aberration** and the neural capabilities of the visual system are more important than defocus blur, and the MAR exceeds that predicted by the above equation.

The natural pupil diameter is chiefly dependent on the ambient light level. Pupil diameters at any light level tend to decrease with age (senile miosis) and with accommodation, as well as varying with a variety of emotional and other factors.

Reducing the pupil size results in smaller amounts of blur in the retinal image for any given level of defocus. Thus an uncorrected low **myope** may experience minimal levels of distance blur under good photopic levels of illumination, but may notice considerable blur when driving at night, when the pupil is large (Figure P.24).

puncta
See lacrimal drainage system.

push-up test, soft lens
See fitting soft lenses.

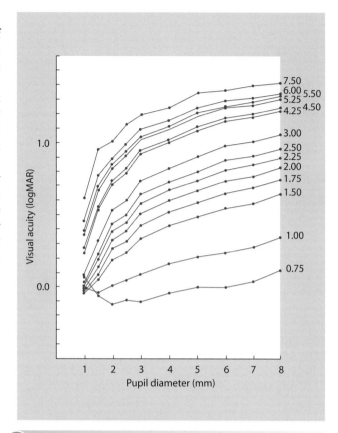

Figure P.24 Effect of pupil diameter on visual acuity (logMAR) for uncorrected myopes at a constant retinal illuminance of 2150 trolands.

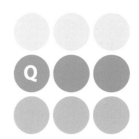

quality, soft lens

Defects can sometimes be detected in **soft contact lenses** when observed at ×10–×20 magnification. These defects can be divided into two broad categories – edge defects and non-edge (body) defects (Figure Q.1) – and four sub-categories, as follows:

1. *Edge defects*
   - nick – small piece of lens material missing from lens edge
   - tear – partial or full separation of lens material continuous with lens edge
   - roughness – uneven edge profile
   - excess material – lens mass or surplus material extending beyond lens circumference.

2. *Non-edge (body) defects*
   - split – partial or full separation of lens material that is not continuous with lens edge
   - blemish – hazy, low-transparency region of lens; may be on lens surface or within lens (Figure Q.2)
   - eccentric optic zone – optic zone not concentric with lens perimeter
   - multiple pieces – lens separated into sections.

Some lenses may contain more than one defect. Patients using disposable lenses should be urged to examine lenses on the tip of their finger to check for obvious defects.

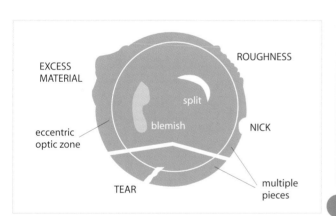

Figure Q.1 Types of defects that can be observed on soft contact lenses. Edge defects are indicated in upper case and body defects in lower case.

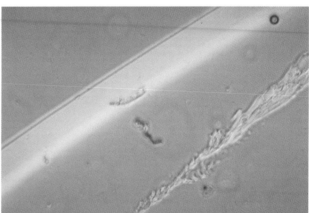

Figure Q.2 Blemish on the surface of an early generation disposable soft lens, in the form of an irregular strip of excess lens mass lying parallel with the lens edge. Lenses containing such blemishes should be discarded.

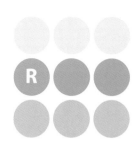

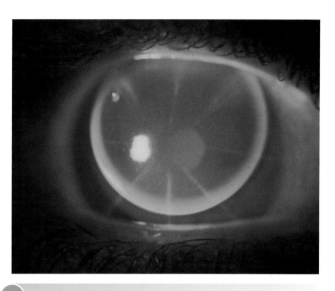

radial edge lift
See edge lift.

radial keratotomy, contact lenses following
Radial keratotomy (RK) is largely being phased out in favour or more sophisticated and predictable laser surgical procedures. Nevertheless, this technique is still indicated in certain circumstances, and patients may therefore occasionally present for supplementary contact lens correction having had RK performed some time previously.

When radial incisions are placed into the mid-peripheral **cornea**, the wounds gape open under the force of the intraocular pressure and stresses from within the corneal tissues. The gaping incisions are first filled with an epithelial plug, which is eventually replaced by a permanent wedge of fibroplastic scar tissue. This results in an overall increase in corneal surface area although the corneal diameter remains unchanged. There is a common misconception that the mid-peripheral cornea steepens following radial keratotomy. However, as the anterior cornea displaces to accommodate the gaping incisions, virtually the entire cornea, from limbus to limbus, flattens. The flattening effect is simply greater in the central cornea than in the periphery, resulting in the false impression of mid-peripheral steepening.

The degree of wound gape and the resultant amount of corneal flattening are dictated by a number of surgical and biological factors including the following:

- the number, depth and length of the incisions
- intraocular pressure forces
- stresses and biochemical properties within the corneal tissue
- patient age at the time of surgery
- individual wound healing responses.

Following RK, the cornea may exhibit significant corneal flattening with only minimal mid-peripheral flattening (approximately 0.1–0.2 mm flatter than its pre-operative curvature). Therefore, in the fitting of a **rigid lens** (Figure R.1), a **back optic zone radius** (BOZR) should be selected to align with the 'more normal' mid-peripheral cornea, approximately 4.0 mm from the centre, along the horizontal meridian. The radius of the post-operative mid-peripheral cornea can be determined through corneal mapping or peripheral **keratometry**. Alternatively, the fit of a

Figure R.1 Rigid lens fitted to a patient post-RK.

diagnostic lens with a BOZR that is 0.1–0.2 mm flatter than the preoperative flat 'K' reading can be evaluated. The appropriate BOZR should result in a **fluorescein** pattern that displays apical clearance over the flatter central cornea and a zone of mid-peripheral bearing at the 3 and 9 o'clock locations. The lens should display unobstructed movement along the vertical meridian.

Lens decentration is a common problem following RK. It is often the result of uneven wound healing, which creates geographic surface elevations on which the lens pivots. Lens decentration is best resolved by increasing the overall lens diameter to 10.0 mm or larger. Final lens power is best determined by performing a sphero-cylinder refraction over a well-centred diagnostic lens. The cornea is malleable and prone to warpage for a period of up to 3 months following RK. Rigid lens fitting should not be carried out during this period unless it is medically necessary for short-term use to aid wound healing.

Several months should be allowed to elapse after RK surgery before fitting soft lenses, to allow the cornea to stabilize; loose-fitting, high water content lenses are the best option. A flat lens fit will tend to align more closely with the corneal contour and will avoid corneal compression following RK.

Incisional **neovascularization** is a common complication associated with the use of **soft contact**

lenses following RK. This is especially true in the case of incisions that extend to or beyond the limbus. More modern surgical techniques in which the incisions terminate short of the limbus may be less prone to this complication. Today, incisional neovascularization can be minimized through the post-surgical fitting of high oxygen permeability **silicone hydrogel lenses** used on a daily wear basis.

radiuscope

The radiuscope (microspherometer) is the standard instrument for checking the **back optic zone radius** (BOZR) (Figure R.2). In Figure R.3, rays from an illuminated target are focused on a point A, and a travelling microscope is focused on this same point. The rays are directed towards the back surface of a **rigid lens**. For a spherical surface, a sharp clear image of the target will be observed in two conditions – when the travelling microscope is focused on the back surface of the lens, and when the lens is moved away from the microscope and the incident rays are perpendicular to the surface.

For the former condition, the reflected light again passes through point A and the distance AB is the BOZR of the lens. To reduce the effects of unwanted reflections, the lens front surface reflectivity is greatly reduced by immersing the lens in water. This optical arrangement, known as the Drysdale method, is employed in most contact lens radiuscopes. Using cross-shaped targets, the radiuscope can measure both spherical and **toric** surfaces. This technique is valuable not just for checking new lenses, but also for monitoring changes in lens shape due to flexure.

For **aspheric** surfaces, the measured BOZR is the radius over the chord diameter. By extending the size of the target, it is possible to focus different parts of the reflected image, thus allowing a rapid check for asphericity. This is not the best quantitative method for numerically evaluating an aspheric surface; nevertheless, it is useful as a quick check for regularity. Peripheral curves can be assessed in multicurve lenses by tilting the lens.

The device used to hold the lens could inadvertently distort the lens and affect the regularity of lens surface and quality. This can cause the reflection to appear fuzzy, which will in turn affect radius measurement. The radiuscope can also be used for checking the front surface of the lens.

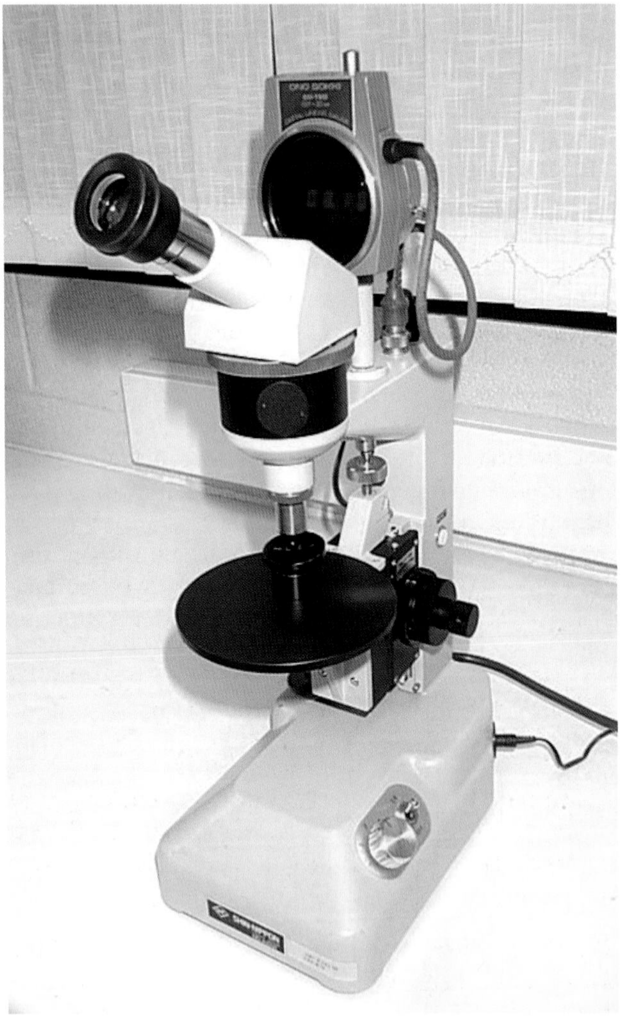

Figure R.2 Radiuscope.

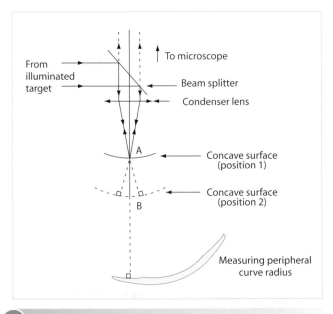

Figure R.3 Basic optical arrangement of the radiuscope (Drysdale method) for measuring a concave (back) lens surface.

re-branding
See lens supply routes.

recurrent erosion syndrome, therapeutic lenses for
Minor trauma to the **cornea** may predispose to this condition. Very often, corneal epithelial basement membrane dystrophy (such as Cogan's microcystic dystrophy or map–dot–fingerprint dystrophy) is found to be present; this is a bilateral condition, so both eyes should always be carefully examined. The eye with the erosion often becomes acutely painful when the eyes are opened during the night or when waking. At these times tear production is minimal and friction is maximal, and so the lid margin pulls on the unstable patch of epithelium, sometimes causing epithelial disruption. A contact lens interposed between cornea and lid can reduce the friction (Figure R.4).

record keeping
During the whole process of the initial assessment, history taking, ocular examination, fitting, and aftercare, information is being gathered upon which clinical decisions as to patient suitability and well-being with respect to contact lens wear will be made. As with all clinical processes, suitable records are essential. These records not only offer insight into the status of the patient, but also give credence to the clinical decisions being made. In the event of a dispute with the patient, clinical records can be invaluable in showing the maintenance of good clinical management and the provision of the standard of care expected.

In essence, record keeping should include all relevant patient information relating to the primary and significant secondary complaints, as well as all the tests conducted in response to that information. The records should clearly indicate the clinical decision being made and the basis of that decision (i.e. diagnosis). A written record of all the advice offered to the patient should be included. As a general rule, it should not be forgotten that potential and existing contact lens wearers are just as prone to general ophthalmic problems as the rest of the population, and non-contact lens causes of visual and ocular problems should not be overlooked.

Practitioners should conduct all the appropriate examination procedures necessary to test their working clinical hypothesis about the cause of the presenting problems. Where testing suggests that the hypothesis is flawed, the data should be re-examined and other possibilities assessed through further testing. At a minimum, the records should reflect this process and include all test results that rule a probable or possible diagnosis in or out of consideration. If this procedure is followed, there can be no doubt about whether the standard of care has been delivered.

red eye, investigation of
Conjunctival redness is so obvious and easily observed that it is perhaps the only sign of contact lens wear that is also reported as a symptom by patients (Figure R.5). Indeed, excessive eye redness is cosmetically unsightly and is generally perceived as a potential disadvantage of wearing contact lenses. It is recognized in eye care that the clinical presentation of a 'red eye' can be one of the most difficult cases to solve, due to the numerous possible known causes. This problem may be even more complex in a contact lens wearer because there are also many other contact lens related causes of red eye.

Throughout the literature, the terms hyperemia, injection, vascularity and redness are used as synonyms. These terms are defined as follows:

- hyperemia – increased blood in a part, resulting in distension of the blood vessels
- injection – a state of hyperemia
- vascularity – the quality of vessels
- redness – of or approaching the colour seen at the least-refracted end of the spectrum, of shades varying from crimson to bright brown and orange.

Strictly speaking, 'hyperemia' or 'injection' is the *cause* and 'redness' is the *effect*. That is, an increased volume of blood in the conjunctival vessels (hyperemia or injection) causes an increased appearance of redness. The term 'vascularity' is

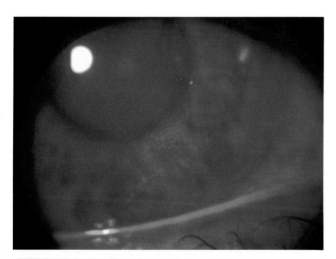

Figure R.4 Recurrent corneal erosion in soft contact lens wearer with dry eye symptoms.

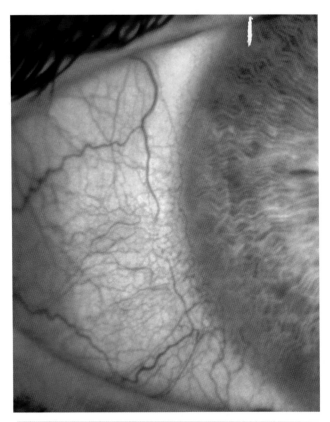

Figure R.5 Bulbar conjunctival redness caused by a defective soft lens irritating the ocular surface.

somewhat ambiguous, and could represent both the cause and effect.

When a contact lens wearing patient presents with a red eye as a primary complaint, the initial diagnostic step is to determine whether or not the problem is related to lens wear. This can often be established by simply removing the lens; eye redness should dissipate rapidly if the problem is purely lens-related. However, the possibility that the lens was somehow exacerbating a complication unrelated to lens wear itself should not be discounted.

Another differential diagnosis that may be necessary when presented with an extremely red eye is to determine to what extent the redness is due to conjunctival injection or ciliary flush. Two simple tests can be applied. A sterile cotton bud can be held lightly against the bulbar **conjunctiva** in the region of redness and gently moved from side to side. The conjunctival vessels will move, but the ciliary vessels will remain in a fixed position. It can then be determined whether the redness relates primarily to the 'moving' vessels (indicating conjunctival involvement) or the 'static' vessels (indicating ciliary involvement).

An alternative test is to instill a decongestant into the eye. The effect of a decongestant is limited to the superficial conjunctival vessels; these drugs have no effect on the deeper ciliary vessels. Thus, if the instillation of a decongestant alleviates eye redness, the condition is primarily conjunctival. If the decongestant has no impact on eye redness, then the redness can be attributed to excessive ciliary flush.

A subconjunctival haemorrhage can be easily differentiated from conjunctival and/or ciliary hyperemia because of the stark appearance of an intensely 'blood-red' eye and the lack of hyperemia around the limbus. Small haemorrhages of individual conjunctival vessels can also increase conjunctival redness, but again these are self-evident and differential diagnosis from vascular engorgement is clear.

Assuming that a given case of eye redness is lens-related, it is necessary to determine whether the source of the problem is the **cornea** or conjunctiva. Conjunctival redness associated with a quiet limbus and absence of pain indicates a primary conjunctival problem. Conjunctival redness associated with an injected limbus and corneal pain indicates corneal involvement, or indeed a problem that is related *exclusively* to the cornea. Redness of both the limbus and bulbar conjunctiva may indicate the co-existence of corneal and conjunctival pathology. Careful examination of the anterior ocular structures with a **slit-lamp biomicroscope**, and inspection of the lens at high magnification, will generally reveal the cause of the problem. It may also be necessary to prescribe different care systems and differentially diagnose the effects of various solutions over time.

If the red eye is deemed to be unrelated to lens wear, then all other possible causes must be investigated. This may involve a full ocular examination, involving the use of direct and indirect ophthalmoscopy, tonometry etc.

refraction
See subjective refraction.

refractive index
In **soft lenses**, refractive index decreases progressively with increasing **water content** (Figure R.6). The variation is almost linear with water content, and the results for **hydrogels** of the various types used in contact lenses lie within a fairly narrow, almost rectilinear band, decreasing from 1.46–1.48 at 20% water content to 1.37–1.38 at 75% water content. It is for this reason that refractive index measurement can be used as a rapid method of determining the approximate water content of an unknown gel. *See* refractometer, soft lens.

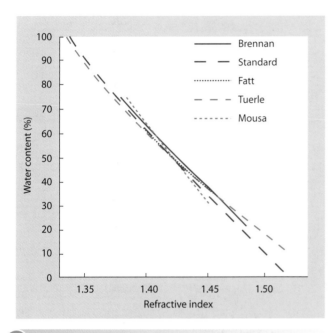

Figure R.6 Relation between water content (%) and refractive index for hydrogels, as determined by various authors.

refractometer, rigid lens

Refractometers are commonly used to measure the **refractive indices** of solids and liquids. In the case of solids, the sample material should have a flat surface which is placed in contact with the refractometer measuring prism. A contact fluid can be used when the surface is irregular. It may not be desirable to introduce a contact fluid beneath a finished contact lens because it may prove difficult to remove due to its steep curvature; however, by placing the convex surface of the lens onto the measuring prism and applying gentle digital pressure, the surface will flatten slightly and create an area of contact sufficient for measurement. This can be achieved using a hand-held refractometer, with a precision of ± 0.001 (Model N3000 Refractometer; Atago Co. Ltd, Japan).

Fluorosilicone acrylates tend to have refractive indices lower than 1.458, and some silicone acrylates and fluorosilicone acrylates have refractive indices between 1.458 and 1.469. Refractive indices greater than 1.469 indicate silicone acrylate materials.

refractometer, soft lens

The **refractive index** of a **hydrogel** is directly related to its **water content**. In theory, this is based on the simple Gladstone–Dale Law. The Gladstone–Dale law, originally proposed for liquid mixtures, is a simple way of predicting the final refractive index of a solution (N) based on the refractive indices of the solvent (N_1), the solid (N_2), and their relative proportions, as follows:

$$N = N_1 \cdot X_1 + N_2 \cdot X_2$$

where X_2 is the relative proportion of solid present in the mixture as a percentage (a), and X_1 is the relative proportion of solvent in the mixture $(100 - a)$.

Measurement of **soft lens** refractive index to infer water content is an accepted simple, rapid, nondestructive technique with universal appeal. Of the several ways one can measure refractive index, a hand-held optical refractometer is probably the simplest and most economically viable (Atago Soft Lens Refractometer, Atago, Japan; Figure R.7). The resolution of refractometry to indirectly infer lens water content can be very high. A +0.001 unit increase in refractive index is equivalent to a −0.7% drop in water. Because this is a surface measuring technique, it is assumed that the refractive index at the surface is the same as the refractive index throughout the lens matrix. However, it is not possible to measure the water content of certain types of cast moulded lenses which, as a result of the curing process, end up with a slight refractive index variation throughout the lens matrix.

regulation
See Food and Drug Administration; General Optical Council; Medical Devices Directive.

Reis–Bückler's dystrophy
See dystrophies of the corneal epithelium, therapeutic lenses for.

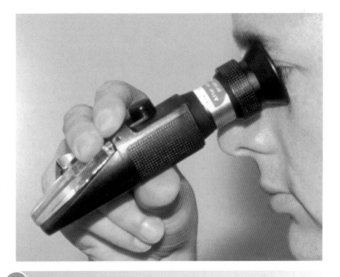

Figure R.7 The Atago CL-1 Soft Contact Lens Refractometer, which is used to determine the water content of soft contact lenses.

relative spectacle magnification

The relative spectacle magnification (RSM) is the ratio of the retinal image size in the corrected **ametropic** eye to that in a specified **emmetropic** schematic eye. Theoretically, the specification of RSM has the advantage of putting retinal image size on an absolute basis. However, in most clinical work it is the changes described by **spectacle magnification** that are of interest, and RSM is of limited practical use.

relief of pain, therapeutic lenses for

Corneal epithelial pain can be severe and disabling. A simple corneal abrasion usually heals quickly and needs no help from the clinician, but a persistent or recurrent epithelial failure may benefit from the fitting of a soft 'bandage' lens, which acts as a barrier between the injured corneal surface and the lid.

removal of lens

See insertion and removal, rigid lens; insertion and removal, scleral lens; insertion and removal, soft lens.

replacement frequency, disposable lens

The ideal lens replacement frequency would be one selected on the basis of the rate of lens spoilation of each patient, and would be such that comfort and vision does not deteriorate throughout the life of the lens. This rate will depend upon the lens material and the **tear film** quality of the patient. In general, a high water content ionic material (FDA Group IV) requires at least monthly replacement, and a high **water content** non-ionic material (FDA Group II) requires at least 3-monthly replacement. These are guidelines only, as individual patient variation can have a significant impact. Monthly or more frequent replacement ensures consistent performance over the period of use of the lens in terms of subjective comfort and visual performance for FDA Group I and Group IV lenses.

In practice, it is not straightforward to identify the ideal lens replacement frequency for a given patient. Instead, an appropriate replacement interval can be chosen from one of the seven 'standard' replacement intervals (generally based on convenient and easily remembered calendar intervals) formulated for various products by contact lens manufacturers – that is, 1 day, 1 week, 2 weeks, 1 month, 3 months, 6 months and 1 year. Such a decision is made after consideration of the desired pattern of wear and the contact lens history of the patient. Monthly and daily lens replacement are the most popular replacement frequencies in the United Kingdom (Figure R.8).

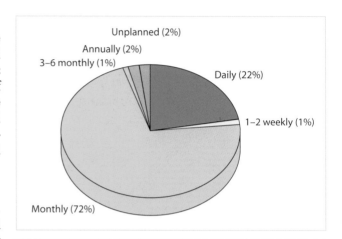

Figure R.8 Replacement frequency of soft lenses fitted to new patients in the United Kingdom in 2001.

reproducibility, soft lens

Practitioners who prescribe lenses that have been manufactured using mass-production technology, and patients who wear such lenses, need to be assured that a series of lenses of identical specifications are indeed all the same, or very nearly so; this characteristic can be described as 'reproducibility'. Studies that have examined this characteristic have all found lenses to be within acceptable tolerance ranges for providing wearers of these lenses with consistent vision and fit. Reproducibility is generally slightly worse for lenses of higher power, but is still clinically acceptable.

residual astigmatism with rigid toric lenses

The term 'residual astigmatism' is often used loosely, and is frequently confused with induced astigmatism or corneal **astigmatism**. Residual astigmatism has been defined in various ways, but the simplistic definition states that residual astigmatism is the component of the spectacle (ocular) astigmatism that is not due to the **cornea**. In the context of rigid lens fitting, a better definition would be that residual astigmatism is the astigmatic component of a lens required to correct fully an eye wearing a **spherical powered rigid contact lens** with a spherical **back optic zone radius**.

Sometimes the axis of the residual astigmatism does not correspond exactly with one of the principal meridians of curvature of the cornea. If the difference between the axes of the spectacle refraction and the principal meridians of the cornea is marginal (less than 20°), it can be assumed that the axes of the spectacle refraction over the lens *do* correspond with the principal meridians of corneal curvature. By doing this, the need for any complex oblique cylinder calculations is obviated and the resulting error in the power calculations is usually not significant. If there is a large difference between the cylinder axis of the ocular refraction and the axis of the corneal astigmatism, then an oblique bitoric lens (where the principal meridians of the toroidal front and back surfaces are not parallel) will be required. *See* compensated rigid bitoric lenses; cylindrical power equivalent rigid toric lenses; induced astigmatism with rigid toric lenses; stabilization of rigid toric lenses; toric lens design, rigid; toric lens, rigid.

retainer lenses
See orthokeratology.

retinoscopy
Retinoscopy is an objective technique for determining the refractive status of a patient. The test is performed by shining a light across the eye of the patient and observing the movement of the light reflex from the pupil; ophthalmic lenses of various power are interposed before the eye until 'neutralization' (no reflex movement) is achieved. While not necessarily performed routinely, retinoscopy also allows qualitative assessment of the optics of the eye. Possible indications for retinoscopy include:

- vision, with spectacles, of less than 6/6
- **astigmatism** of higher levels, or changing magnitude or direction of astigmatism, where **keratoconus** may be suspected
- when looking for clues of **corneal** irregularity, such as a scissors reflex
- pseudo-**myopia**, whereby less minus may be revealed.

retinoscopy assessment, soft lens
See fitting soft lenses.

reverse-geometry lenses
Such lenses were originally developed for the fitting of eyes with **keratoconus**; they have a secondary curve radius that is steeper than the **back optic zone radius** (BOZR). When used for the purpose of **orthokeratology**, these lenses offer the prospect of improved centration (and hence less corneal distortion), and a capacity to induce significant corneal shape change.

Reverse geometry lenses have secondary curves that are steeper than the BOZR (Figure R.9). These lenses are manufactured in a range of optic zone diameters and with secondary curves that are of variable width and steepness compared to the BOZR. This design allows for the lenses to be fitted with a much flatter central **cornea** relationship than

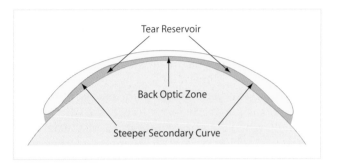

Figure R.9 Reverse-geometry lens design, showing the steeper secondary curve and related tear reservoir.

usual, while maintaining good lens centration. The fitting of these lenses is based on corneal sagittal height measurement so that an improved balance between central touch and tear layer thickness can be established.

re-wetting solutions, soft lens
Contact lens wearers can complain of numerous symptoms, including **dryness** and general discomfort; such symptoms are the primary reasons for the discontinuation of contact lens wear. A common method of the clinical management of ocular discomfort is the prescription of **soft lens** re-wetting solutions, which are also known by the synonyms of 'lubricants' and 'comfort drops' (Figure R.10). Although these products are often well received by wearers, and comfort is improved for at least 6 hours after their instillation, their effect is not much different from that of **saline**. Furthermore, the mechanism of symptomatic relief is unclear, and does not seem to be due to an enhancement of the pre-lens **tear film**.

Some re-wetting solutions are in 'unit-dose' form, which can be advantageous in clinical situations where the introduction of solution preservatives to the ocular surface is contraindicated. The packaging required for this approach is relatively expensive.

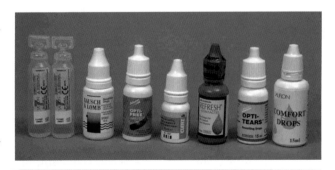

Figure R.10 Soft lens re-wetting solutions.

Most re-wetting solutions are supplied in multi-use bottles, and therefore contain preservatives to prevent contamination of the solution. These preservatives are similar to those found in other soft lens solutions.

A number of products contain viscosity-increasing agents, such as methylcellulose, which promote the adherence of the solution to the lens and enhance the contact time of the solution at the ocular surface. Other components that are commonly found in re-wetting solutions include sodium chloride and buffering agents.

RGP lens
See rigid contact lens.

rheumatoid arthritis
See systemic disease, contact lens wear in.

rigid contact lens
A rigid contact lens is a contact lens made from a rigid or inflexible material that is incapable of being folded so that opposite edges can touch together. The diameter of such lenses is smaller than that of the **cornea** (12 mm; *see* Figure R.11). All rigid lenses, apart from **PMMA**, are made from materials that are permeable to gases. Prior to the demise of PMMA as a contact lens material that is prescribed to patients, non-PMMA rigid lenses were referred to as 'rigid gas-permeable' or 'RGP' lenses – a term that is now redundant.

The readily discernible trend in the development of rigid contact lens materials described in the patent literature is one of increasing **oxygen permeability** balanced against the retention of acceptable dimensional stability and ocular compatibility (characterized by wettability and deposit resistance). The essential structural developments have centred on three areas. The first is the TRIS component, characterized by attempts to incorporate higher proportions of more highly branched siloxy derivatives, giving rise to silicone acrylates. The second is the use of fluorocarbon comonomers in the place of hydrocarbon-based components such as methyl methacrylate, giving rise to fluoro-silicone-acrylates. The third is the improvement of wettability by incorporation of hydrophilic co-monomers, or subsequent surface modification of the formed lens. Because rigid lens

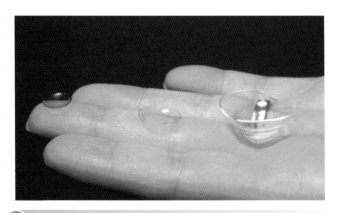

Figure R.11 A rigid lens (left), shown in comparison to a soft lens (centre) and scleral lens (right).

materials necessarily contain much higher levels of cross-linking agents than do **soft lenses**, it might be reasonable to add the development of cross-linking technology as a fourth area. Such materials have *Dk* values many times greater than that of PMMA.

Terms, symbols and abbreviations used to describe rigid (and soft) contact lenses are given in Appendix F.

rigid gas-permeable lens
See rigid contact lens.

rosacea keratopathy
See degenerations of the corneal epithelium, therapeutic lenses for.

rose bengal stain
A purple-red dye that can be introduced into the eye as a drop or from an impregnated paper strip. Staining occurs wherever there is poor protection of the surface epithelium by the **tear film** and/or a dysfunctional mucus layer. Rose bengal is also useful in identifying filaments. It is especially useful in detecting and evaluating damage to the ocular surface in patients with severe **dry eye** conditions such as keratoconjunctivitis sicca.

rotation of toric lenses, soft
See toric lens rotation, soft.

rust spots
See deposits, lens.

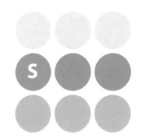

sag

The radius of curvature of a circle can be calculated by measuring the height, or sag, of the curve over a fixed chord diameter. In Figure S.1,

$$R = (y^2 + s^2)/2s$$

where R is the radius, s is the sag height and y is half the chord diameter. By differentiating this formula, the minimum change or difference in s required to detect a change or difference in R of $+0.05$ mm can be calculated as:

$$dR/ds = 0.5 - (y^2/2s^2)$$

For $y = 5$ mm and $s = 2$ mm, $ds = -0.019$ mm. Hence, 'sag' methods should be capable of measuring apical height to within a tolerance of 0.019 mm. Clearly, if y is reduced, then ds will also reduce in order to maintain the tolerance in R.

Instrument manufactures have used this approach to develop several devices for determining lens back surface radius. Using an appropriate calibration curve, the **BOZR** can be estimated. The apical height can be measured using mechanical or ultrasonic

probes, either in air or **saline**. In ultrasonic devices, the sound beam is reflected from the back surface; the BOZR of mass-produced **disposable lenses** can be measured to within ± 0.1 mm of the stated value using this technique.

Sag can be measured using a mechanical probe. The lens is immersed in temperature-controlled saline, and a magnified side view profile of the lens is projected on to a viewing screen. The mechanical probe is manually raised until the observer witnesses slight lens movement, indicating that the probe has come into contact with the posterior pole of the lens. This device tends to measure BOZR slightly less than stated when used on most lenses. In a variation of this approach, the lens is placed on a cylindrical column and a central probe is gently raised until it touches the back surface of the lens. On contact, an electrical circuit is completed. The height of the probe is electronically monitored and displayed; once the probe touches the lens back surface, the displayed figure is 'frozen'. This figure is the sag height of the lens, and by using a calibration chart the BOZR corresponding to the recorded sag height can be determined.

The sag method assumes that the lens back surface is spherical over the chord diameter of measurement. If the surface is aspheric, the estimated BOZR can be noted as the 'equivalent sphere'. If it is suspected that a particular lens design has an aspheric back surface, it is possible to estimate the asphericity of the surface by measuring the apical height over more than one chord diameter.

saline solutions

Many contact lens wearers are prescribed a **saline** rinsing solution when they commence lens wear. These products are particularly helpful to the new wearer, who tends to handle lenses more frequently and requires more attempts at lens insertion, leading to increased contamination from the fingers. Some **hydrogen peroxide** users remove any residual hydrogen peroxide with a saline rinse to reduce any stinging on insertion. The rinsing process can also play a significant role in the removal of micro-organisms from the lens surface.

Home-made and unpreserved saline have been associated with serious ocular surface infections and are not recommended. There are three types of saline solutions available on the market: aerosol,

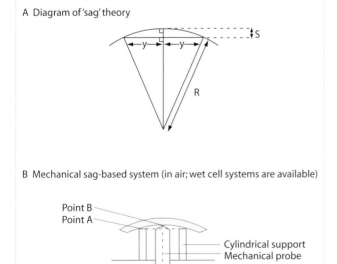

A Diagram of 'sag' theory

B Mechanical sag-based system (in air; wet cell systems are available)

Figure S.1 Sag method for determining back optic zone radius (BOZR). (A) Sag theory. (B) Mechanical sag-based system.

unit-dose and 'squeezy' bottle formats (Figure S.2). The pressure within aerosol saline canisters prevents contamination, although it is recommended that the user eject a small amount of saline before use as contamination of the spray tip has been associated with **corneal** infections. These are usually buffered to retain a consistent pH, and tend to be relatively expensive and bulky. Unit-dose products are non-preserved and can be useful in some circumstances, such as travel to warm climates or in-practice use.

More recently, preserved saline solutions have gained popularity in their 'squeezy' bottle format. With these products, the active ingredient serves only to prevent contamination of the solution, rather than play any role in contact lens disinfection. Examples of these products include Purite saline (**Allergan**), which contains chlorine dioxide; **Bausch & Lomb** saline, which contains sorbic acid; and **CIBA Vision** saline, which contains 60 ppm hydrogen peroxide.

Salzmann's nodular degeneration
See degenerations of the corneal epithelium, therapeutic lenses for.

Sauflon Pharmaceuticals
This company was formed in 1985, and manufactures contact lens care products. It is an international operation, with its headquarters in Twickenham, UK.

scheduling of patients
See patient scheduling in contact lens practice.

scleral lens
Scleral lenses have retained a small but valuable place in modern contact lens practice four decades after the introduction of corneal and hydrogel lenses (see Figure R.11). Originally they were made from glass, until **polymethyl methacrylate** (PMMA) was introduced in the 1940s. From the mid-1980s, rigid gas-permeable materials transformed scleral lens practice, allowing simpler fitting processes and improved patient tolerance, and expanding the therapeutic application of these lenses so that they could be used for more subtle forms of ocular pathology. The essential advance is that gas-permeable scleral lenses can be 'sealed' in most cases; that is, there is no need to introduce small holes (known as '**fenestrations**') into the lens to aid tear exchange and corneal oxygenation.

Advantages of scleral lenses include the following:

- they fit on the sclera and are held in place by the **eyelids**, and therefore can be used for almost any **corneal topography**
- high powers are possible
- they are robust and easily maintained
- handling may be easier for patients who have difficulties with **soft** or **rigid lenses**
- they are surprisingly comfortable because the lids are never in contact with the lens edge
- foreign bodies under scleral lenses are rare.

The primary disadvantages of scleral lenses are as follows

- full coverage of the anterior eye reduces the oxygen available to the **cornea**
- scleral lens manufacture is labour intensive and therefore expensive
- there may be a subjective feeling of bulk in the eye
- scleral lenses can induce a slightly proptosed appearance during wear
- the lens size intimidates some patients.

The two primary indications for fitting scleral lenses relate to vision and therapeutic applications:

1. *Vision*. **Keratoconus** or other primary corneal ectasia is the largest single group for which scleral lenses are indicated. Other applications for which scleral lenses can provide significant improvements in vision include **post-keratoplasty**, high refractive errors and the correction of high **astigmatism**.
2. ***Therapeutic*** *applications*. The pre-corneal fluid reservoir (Figure S.3) maintains corneal hydration in serious **dry eye** conditions such as Stevens–Johnson syndrome and cicatricizing pemphigoid, and creates a favourable environment for corneal healing in some situations. **Tear**

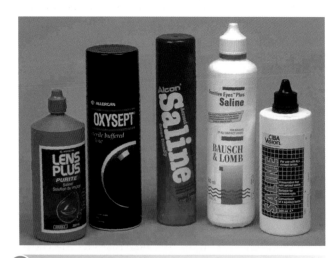

Figure S.2 Examples of saline supplied in aerosol cans and 'squeezy' bottles.

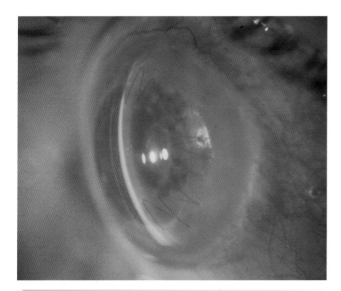

Figure S.3 The extent of corneal clearance is revealed by the thickness of fluorescein-stained tears between the scleral lens and the cornea.

film evaporation is prevented when lid closure is poor or if the lids are absent, and there is excellent corneal protection from trichiasis or lid margin keratinization. Some ocular surface disorders – e.g. **Salzmann's nodular dystrophy** – cause gross corneal irregularities, which can be optically neutralized to improve vision. 'Ptosis props' can be fixed onto scleral lenses to assist in management of ocular myopathy or other causes of poor lid elevation. A painted iris can be encapsulated into a scleral lens to cover an unsightly blind eye, or to relieve intractable diplopia.

SCLS
See Scottish Contact Lens Society.

Scottish Contact Lens Society (SCLS)
This is a body of opticians with a special interest in contact lens supply. The SCLS hosts periodic local meetings, and an international meeting every 2 years in Scotland.

sealed scleral lenses
See fitting scleral lenses.

services, contact lens
See products and services, contact lens.

sessile drop measurement
The wettability (or surface affinity for water) of a biological polymer can be measured using the sessile drop method (*see* Figure C.1). This is one of the simplest laboratory tests to perform, and is also com-

monly referred to as the 'water in air' method (when water is used as the probe liquid). It involves introducing a drop of water (or **saline**) onto the material or lens surface and measuring the angle at the solid/liquid/air interface. The introduction and measurement are both carried out in air, which means that the liquid will be in equilibrium with its vapour.

In theory, measurement of the contact angle by this method requires minimal specialist equipment, since the drop produced can be photographed or projected and the angle readily measured from the image produced. In practice, a fairly inexpensive piece of equipment named a goniometer is usually used. The goniometer consists of a telescope at the end of which is a platform where the sample is placed. The telescope has a crosshair in the eyepiece, which is rotated until it corresponds to an imaginary tangent to the profile of the droplet. The value of the contact angle is then simply read from a graticule to the nearest 1°.

This laboratory test is difficult to perform in a *clinical* environment, and it does not predict how well a material will perform on a specific eye.

settling time, contact lens
Soft lenses alter their fitting characteristics during a period of equilibration due to differences in temperature, pH and osmolarity between the lens storage solution and eye. Lenses tend to show less movement after this period of settling. In some cases, lenses exhibit gross **tightness** immediately after insertion and are unlikely to show sufficient improvement on settling. Many fitting guides recommend a long settling period before assessing lens fit, particularly in the case of high water content lenses (e.g. 30 minutes); however, this is frequently impractical and unnecessary. High **water content** ionic lenses stabilize within a 10–15-minute period. In most cases, lens fit can be assessed 5 minutes after lens insertion. A fast blink rate appears to quicken lens settling.

The initial reaction of new patients to rigid lenses can give an indication of how easily they are going to adapt to **rigid lens** wear. Clearly, those showing little or no lacrimation, and who are able to move their eyes without apparent discomfort, are the most promising candidates for successful rigid lens wear. In these cases, the lens fit can be assessed immediately. However, in most cases it will be necessary to wait 5–10 minutes for excess lacrimation to subside. This period can be used to discuss aspects of the process, such as costs, hygiene, lens maintenance etc., and to answer any questions.

In a few cases when fitting either soft or rigid lenses, it may be some time before lacrimation subsides enough to allow examination. It is necessary, however, to consider other possible reasons for the discomfort. This might be due to a foreign body attached to the lens (the **tears** usually clear any loose foreign bodies), or the fit might be so poor as to be causing some mechanical trauma to the **cornea** or **conjunctiva**. Having ruled out other causes of discomfort, it might be necessary to allow a longer settling period, e.g. 10–30 minutes. It is preferable that the patient does not leave the practice during this period.

silicone acrylates
See rigid contact lens.

silicone elastomer
See silicone rubber.

silicone hydrogel contact lenses
Owing to their silicone content, these **soft lenses** have **oxygen permeability** values that are far in excess of conventional **hydrogel** lenses. A major hurdle in developing these lenses was to work out how to combine the elements of hydrophobic **silicone rubber** with those of a typical hydrophilic hydrogel-forming monomer such as **HEMA**, to form a co-polymer that combines the properties of both. The logical answer was to combine HEMA with the monomer that has been so successfully used in the preparation of rigid lens materials, commonly referred to as TRIS; however, this presented the same fundamental difficulty as trying to combine oil and water to form an optically clear product. Phase separation occurs and the optical clarity of the product is impaired.

PureVision (balafilcon; **Bausch & Lomb**) is based on a substantially homogeneous co-polymer of a vinyl carbamate derivative of TRIS (Figure S.4), giving a water content of 35%, a *Dk* of 110 Barrer, and a water transport slightly (10%) in excess of that of polyHEMA. Focus Night & Day (lotrafilcon; **CIBA Vision**) is described as a lens that contains both ion transport and oxygen transport phases running from the anterior to the posterior surfaces. The biphasic structure of the material is produced by co-polymerizing a fluoroether macromer with TRIS monomer and N,N-dimethyl acrylamide (which acts both as a hydrophilic monomer and a polymerizable solvent) in the presence of a non-polymerizable diluent. The resultant material is a fluoroether-based silicone hydrogel with a water content of 24% and a *Dk* of 140 Barrer.

Both of the lenses described above are treated using gas plasma techniques, but whereas Bausch &

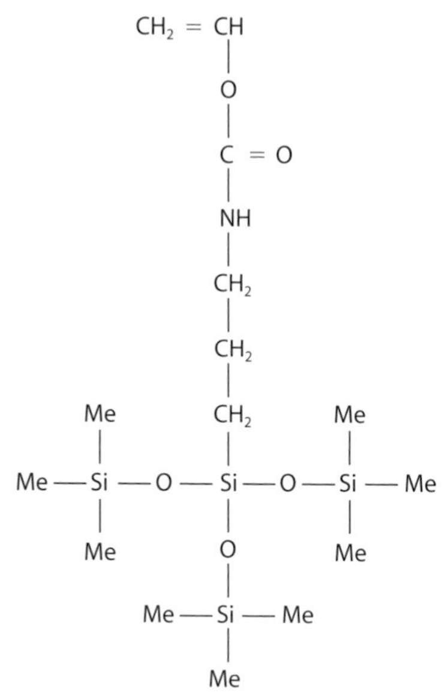

Figure S.4 Vinyl carbamate derivative of TRIS molecule (TRISCV). Me = CH_3.

Lomb has opted for plasma oxidation, CIBA Vision has chosen to apply a plasma coating. In the former case (PureVision), oxidation of TRIS produces hydrophilic glassy silicate islands on the surface, whereas the surface of Focus Night & Day is coated with a 25-nm thick, dense, high **refractive index** coating. These differences are at an atomic level, and are not evident on clinical inspection of the lenses.

Because of their extremely high oxygen performance, silicone **hydrogel** lenses can be used for **extended wear** without inducing excess **oedema** – a factor that has severely limited the application of hydrogel materials as **extended-wear** lenses.

silicone rubber
Silicone rubber belongs to a group of materials, known as synthetic elastomers, that are not only flexible but show rubber-like behaviour – i.e. they are capable of being compressed or stretched, and when the deforming force is removed they instantaneously return to their original shape. They consist of **polymer** chains that possess high mobility and are cross-linked at intervals along the polymer backbones. Because of this chain mobility, oxygen is able to diffuse rapidly through the structure. These polymers have **oxygen permeabilities** more than 100 times greater than that of **PMMA**. Silicone rubber is the most significant member of the group, with an

oxygen permeability around 1000 times greater than that of PMMA. This extremely high oxygen permeability arises from the backbone of alternate silicone and oxygen atoms, which confers not only great freedom of rotation but also a much higher solubility for oxygen than rubbery polymers with simple carbon backbones.

Silicone rubber lenses, surface treated to enhance wettability, were developed in the mid-1960s and found clinically to have little deleterious effect on corneal respiration. However, the problems of maintaining adequate surface properties (Figure S.5), which were initially encountered during routine clinical use, have never been fully overcome. Furthermore, silicone rubber lenses tended to develop tremendous suction forces and were very difficult to remove from the eye. As a result, silicone rubber lenses are used only rarely today. The uniquely high oxygen permeability of the silicon–oxygen backbone has, however, been harnessed in two distinct types of contact lens material: **silicone hydrogel lenses** and **rigid lenses**.

simultaneous vision lenses for presbyopia

A variety of simultaneous lens designs are available in both rigid and soft materials. The recent availability of single-use disposable soft trial lenses and empirically ordered individually based **aspheric rigid lenses** has resulted in increased prescribing of this form of lens correction.

In simultaneous vision designs, the distance and near correction zones are both positioned in front of the pupil in every direction of gaze so that light from either a distant or near object passes through both zones. As fixation is directed to either a distant or a near object, one zone produces a focused image while the other produces a blurred image that overlaps the same retinal elements as the focused one. The simultaneous images placed on the retina by any optical system rely on the visual system being able to select the clearer picture and to ignore the out-of-focus image, whether a distant or near object is being viewed.

The spread of light from the defocused image reduces the contrast of the focused image. As a result, the fitting of a simultaneous vision lens is likely to result in a reduction in image quality in comparison to that resulting from a single vision correction. The extent of contrast loss will depend upon the relative amounts of in-focus to out-of-focus light striking the retina. If equal contrast is to be achieved for both near and far viewing, the refractive system should allow approximate equality of the area of the two portions of the lens transmitting to the pupil. Lens performance may be affected by many factors, which include **pupil** size, lens design and centration of optics relative to the pupil.

The following simultaneous vision lens designs are available:

1. *Bi-concentric designs*. Early soft and rigid simultaneous vision **bifocal lenses** were bi-concentric in design, consisting of two discrete zones of distance and near power. A centre–distance design has the central portion of the optical zone for distance vision, which is surrounded by an area containing the near power. The ratio split between light forming the distance image to that forming the near image can be controlled for a given **pupil** size by altering the diameter of the central segment. As the pupil is a dynamic structure, a fundamental concern with such a design is its dependency on the pupil size. The near pupil reaction means that, as a near object is brought into view, proportionally less of the pupil allows light in from the near zone of the centre distance design. In addition, as the eye ages the pupil naturally decreases in size, resulting in less light from the near portion of the lens and a reduction in near-vision quality. In low luminance levels the pupil naturally dilates, resulting in more light proportionally from the near zone and a reduction in the quality of distance vision. In centre–near designs the optical principle is the same as for the centre–distance lens but reversed, so that the central portion of the lens focuses the light from close objects and this is surrounded by a distance powered area. The design remains pupil-dependent; therefore,

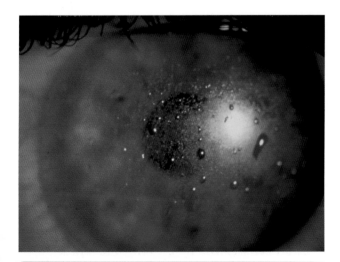

Figure S.5 Poorly-wetting surface of a silicone elastomer lens.

in bright conditions giving pupil constriction, distance vision becomes progressively less clear. Bi-concentric designs in both soft and rigid materials are still available, but are now used less frequently due to the availability of more advanced, easier to fit designs, and single-use **disposable lenses**.

2. *Multi-zone concentric designs*. A consequence of the above discussion is that benefits should be possible if the dependency of lens function on pupil size could be minimized, especially in relation to different lighting conditions. One approach is to increase the number of concentric zones and to power these zones alternatively for distance and near vision. The width and spacing of the zones is based on the variation of pupil size in different illuminations within the presbyopic population. Theoretically, this lens design favours distance vision in extreme high and low lighting conditions, and provides a more equal ratio of light division in ambient illumination conditions.

3. *Diffractive bifocal contact lenses*. These use refraction to correct distance vision, and a combination of refraction and diffraction to correct near vision. This is achieved by a diffractive 'zone plate' on the back surface of the lens, which is able to split the incident light passing through into two discrete focal points. Individual facets ('echelettes') are etched in a concentric ring pattern onto the posterior lens surface (Figure S.6). Each facet is only 2–3 μm deep and therefore will not traumatize the epithelium. As with any simultaneous vision lens, incident light is divided between the distance and near foci so that the intensities of these images are reduced and the images are superimposed on each other,

resulting in a reduction in retinal image quality. In addition, approximately 20% of incident light is lost to higher orders of diffraction, leaving 40% of light to make up each image. This may explain the greater reduction in low-contrast acuities with such lenses when compared to **monovision** correction. Diffractive lenses are largely independent of pupil size; however, like aspheric designs, they are dependent on lens centration.

4. *Aspheric designs*. With **aspheric designs**, the refractive power gradually changes from the geometric centre of the lens to the more peripheral area of the optic zone. Such lenses are best described as 'multifocal' due to the progression of powers, but can also be considered as a type of concentric design as the power distributions are concentric around the centre of the lens. By the nature of their design, lens function will vary with changes in pupil size. This will lead to variation in distance- and near-vision image contrast similar to that described previously for bi-concentric designs. Power distribution is produced by the use of a continuous aspheric surface of fixed or variable eccentricity. As with bi-concentric designs, aspheric lens designs can be subdivided according to whether the power distribution is most plus (least minus) centrally, resulting in a centre–near design, or most minus (least plus) centrally, resulting in a centre–distance design. Both options are available in soft and rigid materials.

single-use lenses
See daily disposable lenses.

slit-lamp biomicroscope
The slit-lamp biomicroscope plays an essential role in the **preliminary assessment** and **aftercare** of the prospective and existing contact lens wearer. The instrument consists of a separate illumination system (the slit lamp) and viewing system (the biomicroscope), which have a common focal point and centre of rotation (Figure S.7). A height control moves both systems simultaneously, and focusing and lateral movements are achieved via a joystick. This common control feature facilitates rapid and accurate positioning of the slit beam on the area of interest, and ensures that the microscope and illumination system are simultaneously in focus.

Virtually all slit-lamp manufacturers have adopted the Koeller illumination system, which is optically almost identical to that of a 35-mm slide projector. A bright illumination system (producing approximately 600 000 lux) is a fundamental

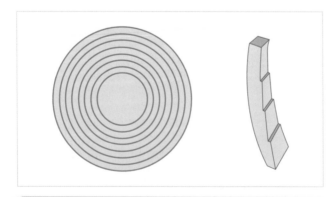

Figure S.6 Diffractive design of simultaneous vision lenses for the correction of presbyopia. Left: concentric design of facets. Right: Each facet is 3 μm deep.

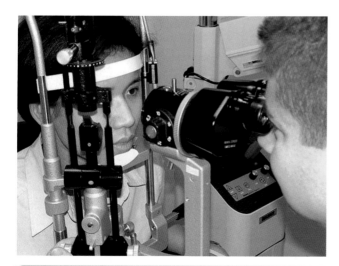

A key prerequisite for a slit-lamp biomicroscope is a viewing system that provides a clear image of the eye and has sufficient magnification for the practitioner to view all structures of interest. Ideally magnifications of up to ×40 should be possible, and this may be achieved through interchangeable eyepieces and/or variable magnification of the slit-lamp objective. Zoom magnification systems have the advantage of allowing the practitioner to focus on a particular structure without losing sight of it during changes in magnification. *See* slit-lamp biomicroscopy.

slit-lamp biomicroscopy
Slit-lamp biomicroscopy refers to the technique of using the **slit-lamp biomicroscope**. In the preliminary examination, biomicroscopy is used to assess the health of the anterior eye, and more specifically to screen for conditions or features that may be relevant to contact lens wear. Any observed signs should be reconciled with symptoms and assessment of the corneal curvature. Characteristics of the normal anterior eye, and the severity of any abnormalities that are detected, can be recorded with the assistance of **grading scales**. In fitting and aftercare examinations, slit-lamp biomicroscopy is also used to assess the fit of contact lenses and the effect of lenses on the anterior ocular structures. A normal technique is to use a variety of illumination methods – such as **direct focal illumination**, **indirect illumination**, **optic section**, **parallelepiped**, **retro-illumination**, **sclerotic scatter**, and **specular reflection** – and cobalt blue light for fluorescein staining.

requirement for a slit lamp if subtle conditions are to be seen clearly. While halogen or xenon lamps are more expensive than tungsten lamps, they are the preferred illumination source as they provide a brighter light, last longer, have better colour rendering, and generate less heat. Illumination brightness is controlled by a rheostat or multiposition switch that allows brightness to be adjusted to obtain the correct balance between patient comfort and optimal visibility of the area of interest. The slit within the illumination system must have sharply demarcated edges, and desirable features include the ability to:

● adjust slit width and height
● graduate the slit width
● rotate the lamp housing
● offset the slit beam.

A number of filters can be incorporated into the illumination system, which serve to enhance the visibility of certain conditions. These include:

● a green ('red-free') filter, which enhances contrast when looking for corneal and iris vascularization
● a neutral density (ND) filter, which reduces beam brightness and increases comfort for the patient
● a polarizing filter, which reduces unwanted specular reflections
● a diffusing filter, which diffuses the illumination source over a wide area
● a cobalt blue filter, which provides a suitable means of exciting sodium
● a Kodak Wratten 12 (yellow) filter, which is placed in front of the viewing system to enhance the contrast of any fluorescent staining observed with the cobalt blue light.

slit-lamp digital image capture
The basic principle of digital imaging is that a light-sensitive silicon computer chip is used instead of film in a camera. The silicon chip is known as a 'charge-coupled device' (CCD), and forms the light-sensitive element in video and digital cameras. The image can be instantly displayed on a computer screen, viewed by the practitioner and patient, then stored or printed (Figure S.8). The image digitization can take place at the camera or computer.

A digital image may be characterized in three main ways:

1. *Image resolution.* This refers to the image dimensions (width × height) in units of the number of dots (pixels). Common resolutions are 640 × 480 or 800 × 600, although a smaller image to fit into a digital record card – such as 320 × 240 – may also be acceptable.
2. *Colour depth.* This is the number of colours that may be specified for each pixel. For true colour, this should be in the thousands or millions.

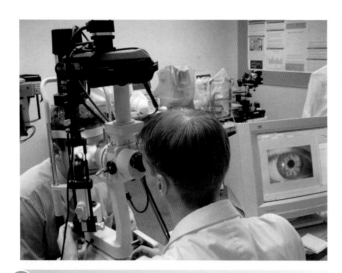

Figure S.8 Equipment for slit-lamp digital image capture.

3. *File format.* This describes the way an image is saved on disk and affects its compatibility with different programs for viewing, e-mailing etc. The Internet standard image file format is JPEG, and carries the benefit of small file size, high definition and broad compatibility with Internet e-mail and browser software.

There are numerous advantages to using digital photography instead of conventional 35-mm film photography. These include the following:

- reduced cost – once a digital imaging system is set up, an image can be captured instantly and at no additional cost
- instant imaging – digital imaging avoids the delay required for film processing in conventional photography, and thus any error in image focus or exposure can be immediately corrected
- patient education – there is a benefit in patients immediately seeing their own condition (for example, limbal **neovascularization**)
- live preview – with a video-based system the image may be previewed on screen and if necessary optimized before it is saved onto a hard disk
- no media costs – with digital imaging there is no ongoing cost for film or processing; although Polaroid photography gives a virtually instant result, it is relatively costly per print and the quality is limited
- ease of upgrade – many conventional slit lamps can be modified for digital imaging, by the addition of a beam splitter and camera; a normal **slit lamp** may be used with a flash rather than needing a specialized photographic slit lamp.

Digital image capture has a distinct advantage in that the captured images are in an electronic format; this opens up the following possibilities:

1. *Image transfer.* Increasingly, clinicians are communicating by electronic mail. A digital image is already on the computer, and this makes attachment to an e-mail easy. Images can be transferred by computer and modem to anywhere – this is the basis of 'telemedicine'.
2. *Presentations.* Images can be transferred to computer presentation programs, which are used for training and delivering lectures.
3. *Web pages.* Digital images can be readily transferred onto Internet web pages, and a similar approach used for storage and retrieval via an internal practice intranet.
4. *Video movies.* Dynamic conditions such as contact lens fittings or certain dynamic forms of pathology evaluation can be captured as a short movie on the computer. For example, a movie enables recording of the intricacies of lid interactions and the effects of lens centration on **fluorescein** patterns. *See* slit-lamp photography.

slit-lamp photography

Traditionally, the imaging system of choice for contact lens practice was a photographic slit-lamp biomicroscope using 35-mm or Polaroid film. A photographic slit lamp differs from a conventional slit lamp in that a flash tube is built in to the illumination system. The flash is necessary to provide sufficient illumination for correct exposure of photographic film. The camera is mounted on the slit lamp with a beam splitter attached to the observation system. *See* slit-lamp digital image capture.

soft contact lens

A small, circular transparent device that is placed directly onto the **cornea** to correct optical defects of vision. It is soft, it can be folded in half, and it is made from **hydrogel** materials. *Syn:* hydrogel lens.

soft lens on-eye power changes

When a **soft lens** is worn, its inherent flexibility allows it to 'drape' so that the shape of the posterior surface approximates closely to that of the anterior **cornea**. Although this greatly simplifies fitting, any associated changes in the curvatures of the lens surfaces and lens thickness may result in the on-eye power of the lens differing slightly from that measured off-eye.

Although draping implies that the **tear lens** between the contact lens and the cornea ought to have zero power, this may not always be the case. A tear lens of about 10 µl in volume may sometimes exist and contribute about −0.15 D of power to the combined lens–eye system. Although low minus lenses may entrap only a small volume of tears (about 5.5 µl), thicker, low plus lenses may entrap a greater volume (about 9.5 µl), giving a correspondingly greater tear lens effect (up to −2.00 D).

Changes in hydration – which are a function of the lens design and material, the wearer, the visual task and ambient environmental conditions – will affect the **refractive index** and geometry of any soft lens, and hence its power. Typically, hydration may fall by up to 8% after the first hour of lens wear. Thinner lenses reach equilibrium after about 5 minutes, whereas thicker, high-power positive lenses may continue to dehydrate for 30 minutes or more after insertion. Effects appear to be material-dependent; in particular, high water content lenses dehydrate more and reach equilibrium sooner than lower water content lenses of comparable thickness. Greater dehydration may occur during near work, due to reduced blinking, and when atmospheric humidity is low. Water loss can occur by several pathways, including evaporation into the atmosphere, drainage into the nasolacrimal system, and, possibly, absorption into the **conjunctival** capillaries.

As the corneal temperature is around 32–35°C, while the room temperature is normally about 20°C, there is a change in temperature when the lens is put on the eye; this affects all the lens parameters, including hydration and the refractive index. However, the associated power change would only be about 0.25 D for a ±10.00 D lens.

Theoretical and empirical models have been developed to allow overall on-eye power changes to be predicted. Among the more mathematically sophisticated models of flexure alone are those based on the concept that the flexed lens always retains constant volume or that the arc length of the back optic zone of the lens remains constant. Any power changes are small for negative lenses, but larger, clinically significant changes, which increase with the lens power, occur for positive lenses. For practical work the most sensible approach is to conduct a trial lens fitting, since, after suitable equilibration, the trial lens will display similar on-eye effects to those of the ordered lens of the same design and power.

soilation
See deposits, lens.

specific gravity, rigid lens
The specific gravity (SG) of a material is a ratio defined as its density divided by the density of water (thus, the SG of water is unity).

The density of **hydrogel** polymers depends upon both the water content and the monomer composition. Typical contact lens co-polymers containing **HEMA** and the more hydrophilic monomers decrease progressively from a specific gravity around 1.16 at 38% water content to around 1.05 at 75% water content (all at 20°C).

If a **rigid lens** is placed in a saturated saline solution, it will float on condition that the SG of the lens is less than that of saturated **saline** (1.197). Adding distilled water to the saline reduces the SG, and the lens will sink when the SG falls below the SG of the lens material. By adding saturated saline to the solution the SG will gradually increase and the lens will start to float again. At this point, no more saline is added. The SG of the lens material is the same as the SG of the surrounding saline. Using a hygrometer, the SG of the saline (and hence that of the lens material) can be measured, and the material identified from a table. This simple technique, which is referred to as 'densitometry', is dependent upon ambient conditions, and is limited by the available range of SG of the saturated immersion fluid.

An alternative approach is to use 20 tubes containing progressively changing concentrations of calcium chloride solution to give specific gravity readings between 1.00 and 1.20. The principle underlying these techniques is shown in Figure S.9.

spectacle magnification
Spectacle magnification, as its name implies, describes the ratio of the image size in the corrected **ametropic** eye to that in the uncorrected eye. It is

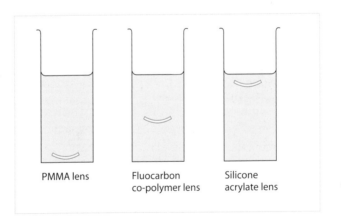

PMMA lens   Fluocarbon   Silicone
                   co-polymer lens   acrylate lens

Figure S.9 The three tubes each contain a solution with a specific gravity (SG) of 1.1. The lens in the centre tube has a SG of 1.1 and displays 'equiflotation'. The PMMA lens in the left tube has a SG of 1.2 and sinks to the bottom. The silicone acrylate lens in the right tube has a SG of less than 1.1 and floats to the top.

particularly significant in cases of **anisometropia** (where after correction the differential magnification of the two retinal images may give rise to symptoms of **aniseikonia**) and with cylindrical errors (where the different magnifications in the two principal meridians caused by the correction may lead the patient to complain of distorted images).

The retinal images of any object in the eyes of an uncorrected ametrope have a size that is governed by the chief rays passing from the extremities of the object through the centres of the entrance and exit pupils of the eye. Each image point will, of course, be blurred. While placing a contact lens on the cornea does not affect the course of the chief ray, and hence does not alter the size of the retinal image, this is not the case with a spectacle lens. A positive correction increases the angle that the chief ray makes with respect to the axis, whereas a negative correction reduces it.

The spectacle magnification will be unity for contact lenses (vertex distance = 0), less than unity for negative, **myopic** spectacle corrections, and greater than one for positive corrections. Spectacle correction is often expressed as the percentage by which it differs from unity, so that a spectacle magnification of ×1.05 would be described as '5% magnification'.

In practice, corrections cannot strictly be treated as thin lenses and the entrance and exit pupils do not lie at the **cornea**. For practical purposes, the pupils may be taken as being situated about 3 mm behind the cornea. Magnification is a function of both lens design and vertex distance (Figure S.10). Spectacle magnification is always close to unity for contact lenses, so that there are likely to be few magnification-related complaints from patients when moving directly from no correction to a contact lens correction, or from one contact lens correction to another. Casual contact lens wearers who normally wear spectacle corrections may theoretically notice spatial distortion, although for myopes this is counterbalanced by the benefit of relatively larger retinal images, which may improve acuity. Spectacle magnification effects after corneal refractive surgery are similar to those with contact lenses.

specular microscope

The specular microscope allows viewing of objects illuminated from the same side as the light source, and the objective lens also acts as the condenser lens. Light passes from inside the microscope out through the objective lens to arrive at a focus near the focal plane of the lens. If this position coincides with a reflecting surface, the focused light is reflected back through the objective lens and is

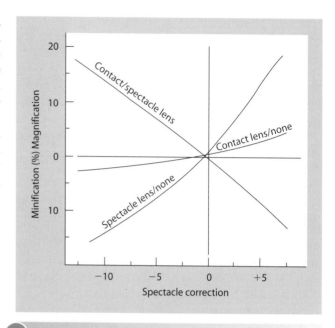

Figure S.10 Typical values for spectacle magnification obtained with spectacle lens and contact lens corrections. The ratio of the two spectacle magnifications is shown. Effectivity has been allowed for, so that points on any vertical line refer to the same ametropia. Adapted from G. Westheimer (1962) The visual world of the new contact lens wearer. *J. Am. Optom. Assoc.* **39**, 135–138.

viewed through the eyepiece of the microscope. This technique enables high magnification images of the **corneal epithelium and endothelium** to be made, which would otherwise be difficult due to their transparency.

Early versions of the specular microscope used a contact dipping cone objective lens that was optically coupled to the **cornea** to provide higher magnification and resolution; however, most modern clinical specular microscopes can achieve equally high magnification without the need for ocular contact (Figure S.11). These instruments are primarily used to view and photograph the corneal endothelium and to monitor its morphology. By direct viewing with the specular microscope, an overall impression of the condition of the endothelium can be established immediately. In addition, some of these instruments allow corneal thickness to be determined by measuring the distance between the epithelium and endothelium.

Typically, the features looked for are the regularity of the endothelial mosaic, the size of the individual cells, the presence of intracellular vacuoles, and abnormal features such as corneal guttae and keratic precipitates. From the images obtained, factors such as the number of cells per unit area, cell shape and

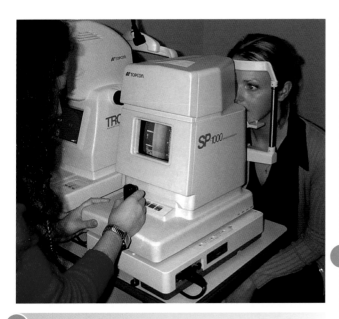

Figure S.11 Specular microscope used for endothelial evaluation.

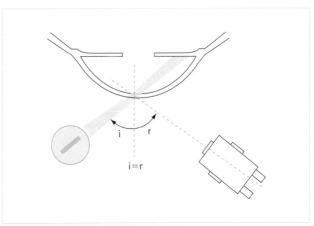

Figure S.12 Specular reflection slit-lamp technique. Adapted from L. W. Jones and D. A. Jones (2001) Slit lamp biomicroscopy. In *The Cornea: its Examination in Contact Lens Practice* (N. Efron, ed.), pp.1–49, Butterworth-Heinemann.

cell area can be calculated, enabling the clinician to assess the endothelial appearance compared with that expected of normal age-matched individuals. This instrument can be used to investigate endothelial changes in a number of disease conditions, including posterior polymorphous dystrophy and Fuch's dystrophy, and in corneal surgery, refractive surgery and contact lens wear. In addition, **deep stromal opacities** such as glass foreign bodies, pigment deposits and corneal dystrophies can be imaged.

specular reflection, slit-lamp technique of

This is a specific case of a **parallelepiped** set-up, where the angle of the incident slit beam is equal to the angle of the observation axis through one of the oculars (Figure S.12). At this angle (typically 40–50°) the illumination beam is reflected from the smooth surfaces of the anterior segment and provides a mirror-like reflection. Such specular images occur at every interface between structures of different refractive indices. The technique of specular reflection is typically used to view the endothelium, and may reveal changes such as **endothelial blebs**, guttae and **polymegethism**. However, even at ×40 magnification only a gross clinical judgement of the endothelium can be made as individual cells can be barely seen. The **tear film** lipid layer and the inferior tear meniscus can also be readily examined, as well as the anterior surface of the crystalline lens. If a contact lens is being worn, front surface wetting can be assessed and the post-lens tear film may be observed using specular reflection.

spherical power equivalent rigid bitoric lens

See compensated rigid bitoric lens.

spherical rigid lens designs

Spherical designs incorporating a spherical back optic zone with a number of flatter spherical peripheral zones are the most widely used and readily understood form of **rigid lens**. The peripheral zone is generally 1–2 mm in width and is composed of one to four peripheral curves. Tricurve designs (i.e. a central curve plus two peripheral zones) are probably the most commonly used lens form. Bicurve designs are occasionally used with small lenses (e.g. < 8.5 mm). Tetracurve and other multicurve designs are used with larger lenses, or where a smoother transition is required between the peripheral zones.

The front surfaces of most spherical designs are bicurve, incorporating an optic zone slightly larger than the **back optic zone diameter** (BOZD), and a front surface peripheral zone. The curvature of the front optic zone is governed by the required lens power, and that of the peripheral zone by the edge thickness, power and **front optic zone diameter** (FOZD) of the lens; these parameters are invariably calculated by the manufacturing laboratory. Monocurve front surface designs (single-cut) are occasionally used in small, low-power lenses, but most lenses are lenticulated (i.e. made with a thinner peripheral zone) in order to reduce mass and overall thickness. Multicurve front surface designs are occasionally used with higher-power lenses in order to reduce peripheral thickness.

spin casting

This process can be used to manufacture **soft lenses**. A convex 'male-shaped' stainless steel tool, or 'insert', is produced on a high-precision engineering lathe and lapped to provide an accurate surface that matches the dry dimensions of the proposed anterior surface of the contact lens. The final surface shape of the steel master is verified using interferometry. Any given tool can be used to make millions of moulds. The steel tool is impressed against heated liquid polypropylene, which then cools and sets to form a solid plastic concave female mould. A series of about eight tools is used to produce eight moulds simultaneously.

The xerogel lens form is created by pouring liquid monomers into the concave moulds, which spin at a high rate about the central mould axis. This takes place in a controlled atmosphere of carbon dioxide at high temperature. The shape of the mould defines the form of the front surface of the lens. The shape of the back surface is governed by centrifugal force generated by the rate of spin of the mould, surface tension and friction forces between the mould and **polymer**, and the effects of gravity. A greater speed of rotation of the mould will result in more polymer mass being shifted towards the lens periphery, and more negative lens power.

As the mould spin rate stabilizes, a catalytic monomer is added and ultraviolet radiation is introduced to initiate polymerization. The lens is removed from the mould, and the mould is discarded. The edges of the lens are polished, and the lens is inspected, hydrated, re-inspected, packaged and autoclaved. In modern industrial settings (Figure S.13), spin casting can produce a much higher lens yield than **lathe cutting**, but still can not match the high volume of lenses that can be produced by **cast moulding**.

spoilation
See deposits, lens.

sport, contact lenses for
Sport and recreation are often cited as key reasons for seeking contact lenses. With modern contact lens

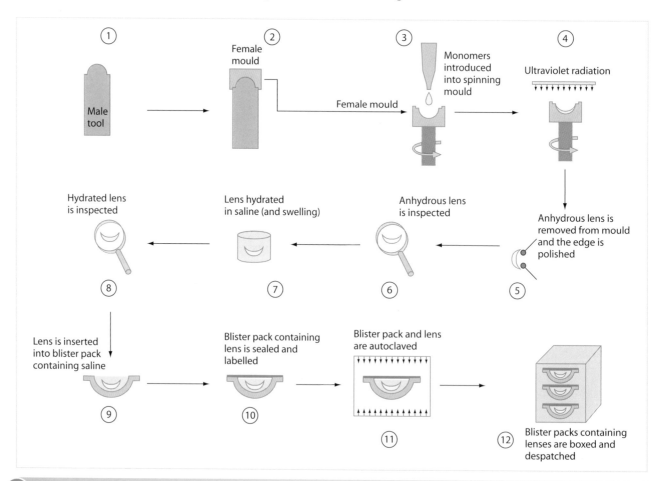

Figure S.13 Schematic representation of a production line for spin cast manufacturing of soft contact lenses.

technology, there is no reason why an **ametropic** sportsperson cannot compete with a normally sighted opponent on an equal basis from the standpoint of visual function. The three primary vision correction options are **soft contact lenses**, **rigid contact lenses**, or spectacles. **Scleral lenses** are sometimes prescribed, but only if circumstances dictate the necessity. A comparison of the key features of the three primary options is presented in Table S.1. Refractive surgery, of course, represents a more radical alternative.

The choice of contact lens for use in a given sport must be made with reference to the length of time that it takes to play the sport, the environment in which it is played, and the general physical demands of the sport. The majority of sports are completed within 2 hours, which equates to a total period of lens wear of 4 hours, allowing for pre- and post-match activity during which lens insertion and removal would be impractical and/or undesirable. Even when these factors are understood, the lens of first choice may not be obvious. The most appropriate lens is sometimes only determined by trial and error.

Sports are played in almost every environment. Perhaps the only environment that is *not* sought for the playing of sport is extreme heat. The most suitable lenses for various environmental conditions are as follows:

- cold – large-diameter, medium **water content** soft lenses
- altitude – high oxygen performance **silicone hydrogel lenses**
- dirt and dust – large-diameter soft lenses; rigid lenses are prone to trap debris beneath the lens and are clearly contraindicated
- aquatic sports – large-diameter, medium water content lenses; goggles worn over contact lenses will, in the same way as worn by a non-lens wearer, ensure good vision, and help to preserve ocular health and reduce lens loss
- sub-aquatic sports – silicone hydrogel lenses, to facilitate the escape of nitrogen gas from beneath the lens; good **blinking** is important
- ultraviolet light – goggles with UV-absorbing tints, to be worn over UV-absorbing contact

Table S.1 Comparison of soft lenses versus rigid lenses versus spectacle lenses for the sportsperson

characteristic	soft lenses	rigid lenses	spectacle lenses
field of view	full	full	restricted
stability of vision (post-blink)	excellent	good	excellent
glare	none	in low light	none
glare protection tint possible	cosmetic only	no	yes
UV protection tint possible	yes	yes	yes
initial comfort	good	poor	good
long-term comfort	good	good	good
adaptation required	very little	yes	sometimes
suitability for intermittent use	yes	not usually	yes
disposability viable	yes	no	no
risk of loss	low	moderate	low
risk of dislodgement during wear	low	moderate	high
risk of damage during wear	low	low	high
risk of damage with handling	high	low	low
ease of care	multiple-step	fewer steps	simple
initial cost	moderate	high	high
ongoing costs	high	moderate	none
cost to correct astigmatism	high	low	low
bifocal correction possible	compromise	very difficult	yes
use in rain	good	good	poor
susceptibility to fog up	no	no	yes
susceptibility to dirt up	no	no	yes
risk of complication	low	negligible	none

lenses, constitute an extra precaution for periods when the mask is removed; skiers should be reminded to also apply UV-protection creams to the remaining exposed skin on the face and neck. *See* prophylactic tints.

The most suitable lenses for various physical situations are as follows:

- extreme body movements – large-diameter soft lenses; rigid lenses are contraindicated
- body contact – large-diameter soft lenses, with supplementary eye and face protection via the use of helmets and masks; rigid lenses are contraindicated
- air flow – large-diameter, medium water content lenses with enclosed goggles; rigid lenses are contraindicated, and good blinking activity is required if goggles are not worn
- gravitational forces – large, **tight-fitting** soft lenses.

The following points are of particular relevance to the prescription and aftercare management of those involved in sport:

- for young sportspersons participating in outdoor sports, prescribe minimum plus power to facilitate sharp far-distance viewing
- **silicone hydrogel lenses** worn on an extended-wear basis are indicated for endurance events of such as rally car driving
- contact lenses are contraindicated (in favour of spectacles) for sports requiring critical static visual acuity, such as archery and shooting
- for routine contact lens care, the best time is immediately following the conclusion of the season
- athletes often come into contact with grip rosin, grease, tape dressings and ointments that are toxic to the eye and highly irritative, as well as dirt, soil or general contaminants; thus, hygiene and general **compliance** must be emphasized
- since contact lenses will not shield the eye from potential trauma, the usual protective eyewear or headgear used in a given sport should also be used by sportspersons wearing contact lenses
- for **presbyopic** sportspersons, monovision is generally contraindicated, and a spectacle over-correction is often the best option.

squamous cells of the epithelium
See corneal epithelium.

stabilization of rigid toric lenses
Three techniques are used to stabilize **rigid toric lenses**:

1. *Toroidal back surface.* With lenses incorporating a toroidal back surface, rotation is generally not a problem due to the stabilizing effect of the toric back surface on the toric **cornea** (provided there is sufficient corneal toricity).
2. *Prism ballast.* This is the most commonly used method of lens stabilization for rigid lenses that have toroidal front surfaces combined with spherical back optic zones. With prism ballasting, the lens is prescribed in the normal manner with the addition of between 1 and 3 Δ. When ordering the lens, practitioners assume that the weight or prism ballast orientates the lens in a certain fixed position on the cornea and order the cylinder axis with respect to this position. To avoid recording the prism base position as 'down along 90' or 'down along 100', its actual location is recorded as being at 270 or 280, respectively. Prism ballast may also be used in combination with a toroidal back surface where the corneal **astigmatism** of the patient is too small (< 2.00 D) to maintain the proper position of a bitoric lens but large enough (> 1.00 D) to cause a front toric lens to become unstable. Prism ballasting can often cause rigid lenses to sit inferiorly, causing patients to experience symptoms of **discomfort** and flare.
3. *Truncation.* A truncation is created by slicing off the bottom of the lens in such a way that when the truncation rests against the lower lid, the lens will adopt the correct orientation in the eye (Figure S.14). Truncations can also be added to front surface toric lenses if prism ballasting is insufficient to stabilize the lens. Truncations can be

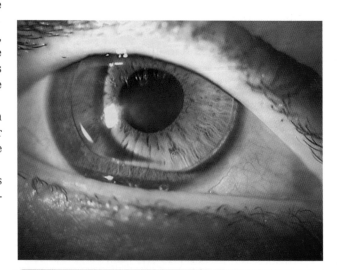

Figure S.14 A prism-ballasted rigid toric lens with a single truncation designed to align with the lower lid.

uncomfortable for the patient, and they are not always successful in preventing lens rotation. Consequently, a **soft toric contact lens** is generally preferred to a rigid toric contact lens when fitting patients who have significant residual astigmatism but negligible corneal astigmatism.

See compensated rigid bitoric lenses; cylindrical power equivalent rigid toric lenses; induced astigmatism with rigid toric lenses; residual astigmatism with rigid toric lenses; toric lens design, rigid; toric lens, rigid.

stabilization of soft toric lenses

All forms of **soft toric lenses** need to be stabilized so that the toric optics of the lens can be maintained in the correct orientation so as to correct the ocular **astigmatism**. The aim is to minimize rotation from the ideal in-eye orientation. The orientation of a soft toric lens on the eye must be predictable and consistent, otherwise sub-optimal vision will result. The following stabilization techniques can be employed:

1. *Toroidal back surface.* It is thought by some that a soft toric lens with a toric back surface will generally locate better than a front surface toric lens, because it is believed that the back toric surface is more likely to align with, or 'lock on' to, the matching toroidal **corneal** surface. However, experience has shown that a toroidal back surface alone is insufficient to achieve lens stabilization.

2. *Prism ballast.* The theory of prism ballast is that base down prism is incorporated into the lens so that the lens will be heavier at the prism base (due to excess lens mass). Gravity then acts to cause the prism base to locate inferiorly. This effect, however, is minimal. Prism ballast lenses work not because of the extra weight of the prism base, but because the thin apical zone is squeezed between the upper lid and eyeball.

3. *Peri-ballast.* This method of lens stabilization features a lens with a minus carrier (peripheral zone), with the carrier being thicker inferiorly. In other words, the prismatic thickness profile changes are confined to the lens carrier, where the carrier is thinner superiorly (prism base down).

4. *Truncation.* Truncation refers to the technique of slicing off the bottom of the lens, so as to form a 'shelf' that will rest upon (and therefore align with) the lower lid. There are problems with the use of truncation in soft toric lens fitting. The truncated edge can make the **soft lens** uncom-

fortable to wear, and the measurement of the lid angle can be difficult and imprecise. Quite often the truncation does not work, with the lid angle appearing to have no effect on the positioning or location of the truncated lens. Instability can occur with oblique cylinders because of the uneven thickness produced by them. For these reasons, soft toric lens truncation is rarely used today.

5. *Dynamic stabilization.* The technique of dynamic stabilization is currently the most commonly used method of stabilization for soft toric lenses (Figure S.15). With this technique, the dominant lens orientation effect is achieved by pressure from the upper lid (primarily) and the lower lid. The pressure exerted on the thin zones of a lens between the upper lid and globe and between the inferior lid and globe causes the lens to orientate correctly, with the thick zone of the lens lying horizontally between the lids.

See toric lens fitting, soft; toric lens rotation, soft; toric lens, soft.

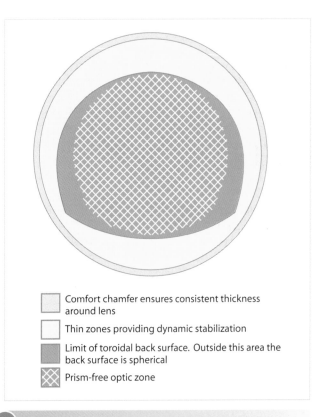

☐ Comfort chamfer ensures consistent thickness around lens

☐ Thin zones providing dynamic stabilization

▨ Limit of toroidal back surface. Outside this area the back surface is spherical

▨ Prism-free optic zone

Figure S.15 Design features of a soft toric lens that help to minimize lens rotation by dynamic stabilization. Note the prism-free optic zone in the toroidal region of the lens.

staff, contact lens practice
See personnel, contact lens practice.

staff training in contact lens practice
Staff training embraces the identification and development of employee potential for job satisfaction, improvement, practice value creation and ultimately improved patient care. It can often be the driver of improvements, and has the potential to bring about reduced costs, increased value and practice profitability. Ultimately, training is about getting people to do different things or to do things differently.

For training to be effective for the practice, however, it must be:

- valid – i.e. relevant to jobs in the practice, and to the overall style of the practice (e.g. a specialty contact lens practice)
- capable of solving problems identified as needing resolution in practice
- focused on objectives, either at the individual or at the job/practice level
- measurable, with results that can be gauged directly or indirectly.

Improvements that training and development bring should result in reduced costs and increased value and profits through (for example):

- improved efficiency – doing the job correctly, accurately and with care at the outset reduces replacements, unplanned rescheduling and revisits to the practice by patients, and this improves utilization of resources and practice output overall
- improved quality – this enhances the reputation of the practice, and reduces complaints, costs of returns, refunds and credits
- less wastage and re-working – this leads to less material being wasted, but the greater cost saving is in the staff costs, the time for which the equipment is occupied, and the ancillary costs in re-working the job by the laboratory (e.g. a complete pair of spectacles, alternative set of contact lenses etc.)
- improved consulting room and equipment utilization – consulting room occupancy and equipment use dictates the capacity of the practice to conduct eye exams and contact lens consultations; an unnecessarily occupied or indeed unoccupied consulting room is costly
- reduced time taken to do jobs – less time taken to produce same or better quality products will translate to reduced staff costs relative to sales revenues
- improved time management – this translates to improved patient scheduling and staff usage, which will lead to reduced staff costs relative to sales revenues
- reduced staff turnover – this means that costs of recruitment, selection, training and reduced efficiency are not unnecessarily incurred
- reduced accidents and equipment 'downtime' – this reduces costs to the practice in terms of sick pay, 'down time' of equipment, compensation claims, insurance premiums, unscheduled service costs and replacements
- reduced sickness and absenteeism – greater job satisfaction means better staff morale and efficient teamwork.

Training alone is not the driver of these benefits. Other factors that affect these issues include economic, political and employment situations locally and in the country. An important decision for the practice owner/manager is to decide what training can be done by the practice itself and what external support will be required.

steep lens fit
A lens that has a curvature greater than that of the anterior eye (especially the **cornea**) is deemed to be fitting steep. The degree of steepness cannot be predicted simply by comparing the **back optic zone radius** of the lens with central corneal curvature, because the curvature of both the lens and the cornea can change dramatically towards the periphery. In general, a steep-fitting lens will appear to be tight. A steep rigid lens fit, when examined using **fluorescein**, will display a broad region of central clearance and substantial peripheral bearing (Figure S.16).

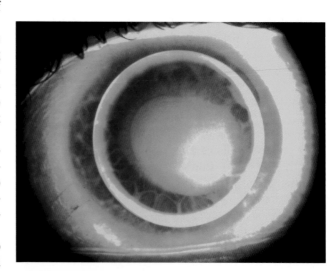

Figure S.16 Steep-fitting rigid lens revealed by fluorescein.

sterile keratitis
See keratitis, sterile.

Stevens–Johnson syndrome
See eyelid pathology, therapeutic lenses for.

stock kept unit
See practice logistics.

stock lenses
See practice logistics.

storage case, contact lens
An important component of the complete lens care system is the case in which the lenses and disinfecting solutions are stored. Surveys have reported that up to 77% of lens cases are contaminated with bacteria and 8% with **Acanthamoeba**. Contamination appears to be unrelated to solution type, and it is now clear that the development of microbial biofilms in contact lens cases can reduce the effect of a disinfecting solution. Indeed, it has been speculated that long-term use of a solution might select a naturally resistant population of microbes that adapt to survive exposure to a disinfectant. Interestingly, some bacteria release catalase when their cell membranes are disrupted; this release could potentially act to neutralize local **hydrogen peroxide** and protect other bacteria within the biofilm.

The careful cleaning of lens cases has been advocated by some practitioners. This can include measures such as manually scrubbing the case (using a cotton-wool bud or new toothbrush) with cooled boiled water, or submersing the case in boiling water on a regular basis. However, with **compliance** acknowledged to be poor in a high proportion of lens wearers, this approach might be unrealistic. Certainly, rinsing the contact lens case with fresh disinfecting solution after lens insertion and leaving the case open to air dry is likely to be helpful. It is clear, however, that the regular replacement of contact lens cases for both **soft and rigid lenses** is an effective method of reducing this potential problem. Many manufacturers assist practitioners in this regard by supplying a new contact lens case with each bottle of disinfecting solution.

stress test
See extended wear.

striae
See oedema.

stroma
See corneal stroma.

stromal edema
See oedema.

stromal microdots
See microdots.

stromal neovascularization
See neovascularization.

stromal oedema
See oedema.

stromal opacities
See deep stromal opacities.

stromal thinning
Although low levels of stromal **oedema** during the day may appear to be harmless, there is a growing body of evidence indicating that chronic oedema may compromise the physiological integrity of the **cornea**. It is now clear that long-term extended wear of hydrogel lenses can induce a slight thinning of the stroma. Whereas the extent of stromal oedema varies with the prevailing level of corneal oxygenation and dissipates upon removal of hypoxic stress, stromal thinning is a chronic and apparently irreversible tissue change observed in patients who have worn lenses for many years.

Extended wear of **hydrogel** lenses causes the stroma to thin at a rate of 2 µm per year (Figure S.17).

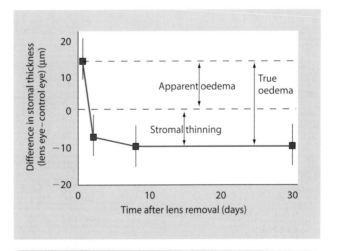

Figure S.17 Change in corneal thickness of lens-wearing eyes (compared with 'normal' non-lens-wearing eyes; the dotted zero line) after ceasing wear of hydrogel lenses that had been worn on an extended wear basis for 5 years. When the lenses were removed (t = 0), the lens-wearing eye was apparently about 14 µm thicker than the normal eye. However, after 7 days, when all oedema had subsided, the cornea of the lens-wearing eye was about 25 µm thinner than it had been originally, representing the true oedema. This suggests that long-term extended hydrogel lens wear induced 11 µm of stromal thinning.

This phenomenon can be of clinical significance; for example, patients who have worn contact lenses for many years may be precluded from undergoing laser ablative refractive surgery if too much thinning has occurred.

The phenomenon of contact lens induced stromal thinning does *not* confound or invalidate interpretation of the clinical signs of stromal oedema. Striae, folds and haze represent a given level of oedema irrespective of whether or not the stroma has thinned.

It is presumed that stromal thinning is due to the effects of chronic oedema, and two mechanisms may be postulated to explain how this might occur. First, stromal keratocytes may lose their ability to synthesize new stromal tissue due to the direct effects of tissue **hypoxia**, and/or the indirect effects of chronic lens-induced tissue acidosis due to an accumulation of lactic acid and carbonic acid. Second, constantly elevated levels of lactic acid associated with chronic oedema may lead to some dissolution of the mucopolysaccharide ground substance of the stroma. Recent evidence obtained using confocal microscopy demonstrates a loss of stromal keratocytes following long-term hydrogel lens wear.

subjective refraction

The subjective refraction may be best performed in a trial frame, since many contact lens patients are young and the trial frame may be less likely to induce **accommodation** than the phoropter. Even if 6/6 vision is achieved, it is useful to check the subjective refraction in each eye with the spectacles or contact lenses that the patient presents with, as they may reveal excess minus power that could account for symptoms unrelated to visual acuity (such as asthenopia or binocular vision problems).

It is necessary with non-**presbyopic** patients to adopt a technique with the refraction so as to relax accommodation. Measuring blur function is one such method, whereby the addition of +0.50 D or +0.75 D lenses is expected to blur the 6/6 line significantly. *See* over-refraction.

superficial cells of the epithelium
See corneal epithelium.

superior limbic keratoconjunctivitis

In its mild form, contact lens induced superior limbic keratoconjunctivitis (CLSLK) is easy to overlook. The condition is confined to the superior limbal area, and as such is hidden by the upper lid in primary gaze. The proper procedure for observing this condition is to lift the upper lid while the patient gazes down.

A myriad of signs are observed in the region of the superior limbus in patients with CLSLK (Figure S.18); these include:

- punctate epithelial **fluorescein** staining
- epithelial **rose bengal** staining
- intra-epithelial opacities
- sub-epithelial haze
- epithelial dulling
- **microcysts**
- infiltrates and irregularities
- stromal fibrovascular micro-pannus
- fine sub-epithelial linear opacities
- limbal **oedema**
- tissue hypertrophy
- vascular injection
- poor wetting, punctate staining, hyperaemia, chemosis and irregular thickening of the superior bulbar **conjunctiva**
- papillary and follicular hypertrophy
- hyperaemia and petechiae of the upper tarsal conjunctiva
- corneal filaments
- **corneal warpage** and **astigmatism**
- corneal pseudo-dendrites.

The tissue compromise progresses from the limbus to the centre of the **cornea** in a V-shaped pattern with the apex directed towards the pupil centre. Symptoms of CLSLK include:

- increased lens awareness
- lens intolerance
- foreign body sensation
- burning
- itching
- photophobia

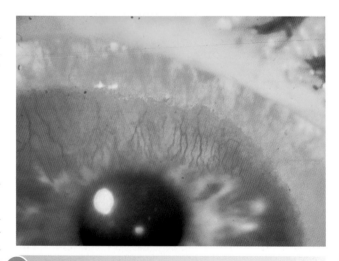

Figure S.18 Superior limbal keratoconjunctivitis.

- redness
- increased lacrimation
- slight mucus secretion
- slight loss of vision.

This condition occurs mostly in **soft lens** wearers, it is almost always bilateral, and the specific signs often display symmetry between the eyes. There is considerable variability in the time course of onset of the condition; signs usually become manifest between 2 months and 2 years of commencing lens wear.

The primary aetiological factor in the development of CLSLK is thimerosal hypersensitivity. Provocative tests in thimerosal-sensitized patients result in general circumlimbal redness (not just confined to the superior limbus), meaning that contact lens wear must be impacting on the clinical presentation of CLSLK, which is confined to the superior limbus. Although other factors perhaps play a minor role by initiating, modulating or exacerbating the condition, it is unlikely that CLSLK will develop in the absence of ocular contact with thimerosal. Other factors implicated in the aetiology of CLSLK include:

- thimerosal toxicity
- mechanical effects
- lens deposits
- **hypoxia** beneath the upper lid.

Patients suffering from CLSLK may be advised to cease lens wear for 2–4 weeks if less than Grade 2, and up to 3 months in severe cases (greater than Grade 2). All previously worn lenses should be discarded. Refitting can be undertaken when the corneal haze has largely resolved and the corneal surface is smooth (less than Grade 1); however, a vascular pannus may be permanent. Lens wear can be resumed in the presence of a vascular **pannus** as long as the patient is monitored closely to check for the absence of further vascular encroachment. Thimerosal and any other potentially allergenic preservatives should be excluded from the care system. Single-use **daily disposable lenses** are the best option. Ocular lubricants in the form of drops or ointments may provide symptomatic relief during the recovery phase, further to affording a positive placebo effect in a naturally anxious patient. Clinical signs and visual acuity will generally resolve within about 4 months of cessation of lens wear, although this can vary from 3 weeks to 9 months.

surface damage, lens

All soft lenses are manufactured with a 'shelf-life', which primarily indicates how long the lens can be guaranteed to be sterile. In addition, there is the possibility of natural **polymer** degradation over time, whereby clinically relevant changes may be noticed – typically on the lens surface – after about 5 years from the time of manufacture.

Physical trauma can also lead to a variety of lens **defects**. If a defect is obvious, such as a large piece of the lens breaking off, then the patient will typically notice this and discard the lens. If such a defect is not noticed, **discomfort** on **insertion** will normally alert the wearer to the problem. However, small defects may not be noticed, and this is potentially problematic because such defects can compromise ocular integrity at a sub-clinical level.

Rigid lenses can develop fine surface scratches over time (necessitating lens polishing), or fine splits (requiring lens replacement) (Figure S.19). Another ageing problem with rigid lenses is the development of crazing; that is, the appearance of interconnecting surface cracks that can extend deep into the lens. Crazing predisposes the lens to the development of secondary deposits, and the lens can become uncomfortable due to the crazing and/or the existence of deposits. Crazing can also be due to problems occurring during manufacture.

surface properties, soft lens

It is apparent that **soft lenses** do not suffer deficiencies in terms of inherent wettability, provided that they are fully hydrated. However, two contributing factors influence their behaviour in the eye. The first is the fact that the anterior surface of the lens will progressively lose water, especially in adverse environmental conditions. The second is that the **polymer** chains are able to rotate rapidly in response to a changed interface. When in contact with aqueous fluids, the hydrophilic groups rotate to the surface. Conversely, when in contact with more hydrophobic

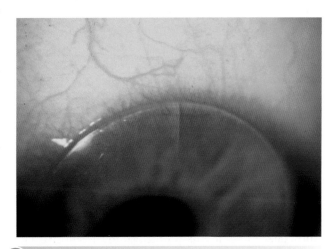

Figure S.19 Split in a rigid lens.

interfaces, such as air or lipids, the hydrophilic groups 'bury' themselves within the gel and a more hydrophobic surface is exposed. Chain rotation is a dynamic process, whereas evaporative water loss is a progressive process. Molecular processes such as protein deposition and denaturation are well able to respond to the dynamic processes, which is why the eye presents such a challenging environment. The progressive dehydration has a more influential effect on the gross surface properties of the **hydrogel**, and is part of the complex process that produces end-of-day discomfort for many wearers.

Two surface properties that can be used to characterize hydrogels are surface energy (which manifests itself as wettability) and the coefficient of friction (which underlies the biotribological behaviour of the lens). Both of these properties are linked to the water-binding ability of the lens. Frictional studies show that both synthetic hydrogels and natural hydrogels (e.g. the **cornea**) are normally lubricated by a hydrodynamic (water) boundary layer. This dominates the dynamic coefficient of friction to the extent that when an intact lubricating layer separates the hydrogel and substrate, it is the properties of the solution rather than those of the material or substrate that govern the value of sliding friction. The simplest analogy is that of a car aquaplaning – the ease of sliding is independent of the rubber from which the tyres have been fabricated. When this water layer breaks down, there is an increase in the resistance to sliding. The surface energy of a hydrogel is a more progressive property. It rises rapidly up to a water content of around 30%, and much more slowly thereafter. As previously stated, however, at a hydrophobic interface the surface energy drops dramatically because of chain rotation.

The clinical consequence of these facts is relatively simple to state, but complex to relate to direct measurement. All conventional hydrogels have very adequate wettability and frictional behaviour when fully hydrated, no matter what the initial **water content**. Problems only arise because of progressive dehydration and the dynamic responsiveness of the lens material to air and lipids (caused primarily by tear break-up). These processes in turn influence the irreversible deposition of tear components and the onset of symptoms such as end-of-day dryness, which are linked to biotribological phenomena.

surface wetting

A stable, uniform tear film over the surface of **soft and rigid lenses** is required to maintain good, stable vision. A surface with poor wetting characteristics will break up the prelens **tear film**, creating sources of light scatter, which will depreciate optical transmission and hence visual quality. High **oxygen permeability** (Dk) silicone-based lens materials have intrinsically poor wetting properties. The wettability of the surfaces of lenses made from these materials can be improved using a variety of manufacturing and chemical techniques, such as plasma treatment. Lens surface wetting properties are measured using a variety of techniques – e.g. the **captive bubble**, **Wilhelmy plate** and **sessile drop** methods. The wettability of a lens is typically expressed as the 'wetting angle' or 'contact angle', which is the angle between the test surface and the tangent of a fluid drop or air bubble in contact with the surface.

The friction from high-speed polishing may singe the lens surface and thus affect wettability. Chemical conditioning solutions may improve lens wettability *in vitro*, but not necessarily *in vivo*. Placing the lens on the eye and checking the stability of the prelens tear film using a **tear break-up** test is a useful *in vivo* clinical measurement of lens wetting. The Keeler **Tearscope** can assess lens wettability quantitatively and allow the clinician to categorize the structure of the pre-lens tear film (Figure S.20).

surfactant cleaning

There are two key reasons why a contact lens should be cleaned with a surfactant solution. First, a wide variety of intrinsic debris (tear-film products such as proteins, lipids and mucus) and extrinsic debris (environmental pollutants and cosmetics) can adhere to the surface of a contact lens. This can lead to lens distortion, **discomfort**, an unsightly cosmetic appearance (as soiled lenses can show marked discoloration clearly visible to an onlooker), ocular sur-

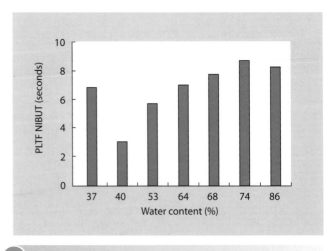

Figure S.20 Pre-lens tear film (PLTF) non-invasive break-up time (NIBUT) of hydrogel lenses of various water content, determined using a Tearscope.

face and **eyelid** pathology, and vision loss. Secondly, a cleaning action supplements the disinfection process by reducing the levels of micro-organisms on the contact lens. The processes of rinsing and rubbing lenses in the course of surfactant cleaning also lead to a reduction in the bioburden on the lens.

A common method of lens cleaning is to use a 'stand-alone' surfactant cleaner. The lens is placed in the palm of one hand, a few drops of surfactant cleaner are introduced into the concavity of the lens, and the forefinger of the other hand rubs the cleaner into the lens (Figure S.21). Agents that contain surfactant cleaners are detergents that solubilize debris from the lens surface. Furthermore, because the surfactant molecules have a hydrophilic end and a hydrophobic end, a monolayer is formed around lipid droplets created after physical dispersion of any lipid spoilation, creating a 'micelle'. With the hydrophobic end of the surfactant molecule 'buried' in the lipid droplet, and the hydrophobic end 'exposed', re-coalescence of the lipid due to repulsion of the electrical charges is prevented. Because the hydrophilic region is water soluble, the lipid spoilation can be emulsified.

Some surfactant cleaning products also contain other agents to assist with the cleaning process. Miraflow (**CIBA Vision**) contains 20% isopropyl alcohol as a lipid solvent. Opti-Free Daily Cleaner (**Alcon**) contains fine polymeric beads that provide a mildly abrasive characteristic, although this is not thought to affect the lens surface.

Most surfactant cleaners contain other agents such as preservatives to prevent microbial contamination after opening. In the case of Miraflow, the isopropyl alcohol acts as a preservative in addition to its lipid-removing characteristics. Other preservatives include sorbic acid and potassium sorbate. Due to the hypersensitivity reactions to thiomersal and **chlorhexidine**, these preservatives are rarely found in modern soft lens cleaners.

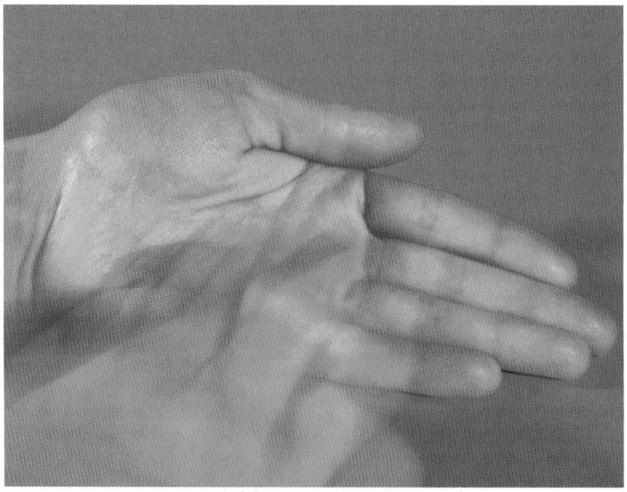

A number of cleaners contain ethylene diamine tetra-acetic acid (EDTA), or one of its salts, as a chelating agent. A chelating agent is a substance comprised of molecules that can form several co-ordinate bonds to a single metal ion. In the case of contact lens care, EDTA removes ions such as calcium, resulting in a lens-cleaning effect (protein can bind to calcium on the lens surface, and therefore increase deposition) and an antimicrobial effect (calcium ions are required for cell wall metabolism by micro-organisms). Phosphate or borate buffers are also included in the cleaner to stabilize solution pH.

Generally, **rigid lenses** are cleaned with a separate solution to the disinfectant and wetting product. An exception to this is Solo-Care Hard (CIBA Vision), which is analogous to a soft lens multipurpose solution because it contains a surfactant cleaner. Rigid lens cleaning solutions can be more intensive than their soft lens equivalents because there is less opportunity for the solution to enter the lens material with the subsequent possibility of toxic reaction. For example, Total Care Daily Cleaner (**Allergan**) contains three cleaning agents and Boston Advance cleaner contains a silica suspension of microscopic beads that act like a gentle polish on the lens; this is beneficial with deposits such as denatured proteins, which can otherwise be difficult to remove. This cleaner also contains an alcohol base, which assists in removing lipid type spoilation.

swell factor, soft lens

Since both the linear swell and volume swell that occur on hydration of **hydrogels** are a direct consequence of the volume of water absorbed, any phenomenon that causes a change in **water content** will cause a change in lens dimensions. The precise combination of monomers used can have a marked effect on the stability of the material.

Extremes of behaviour are observed with respect to the temperature dependence of the water content of hydrogels. Group I materials, particularly poly-HEMA, show little temperature dependence, and Group IV materials show a significant drop in water content between 20°C and 30°C. These thermally induced changes take place rapidly, and the lens will quickly reach its new equilibrium water content on insertion into the eye. All lenses dehydrate over time in the eye, but that process is separate from

Figure S.21 Surfactant cleaning a soft lens.

thermal re-equilibration and is no better or worse for any particular class of hydrogels. The initial drop in water content will, however, significantly reduce the oxygen permeability of the lens material.

The sensitivity of water content to tonicity is similarly affected by monomer structure. In general, hydrogels show some small decrease in water content when the equilibration solution is changed from pure water to isotonic **saline**. Such a change, as with others induced by changing the nature of the storage solution, is much greater than those brought about by tonicity variations in the eye.

Variations in water content with respect to pH are more marked and are monomer-dependent. The pH ranges required to bring about such changes are, however, greater than those found diurnally or on a patient-to-patient basis in the eye, which lie well within one pH unit. High water content anionic hydrogels (FDA Group IV materials) suffer dramatic parameter changes in solutions of different pH; however, this is largely inconsequential if such materials are used to make **disposable lenses**. In order to maintain the stability of lenses during storage and to minimize dimensional changes between the storage medium and the eye, lenses are packed in buffered saline solution, which ensures that both pH and tonicity are controlled.

swimming in contact lenses

Contact lenses can be worn safely in sea water, fresh water and chemically treated water, although swimming should be avoided if it is known that the body of water where the swimming will occur is subject to high levels of pollution (many seaside authorities routinely advise of the ambient pollution levels). Overall, the risk of infection as a result of swimming in lenses is extremely small.

There is a greater risk of lens loss when swimming in lenses; this risk will be minimized if large-diameter **soft lenses** are worn. The use of swimming goggles will prevent lens loss and further reduce the already low risk of infection. It is advisable not to wear contact lenses in spa baths due to the increased risk of acanthamoeba infection.

Swimmers should be advised to follow these guidelines for avoiding lens loss and preserving eye health when not wearing goggles:

- close the eyes on impact with water
- do not open the eyes fully when underwater; instead, squint and maintain the head position in the direction of gaze
- upon surfacing, gently wipe water from the closed lids before opening the eyes

- irrigate the eyes with fresh **saline** upon leaving the water
- remove, clean and disinfect contact lenses as soon as practicable after swimming.

systemic disease, contact lens wear in

Patients with any systemic disease known to affect the anterior eye potentially face problems during contact lens wear. Conditions such as **diabetes**, thyroid deficiency, hyperthyroidism, rheumatoid arthritis, atopic eczema, psoriasis and acne rosacea may affect a patient's suitability for contact lenses. In general, these conditions, when managed, do not *contraindicate* contact lens wear but may influence the lens type or the wear schedule selected. Patients with allergies can achieve success with contact lenses but may require more frequent **aftercare** examinations, since these patients are more susceptible to lens-induced **discomfort** and lid problems. There is no contraindication to fitting contact lenses to patients who are HIV-positive providing the anterior eye is healthy. Practitioners should wear protective gloves if they have open skin lesions. If the patient has progressed to AIDS, the increased risk of opportunistic infection should be considered and contact lens fitting approached with extreme caution.

Restrictions of mobility, as in rheumatoid arthritis or 'diabetic hand syndrome' (Figure S.22), may make the handling of contact lenses difficult. Patients should be encouraged to handle their own lenses whenever possible. When handling becomes impossible, a relative or neighbour may provide assistance and periods of extended or continuous wear may be appropriate.

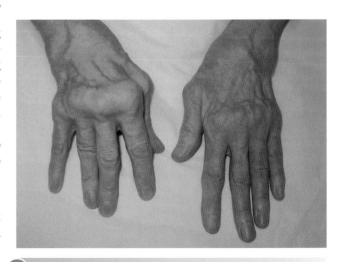

Figure S.22 Deformation of the knuckles and finger joints in a patient with rheumatoid arthritis.

The ocular complications of both prescription and over-the-counter medications – such as decongestants, antihistamines and oral contraceptives – should be taken into consideration in the context of contact lens wear. Possible side effects of medications include **dry eye**, photosensitivity, **corneal** and contact lens deposition, punctate keratopathy, subconjunctival haemorrhage, and discoloration of contact lenses.

When considering whether to proceed with contact lens fitting in patients with systemic disease affecting the anterior eye, the practitioner needs to conduct a risk–benefit analysis. Where an increased risk of ocular complications has been ascertained, the patient should be informed of the risks and the benefits of contact lens wear. The importance of **complying** with recommendations for lens care and maintenance, wearing schedules and attending follow-up visits should also be emphasized. A thorough understanding of the ocular and systemic history, careful examination during fitting and follow-up to exclude the possibility of external eye disease, and the use of superior contact lens products will increase the likelihood of success for all prospective contact lens wearers. *See* diabetes, contact lenses for.

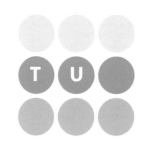

tarsal glands
See meibomian glands.

tarsal muscles (of Müller)
The superior and inferior tarsal muscles are smooth muscles that arise from the lower border of the levator in the upper lid and the inferior rectus in the lower lid, and insert into the orbital margins of the tarsal plates. The role of the superior tarsal muscle is to assist the levator in maintaining the width of the palpebral aperture. A mild degree of ptosis results from damage to its sympathetic nerve supply (Horner's syndrome).

TD
See total diameter.

teaching patients
See patient education.

tear break-up time
Rapid tear break-up can lead to symptoms of **dryness** and discomfort in both lens wearers and non-lens wearers. The tear film break-up time can be assessed by instilling **fluorescein** into the eye and timing how long it takes for breaks in the even fluorescent glow to appear (Figure T.1). One problem with this approach is that it is invasive in that the instillation of fluorescein in itself alters the quality and quantity of the **tear film**. *See* non-invasive tear break-up time.

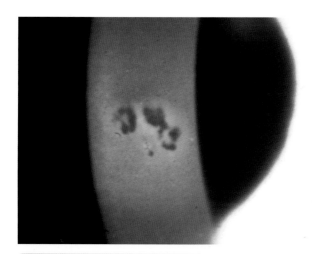

Figure T.1 Dark spots in the illuminated optic section indicate break-up of the pre-corneal tear film.

tear electrolytes
Human **tears** contain approximately the same range of electrolytes found in plasma. During the process of secretion by the **lacrimal gland** there is a process of active electrolyte transport, which is coupled to the passive movement of water by an osmotic process. Acinar-derived fluid is essentially an isotonic ultrafiltrate of plasma. Its composition is altered as it passes along the ductal system, where further chloride and potassium ions are secreted. A variety of ion transport proteins have been identified in acinar cells, including sodium-potassium ATPase and potassium and chloride channels.

tear film
The tear film is a complex fluid which covers the exposed parts of the ocular surface framed by the **eyelid** margins. The physical characteristics of this fluid are summarized in Table T.1. Classically, the tear film has been regarded as a trilaminar structure, with a superficial lipid layer (secreted by the **meibomian glands**) that overlies an aqueous phase (derived from the main and accessory **lacrimal glands**) and an inner mucinous layer (produced mainly by **conjunctival** goblet cells). The tear film performs several important functions, which can be broadly classified as:

- optical
- metabolic support
- protective
- lubrication.

By smoothing out irregularities of the **corneal epithelium** the tear film creates an even surface of good optical quality which is reformed with each **blink**. The air–tear interface forms the principal refractive surface of the optical system of the eye

Table T.1 Physical properties of the pre-ocular tear film

parameter	value
osmolarity	302 (± 6.3) mOsmol/l
pH	7.45
volume	7.0 (± 0.2) µl
rate of production:	
unstimulated	1–2 µl/min
stimulated	> 100 µl/min
refractive index	1.336

and provides two-thirds (43 D) of its total refractive power. Since the **cornea** is avascular, it is dependent on the tear film for its oxygen provision. When the eye is open the tear film is in a state of equilibrium with the oxygen in the atmosphere, and gaseous exchange takes place across the tear interface. The constant turnover of the tear film also provides a mechanism for the removal of metabolic waste products.

Tears play a major role in the defence of the eye against microbial colonization. The washing action of the tear fluid reduces the likelihood of microbial adhesion to the ocular surface. Moreover, the tears contain a host of protective antimicrobial proteins (Table T.2). The tear film acts as a lubricant, smoothing the passage of the lids over the corneal surface and preventing the transmission of damaging shearing forces. To facilitate this, tear fluid displays non-Newtonian behaviour with respect to shear. Newtonian fluids maintain a constant viscosity with increasing shear rates. By contrast, tear fluid has a relatively high viscosity between blinks to aid stability, and with increasing shear rates during the blink process the viscosity falls dramatically, thereby easing the movement of the lids over the ocular surface.

The classical trilaminar model of tear film structure has recently been challenged. Several pieces of evidence have suggested that the mucin contribution to the tear film is much greater than previously thought, and an alternative tear film model, which possesses a substantial mucinous phase, has been proposed. The nature of the mucinous phase has not been fully established, but is thought to consist of a mixture of soluble and gel-forming mucins. There is currently great uncertainty as to the overall thickness of the pre-corneal tear film. Published values, using several different techniques, lie in the range 3–40 μm. Invasive methods (e.g. using fine glass filaments) usually give rise to thickness estimates between 4 and 8 μm. Interferometric measurement gives values of around 40 μm, but these data have been questioned on the basis of methodological and interpretational difficulties.

tear layer
See tear film.

tear lens
The power of the tear lens beneath a **rigid lens**, sometimes alternatively called the liquid, fluid or lacrimal lens, depends on the relative geometry of the optic zone of the back surface of the rigid lens and the anterior surface of the **cornea**. The tear lens may contribute negative, zero or positive power to the overall lens–eye system, depending upon whether the fitting of the rigid lens is **flat**, in alignment or **steep**.

From a clinical perspective it is important to determine the likely magnitude of the power of the tear lens and how it varies as the **back optic zone radius** (BOZR) of the lens is changed. As an approximate rule of thumb, for a rigid lens the tear lens power increases by about +0.25 D for each 0.05 mm that the BOZR of the lens is steeper than the corneal radius. Correspondingly, on any cornea the **back vertex power** (BVP) of the rigid contact lens needs to be changed by −0.25 D for each 0.05 mm that the BOZR is made steeper, to compensate for the extra positive power of the liquid lens. If the lens BOZR is made flatter by 0.05 mm, the BVP needs to be changed by +0.25 D.

Trial or diagnostic lenses are often used to find the BOZR that gives the required fit with a particular lens design – an **over-refraction** then being carried out to determine any additional power needed in combination with the trial lens used to give the patient clear vision. In this case the ordered lens power is simply the sum of the BVP of the trial lens and the over-refraction (assuming that the power of the latter is small enough for effectivity to be ignored). This is because the BOZR and corneal radii will be exactly the same as with the trial lens, so that the tear lens has equal power in both cases.

The situation may arise where a trial lens with a given BOZR is not available, in which case it may be necessary to order a lens with a BOZR that differs from that of the trial lens actually used. Since the BOZR in the two cases differs, so also will the power of the tear lens, and this in turn will influence the required BVP of the ordered lens.

tear lipids
The source of lipids in the **tear film** is the **meibomian glands** embedded within the tarsal plates of each lid. The **blinking** process is an important mechanism in the expulsion of the secretion from the glands. Lipid is delivered directly as a clear oil onto the lid margins, and is spread over the tear film from the inner edge of the lid margins with each blink. The thickness of the lipid layer is variable (60–100 nm) and, depending on thickness, gives rise to characteristic interference patterns when viewed in specular reflection. Meibomian secretion consists of a complex mixture of lipids, including wax esters, sterol esters, fatty acids and fatty alcohols (Table T.2). The primary functions of this secretion are to provide a hydrophobic barrier at the lid margin to prevent over-spill of tears, and to cover the surface of the tear film to retard evaporation.

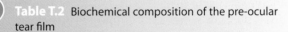

Table T.2 Biochemical composition of the pre-ocular tear film

component	concentration
Electrolytes[a]:	
Na$^+$	135 mEq/l
Cl$^-$	131 mEq/l
K$^+$	36 mEq/l
HCO$_3$$^-$	26 mEq/l
Ca^{2+}	0.46 mEq/l
Mg^{2+}	0.36 mEq/l
Major proteins[a]:	
lysozyme	2.07 g/l
secretory IgA	3.69 g/l
lactoferrin	1.65 g/l
lipocalin	1.55 g/l
albumin	0.04 g/l
IgG	0.004 g/l
Lipids[b]:	
wax esters	32.3% (dry weight)
sterol esters	27.3%
polar lipids	14.8%
hydrocarbons	7.5%
diesters	7.7%
triacylglycerides	3.7%
fatty acids	2.0%
free sterols	1.6%
Mucins[c]:	
MUC1	nd
MUC2	nd
MUC4	nd
MUC5AC	nd

Sources:
(a) Main and accessory lacrimal glands
(b) Meibomian glands
(c) Epithelial cells/goblet cells.
nd = not determined.

tear mucins

Mucins are a family of high molecular weight glycoproteins of which sugars contribute up to 85% of their dry weight. Structurally, they consist of a polypeptide backbone to which chains of sugar molecules attach via O-linkages to the amino acids serine and threonine. Mucins are a heterogeneous group of molecules, which can be subdivided into secretory and integrated-membrane varieties (*see* Table T.2). So far modern molecular biology techniques have identified nine mucin (MUC) genes, although only four of these (MUC1, MUC5AC, MUC4 and MUC2) are expressed on the human ocular surface. The epithelia of the **cornea** and **conjunctiva** express the transmembrane mucins MUC1 and (to a lesser extent) MUC4, which attach to apical microvilli, where they form a hydrophilic base to facilitate the spreading of the goblet cell-derived mucin MUC5AC. A secondary goblet cell mucin (MUC2) is present in only trace amounts. Mucins play a major role in stabilizing and spreading the tear film, and provide protection against desiccation and microbial invasion. The combined aggregation of mucins is known as mucus. *Adjective* mucous.

tear production

The terms 'basic (basal)' and 'reflex' can be used to describe tear flow. The **accessory lacrimal glands** are the basic (minimal flow) secretors, and reflex secretion (i.e. in response to strong physical or emotional stimulation) is mediated by the main **lacrimal gland**. Alternatively, tear output can be thought of as a continuum whereby the rate of production is proportional to the degree of sensory or emotive stimulation. This concept would also mean that a functional distinction between main and accessory lacrimal glands, in terms of basal and reflex tear production, is unnecessary. Rather, it is more likely that tear flow is the combination of contributions from both glands, although the output from the accessory glands alone is sufficient to maintain a stable tear layer.

tear proteins

Tear proteins are thought to originate from three main sources; the **lacrimal gland**, ocular surface epithelia and **conjunctival blood vessels**. The major lacrimal proteins include secretory IgA (sIgA), lysozyme, lactoferrin and lipocalin (formally known as tear-specific pre-albumin). IgA, which is the major immunoglobulin in tears, is secreted as a dimer by plasma cells in the interstices between lacrimal acini. It then binds to a receptor on the basolateral aspect of acinar cells, and is transcytosed across the cell and secreted into tear fluid. IgA is a constitutively secreted lacrimal protein whose rate of secretion is independent of flow rate. During sleep, the levels of IgA increase as sIgA production continues and as acinar secretion declines. IgA plays an important role in the defence of the ocular surface against microbial infection by preventing bacterial and viral adhesion, and inactivating bacterial toxins. Other immunoglobulins (e.g. IgG and IgM) are present in tears at much lower levels (*see* Table T.2).

Lysozyme, lactoferrin and lipocalin, by contrast, originate from acinar cells, and their rate of secretion roughly matches flow rate. Lysozyme is a well-known bacteriolytic protein, which has the ability to lyse the cell wall of several gram positive bacteria. Lactoferrin serves an important bacteriostatic function by binding iron and making it unavailable for bacterial metabolism. It also acts as a free radical scavenger, thereby reducing free-radical mediated cell damage. Lipocalins are a family of lipid-binding proteins with an affinity for a broad array of lipids including fatty acids, phospholipids and cholesterol. It has been suggested that tear lipocalins act as scavengers for a wide range of meibomian lipids, which could spill onto the corneal surface and perturb its wettability. Furthermore, lipocalin may promote lipid solubility at the aqueous–lipid interface to facilitate the formation of a thin layer of lipid on the surface of the tear film.

tears
See tear film.

Tearscope-plus
An instrument known as a Tearscope-plus (Keeler, UK) can be used to observe certain characteristics of the **tear film** non-invasively. This instrument takes the form of a small white dome with a central sight hole, surrounded by a cold cathode light source. It can be held directly in front of the eye, or used in conjunction with a **slit-lamp biomicroscope** to gain more magnification (Figure T.2). The thickness distribution, quality and freedom of movement of the tears can be assessed by observing the reflected light from the featureless white dome, and the integrity of the aqueous and lipid phases can be inferred from colour fringe interference patterns.

template method of BOZR determination
See profile matching, soft lens; back optic zone radius.

theatric tinted lenses
Lenses can be designed and tinted – typically with opaque agents – to create dramatic or theatrical effects (Figure T.3). Such lenses are also known as 'costume' or 'party' lenses. Effects such as wolf eyes, national flags, hearts, stars, smiley faces etc. can be created, and some companies market afocal lenses specifically for this purpose.

Although these lenses are viewed as a fashion accessory, potential users must be advised to have a thorough initial eye examination to check that their eyes are suitable for wearing contact lenses, and that the fit is satisfactory. Regular **aftercare** examinations are also recommended. Users should also be warned that such lenses should never be 'shared' with anyone else because the contact lenses may not fit or may be contraindicated in another person, and because there is a danger of cross-contamination and infection. *See* tinted lenses.

Theodore's superior limbic keratoconjunctivitis
See filamentary keratitis, therapeutic lenses for.

therapeutic lenses
Contact lenses can be of therapeutic benefit in the following situations/conditions:

- **distorted corneal shape**
- **relief of pain**
- **recurrent erosion syndrome**
- **dystrophies of the corneal epithelium**
- **filamentary keratitis**
- **dry eye**
- **degenerations of the corneal epithelium**
- **chemical injuries**
- **cicatricial conjunctivitis**
- **eyelid pathology**
- **post-trauma or post-surgery**

All types of contact lens have therapeutic uses, as follows:

1. *Soft lenses.* When considering the fitting of a 'bandage' lens, it is necessary to define or predict its probable pattern of use. The relevant considerations are:
   - whether **extended wear** is necessary
   - whether the patient (or, failing the patient, a

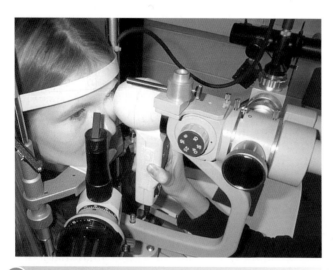

Figure T.2 Tearscope Plus used in conjunction with a slit-lamp biomicroscope.

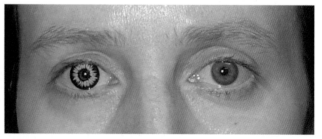

Figure T.3 Theatric 'wolf eye' lens in the right eye.

relative or friend) can be taught to handle (or at least to remove) the lens

- the likely duration of therapeutic lens management
- whether the patient lives within practical travelling distance of the clinic or hospital
- whether the necessary topical medications are available unpreserved
- whether the risks of **hypoxia**, mechanical trauma and infection are outweighed by the perceived benefits of therapeutic lens wear.

Some hospital departments keep sets of 'bandage' lenses, custom made from high **water content** materials, in various radii and diameters. Others use commercially available lenses such as omafilcon A (Proclear, **Biocompatibles–Hydron**) or **daily disposable lenses. Silicone hydrogel lenses** have an important therapeutic role because of their very high gas permeability. In fitting, it is important to cover all anterior ocular areas requiring protection, and to aim for a little movement on blinking. There must be no compression of the limbus.

2. *Silicone elastomer lenses.* These lenses have an important range of therapeutic roles, especially in tear-deficient eyes. The material is tough and durable, and has good optical properties. The main practical problem is the frequent failure of the surface treatment, which confers wettability on a naturally non-wettable material. This results in lens binding and discomfort.

3. *Rigid lenses.* It is frequently necessary to use rigid lenses for a combination of optical and therapeutic indications. Although of less than corneal diameter, they may provide enough cover to protect the **cornea** from abnormal lashes, keratinized lid margins, and other hostile factors. Sometime lenses of large diameters are used (Figure T.4). In cases of ectatic conditions such as pellucid marginal degeneration, the cornea may become highly **astigmatic**, necessitating the fitting of a **rigid bitoric lens**.

4. *Scleral lenses.* These have a host of therapeutic roles. Their advantages include the following:
   - corneal contact can be avoided
   - any eye shape can be fitted
   - complete protection of the **cornea** and bulbar **conjunctiva** is provided
   - sealed fits are possible, using gas-permeable materials, which simplifies the fitting process and minimizes 'settling back'
   - using gas-permeable materials, overnight wear is possible.

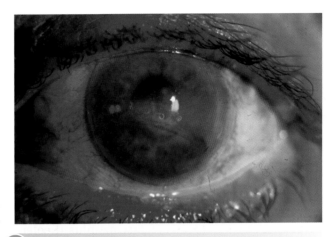

Figure T.4 Large 'limbal diameter' rigid lens used to protect a neurotrophic corneal lesion in the early stages of the healing process.

therapeutic lenses, complications of

The adverse effects of contact lenses used therapeutically are similar to those used for general cosmetic wear, although the diseased or injured eye may be particularly at risk. Complications of particular concern in therapeutic contact lens prescribing include **hypoxia** (with or without neovascularization) (Figure T.5), sterile corneal infiltrates, and suppurative **keratitis**. Careful follow-up is vital after the fitting of a lens for a therapeutic indication, and there is as yet no reason to vary the convention of examining the eye on the day after fitting and not more than 1 week after that. If **unplanned replacement lenses** are used, spoilation may be observed to occur more quickly than with healthy eyes. Any change of the comfort

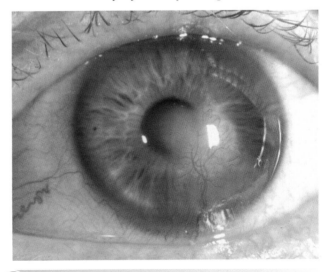

Figure T.5 Neovascularization with lipid leakage following 40 years of PMMA scleral lens wear.

or vision of the patient may be of great significance, and instruction should be given to the patient to remove the lens in such circumstances and to return to the clinic as an emergency if not rapidly relieved of the new symptoms.

therapeutic lenses, tinted

A therapeutic tinted lens can be defined as a lens that is designed to treat an underlying defect or disease. Primary therapeutic applications of contact lenses include reducing excessive photophobia and glare due to aniridia (Figure T.6), eliminating monocular polyopia due to trauma, eliminating binocular diplopia in squint (in cases where surgical and optical intervention is not viable or is contraindicated), and variable nystagmus.

There are often secondary therapeutic benefits of tinted lenses designed for prosthetic use. These include the following examples:

- a lens with an opaque pupil masking a cataract but also eliminating disturbing light in a near-blind eye
- a **rigid lens** with an opaque iris pattern fitted to a **distorted cornea** in a sighted eye also having the effect of improving vision by neutralizing corneal optics, and the incorporation of appropriate lens power to correct vision
- a lens with an opaque iris pattern to mask aniridia in a sighted eye also reducing glare.

The prescription of tinted lenses to supposedly enhance colour vision in colour-defective patients, to cure dyslexia and to alleviate migraine can also technically be described as therapeutic applications, although in most cases improvements are attributed to a placebo effect rather than a true therapeutic effect. *See* tinted lenses; ChromaGen lenses.

thickness caliper, rigid lens

Knowledge of **lens centre thickness** is required for calculation of gas transmissibility and lens flexibility. The central and peripheral thickness can be measured using a contact lens thickness caliper; this may be a mechanical device where lens thickness is read off an analogue scale (Figure T.7), or it may be an **electromechanical device** where the thickness is displayed as a digital readout. Care must be exercised when touching the lens surfaces with the calipers, which depress the surface and give a lower reading than the true thickness.

thickness measurement, soft lens

See electrical contact thickness gauge, soft lens; electromechanical thickness gauge, soft lens.

thimerosal disinfecting solution

See chlorhexidine-thimerosal-preserved disinfecting systems.

Thygeson's superficial punctate keratopathy

See dystrophies of the corneal epithelium, therapeutic lenses for.

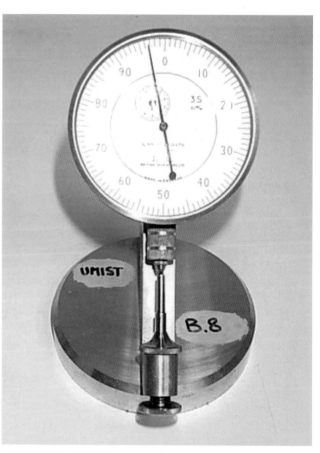

Figure T.7 Rigid lens thickness caliper.

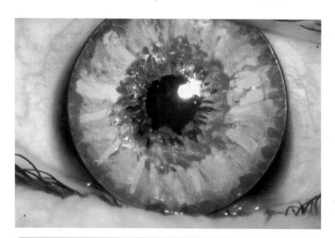

Figure T.6 Large-diameter rigid lens with hand-painted artificial iris.

thyroid deficiency

See systemic disease, contact lens wear in.

tight lens fit

A lens that moves or lags very little or not at all is deemed to be fitting tightly. Tight-fitting lenses induce greater levels of **corneal staining** than well-fitting lenses, and the prevalence of this staining increases with increasing tightness. **Conjunctival staining** corresponding to the lens edge may also be evident. Tight-fitting lenses tend to be comfortable, but patients occasionally complain of aching eyes later in the wearing period. Switching to a similar lens of flatter **back optic zone radius** or changing to a lens with a tendency towards tight fitting may solve the problem.

tight lens syndrome

See contact lens induced acute red eye (CLARE).

tinted lenses

A wide variety of manual (Figure T.8) and automated techniques can be used to apply translucent or opaque tints to **soft and rigid lenses**. An important initial consideration in deciding on the most appropriate tinted lens for a given patient is whether to use a soft or rigid lens. A particular lens type may be indicated for clinical reasons; for example, a rigid lens would be required in the case of a sighted eye with **corneal distortion**.

Soft lenses have the advantage of offering full corneal coverage and stability on the eye, and are thus particularly suited for cosmetic use. An advantage of rigid lenses is that it is possible to paint unique designs and so effect a more realistic iris appearance in terms of a more precise match of colour and iris features. However, full corneal coverage is not possible, and rigid lenses move on the

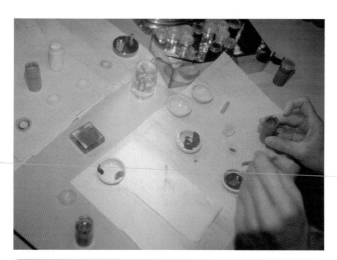

eye. These effects can be minimized by fitting slightly **tight**, large-diameter lenses. In general, rigid lenses are best suited for prosthetic use. In certain cases of extensive ocular disfiguration, painted **scleral lenses** may give the best result.

The applied tint can be translucent or opaque. The resulting lens may be wholly translucent if translucent tints alone are applied, semi-opaque if opaque tints have been used on portions of the lens, or completely opaque if opaque tints have been applied across the entire lens surface. A translucent tint allows certain wavelengths of light to pass through, thus effecting a colour change. Light passing through such a tint, and reflecting back off the iris, will be further modified such that the cosmetic effect is a combination of the colour of the translucent tint and iris. Translucent tints can therefore be said to enhance or modify natural iris colours. This effect is only successful with relatively light coloured irides.

Opaque tints can substantially or completely block the passage of light. A coloured pattern can be applied over a totally opaque base to effect a complete change of eye colour while at the same time, for example, masking out underlying iris disfigurations. Thus, the primary cosmetic application of opaque tints is to change the colour of dark irides or have the prosthetic effect of restoring a normal appearance to a disfigured eye.

Tinted lenses are used for a variety of purposes, including **lens handling, cosmetic, prosthetic, therapeutic, prophylactic** and **theatric** applications.

Translucent tints can be created using four basic techniques; **dye dispersion tinting, vat dye tinting, chemical bond tinting,** and **print tinting**. Opaque tints can be applied using **dot matrix printing, laminate tint constructions,** or an **opaque contact lens backing**.

The procedures for fitting tinted lenses may differ from those employed for fitting non-tinted lenses. Tinted rigid lenses need to be of a large diameter so as to cover as much of the cornea as possible, and to minimize lens movement. Tinted soft lenses are also best fitted marginally more steep than non-tinted lenses to reduce lens movement. A full appreciation of the cosmetic effect of tinted lenses is gained by viewing the lenses in the eyes (using a mirror in the case of the patient) in environments that the patient anticipates being in – that is, both inside under artificial light and outside in natural light.

Chlorine-based disinfecting solutions can cause some lens fading. All other lens care products appear to be innocuous in this regard, including **hydrogen peroxide disinfecting solutions** and alcohol-based daily **surfactant cleaning** solutions. Intensive cleaners that employ acids, bases and oxidizing agents could cause tint fading, and so should not be used on tinted lenses.

Although tinting using laminate construction reduces **oxygen transmissibility** by increasing lens thickness, none of the other tint processes appear to affect lens oxygen performance.

Patients who wear opaque lenses with a clear pupil sometimes complain of haze or a veiling effect in their peripheral vision. This is due to a slight restriction of the visual field during the wear of such lenses. The phenomenon is more noticeable if the lens becomes decentred. In view of the measurable visual impairment when wearing such lenses, patients should be advised against wearing them when undertaking critical visual tasks, such as driving.

Some fashion-conscious patients may possess numerous pairs of lenses of different tint designs. Such patients should be advised to mark their lens cases to avoid repeated opening, thus reducing the risk of contaminating stored lenses. Advice should be given to patients concerning long-term lens storage – such as the desirability of periodic lens cleaning even if lenses have not been worn.

Although disposable tinted lenses are available, some products, such as theatric lenses, are more expensive and are retained for long periods of time. Long-term lens maintenance therefore becomes an important issue. Some tinting processes can alter the lens surface charge. This could facilitate increased protein deposition, the consequences of which may be decreased vision and comfort, sensations of **dryness**, susceptibility to adverse eye reactions, lens distortion, and alterations to lens fitting characteristics.

Tinting processes can alter lens surface chemistry, which in turn can reduce surface wettability and lead to symptoms of dryness. Slight irregularities caused by surface tints may render tinted lenses slightly less comfortable than equivalent non-tinted lenses. Ocular lubricants can help alleviate these sensations.

tolerances

Contact lens manufacture is an inexact science, and manufacturers strive to supply lenses that have dimensions and optical characteristics in accordance with those specified. Manufacturing tolerances are the range of acceptable discrepancies between what is specified and what is supplied. Tolerances are agreed by consensus among a range of stakeholders in contact lens manufacture and clinical practice, with regard to known capabilities of currently available manufacturing techniques, and the likely clinical effects of discrepancies in lens dimensions from those specified. Currently agreed specifications for soft and rigid lenses are given in Appendix E.

topical medication

See concurrent medication with contact lenses.

toric lens design, rigid

Although spherical **rigid lenses** in general may be successfully fitted to **astigmatic** patients, with either apical clearance or apical contact, it is generally more satisfactory to fit such lenses with toroidal back optic zones in or near alignment. The physical fit, as denoted by the **fluorescein** pattern, will be similar to that seen with a well-fitted **spherical lens** in alignment with a **cornea** devoid of clinically significant astigmatism. Conversely, a toric lens aligning too closely with the cornea can lead to poor tear interchange. Consequently, it is advisable to use a toroidal back optic zone with the steeper radius fitted slightly flatter (longer radius) than the corresponding corneal radius so as to assist the interchange of tears. The flatter radius will generally be fitted 'on K' or else a little steeper than its corresponding corneal radius.

The peripheral radii are usually chosen to reflect the type of peripheral fit preferred by the practitioner concerned. Each meridian is considered separately, and the peripheral fittings in the two principal meridians are selected to provide the same difference between back optic and peripheral radii most commonly used by the practitioner in fitting spherical corneas. In addition, the peripheral curves will usually have the same degree of toricity as the BOZR.

For lenses with a spherical back optic zone and a toroidal peripheral zone, the peripheral curve region should be as large as possible to increase the likelihood of alignment with the toric cornea. These lenses are usually fitted fairly small to minimize meridional sag differences and slightly steeper centrally than the flatter corneal meridian to achieve a compromise fit. The meridional difference in the peripheral curves should be at least 0.6 mm to help minimize lens rotation.

For spherical lenses, the power of the contact lens in air plus the power of the tear lens in air should add up to the ocular refraction. With toric lenses, the same rule applies, but here the two separate meridians must be considered. *See* compensated rigid bitoric lenses; cylindrical power equivalent rigid toric lenses; induced astigmatism with rigid toric lenses; residual astigmatism with rigid toric lenses; stabilization of rigid toric lenses; toric lens, rigid.

toric lens fitting, soft

The fitting principles for **soft toric lenses** are very similar to those for **spherical soft lenses**. A well-fitting lens is comfortable in all directions of gaze, gives complete **corneal** coverage, and appears properly centred. On **blinking**, there should be about 0.25–0.5 mm of vertical movement when the eye is in the primary position. On upwards gaze or lateral movements of the eye, the lens should lag by no more than 0.5 mm. Generally, when specifying the lens diameter, the practitioner should err on the large side, as a larger diameter means that more area is available for the stabilization zones to take effect in the periphery of the lens. A well-fitting lens will reveal stable lens orientation with a quick return to axis if mislocated. A **tight-fitting lens** will show stable lens orientation but a slow return to axis if mislocated. A **loose-fitting lens** will demonstrate an unstable and inconsistent lens orientation.

Due to the absence of a tear lens, the **back vertex power** for a soft toric lens should be similar to the spectacle refraction (or ocular refraction if the vertex distance effect is significant). The back vertex power of the lens can be determined either empirically or by performing a sphero-cylindrical **over-refraction** (SCO) over a diagnostic lens. With empirical prescribing, the BVP ordered for the soft toric lens will be equal to the ocular refraction of the patient, based on the assumption of an afocal tear layer under the soft toric lens. For the latter method, a SCO may be performed over a spherical trial lens. The resultant toric lens power is simply calculated by adding the SCO to the BVP of the trial lens. With both methods, some arbitrary allowance for lens rotation may have to be incorporated into the final lens prescription.

Factors affecting the orientation of a soft toric lens in the eye include variations in lid tension (tightness), lid location, lid angle and lid symmetry; the type of fit (steep, alignment or flat); and the thickness profile of the lens. If it is expected that the soft toric lens to be ordered will rotate when placed on the eye of the patient, then an allowance must be made for this rotation, otherwise the cylinder axis of the lens *in situ* will not adopt the correct orientation for the ocular correction.

When allowing for nasal rotation in the right eye, the amount of rotation should be subtracted from the required cylinder axis, and *vice versa* for the left eye. When allowing for temporal rotation in the right eye, the amount of rotation should be added to the required cylinder axis, and *vice versa* for the left eye. Hence:

- if left eye and nasal rotation – add
- if left eye and temporal rotation – subtract
- if right eye and nasal rotation – subtract
- if right eye and temporal rotation – add.

The acronym 'LARS' (left add, right subtract), relating to nasal rotation of the inferior aspect of the lens, can be quite useful.

Many practitioners work on the principle that clockwise rotation necessitates adding the allowance for rotation to the required cylinder axis, and counter-clockwise rotation requires subtracting the allowance for rotation to determine the final cylinder axis. Hence:

- if clockwise rotation – add
- if counter-clockwise rotation – subtract.

If, at the dispensing or **aftercare** visit, the lens rotation is not what was expected (but the lens location is stable), the lens can simply be reordered with the revised allowance for lens rotation. Generally speaking, rotational stability is a more important factor than the degree of rotation. Lenses that give suboptimal but stable acuity are likely to be more acceptable than lenses that give moments of clear vision followed by moments of poor vision as the lens rotates. *See* stabilization of soft toric lenses; toric lens rotation, soft; toric lens, soft.

toric lens manufacture

Either surface of a **rigid lens** will sometimes require a toric form for the correction of **astigmatism** and/or to achieve rotational stabilization. This can be achieved by directly **lathing** a toric surface on to a plastic button (or the xerogel in the case of soft lenses), or by a technique known as crimping. The process of directly lathing a toric back surface onto the lens button is achieved by using a 'fly-cutter', which is a diamond tool that has its cutting tip set at right angles to the axis of its support shank. The position of the fly-cutter and lens blank are reversed, so that the lathe manoeuvres the lens button in an arc around the fly-cutter, which spins in a fixed position. A similar principle is applied for generating a front toric surface.

To generate a toric back surface using the technique of crimping, a spherical back curve is cut into the button in the usual way, except that a stepped rim is also engraved into the base of the blank. The curvature of this surface is the average of the required toric radii of the finished lens. The thickness of the button is machined down to about 0.20 mm thick so that the button can be flexed. The button is placed in a crimping tool with the concave surface facing upwards; this tool is a form of clamp that allows pressure to be incrementally applied to the rim of the button until it bends by a measured amount. The extent of bending is monitored optically using a conventional radiuscope.

The crimping assembly containing the flexed button is fixed to the spindle of a lathe and set spinning. A spherical surface is cut into the rotating flexed button. When the button is eventually released from the crimping tool, it reverts back to its natural shape and the lathed surface assumes a toric form. The lens is blocked and a spherical curve can be generated on the front surface. Crimping is used again to generate a toric front surface if required.

Toric soft lenses can be manufactured using moulding technology by designing the toric form into the moulds.

toric lens orientation, soft
See toric lens rotation, soft.

toric lens, rigid
The use of rigid toric lenses (in preference to **rigid spherical lenses**) is indicated under the following circumstances:

- to improve the vision in cases where a lens employing spherical **front and back optic zone radii** is unable to provide adequate refractive correction.
- to improve the physical fit in cases where a lens with a spherical **back optic zone radius** (BOZR) and spherical back peripheral zone radii fails to sit properly on the **cornea**.

These two applications are not always distinct, and occasionally a toric lens will be used for both physical and optical reasons.

There are many varieties of rigid toric lens available to the practitioner. Most commonly, such lenses will consist of a toroidal back optic zone and peripheral zone. These lenses are generally used in attempting to obtain a good physical fit on a cornea that is too toroidal to allow a good fit with a lens having a spherical BOZR and spherical peripheral radii. Lenses with toroidal back optic and peripheral zones can be produced with or without a toroidal front optic surface. A lens that has a toroidal back optic zone and a toroidal front surface is said to have a 'bitoric' construction. If the principal meridians are not parallel, then the lens is designated as having an 'oblique bitoric' construction.

Occasionally, a rigid toric lens may be prescribed that consists of a spherical back optic zone and a toroidal peripheral zone. This type of lens can also be produced with or without a toroidal front surface, the latter usually being the preferred option. Lenses with spherical back optic zones and toroidal peripheral zones are used as a means of attempting to improve the physical fit of a lens on an astigmatic cornea without the optical complications inherent in the use of lenses with toroidal back optic zones.

A rigid toric lens with a spherical back optic zone and spherical peripheral zone combined with a toroidal front optic surface is required in the situation where there is a significant amount of residual (non-corneal) **astigmatism** but minimal corneal astigmatism. In this case, the residual astigmatism needs to be corrected by means of a toroidal front surface, with a spherical optic zone indicated for the back surface due to the negligible corneal **astigmatism**.

Since rigid lenses with both spherical BOZR and peripheral radii are often used successfully on corneas with medium to high degrees of astigmatism, it is important to decide what degree of corneal astigmatism should indicate the use of toroidal back optic zones. In general, these lenses should only be used when a lens with a spherical BOZR cannot be made to fit successfully. It is rare to find that toroidal back optic zones are necessary unless the corneal astigmatism exceeds 2.50 D (i.e. the difference in the corneal radii, as measured with a **keratometer**, exceeds approximately 0.5 mm).

In cases of uncertainty (for example, where the corneal astigmatism is between 2.00 and 3.00 D), a toroidal back optic zone would be used in preference to a spherical back surface curve when:

- a spherical lens exhibits poor centration or excessive movement
- excessive lens flexure is noted with a spherical lens
- **fluorescein** patterns with a spherical lens reveal excessive bearing along the flatter corneal meridian, regardless of the BOZR that is fitted
- Significant 3 and 9 o'clock staining occurs with a spherical lens
- there is marked **corneal distortion** and spectacle blur upon removal of the spherical lens from the eye; this occurs as a result of poor alignment between the spherical lens and the toric cornea, with the spherical lens subsequently having a moulding effect on the toric cornea
- there is significant residual astigmatism; in this case a spherical back surface may provide an adequate fit, but a toric back surface is utilized to stabilize the lens and prevent rotation, due to the presence of the correction for the residual astigmatism on the front surface of the lens.

A great deal depends on factors other than corneal astigmatism. Lid positions and tension are important. In a case of high with-the-rule corneal astigmatism and a drooping, loose lower lid, a toroidal back optic zone may be needed to obtain a good physical fit and centration. However, a similar eye with a firm, high lower lid may well be successfully fitted using a lens with spherical back surface curves.

The majority of cases of corneal astigmatism are found with the steeper corneal curve in the vertical meridian (with-the-rule). If an attempt is made to fit such an eye with a spherical BOZR, the lens often drops low on the cornea, causing physical discomfort and/or poor vision. The presence of against-the-rule corneal astigmatism usually necessitates the use of a toroidal back optic zone earlier than would be required with an equivalent amount of with-the-rule corneal astigmatism. This is due to the tendency for rigid spherical lenses to decentre laterally on corneas with even just moderate amounts (1.50–2.00 D) of against-the-rule astigmatism. *See* compensated rigid bitoric lenses; cylindrical power equivalent rigid toric lenses; induced astigmatism with rigid toric lenses; residual astigmatism with rigid toric lenses; stabilization of rigid toric lenses; toric lens design, rigid.

toric lens rotation, soft

Soft toric lenses contain markings at a specific reference point so the degree of rotation can be assessed when the lens is on the eye (Figure T.9). The markings may be in the form of laser traces, scribe lines, engraved dots or ink dots. These markings do not represent the cylinder axis; they are simply a point of reference with regard to which the rotation of the lens can be assessed. They may be either at the 6 o'clock position of the lens, or in the horizontal lens meridian at the 3 and 9 o'clock positions. The latter situa-

tion is preferable, as the markings can be then observed without having to retract the lower **eyelid** (which would interfere with the dynamic stabilizing forces that normally act to orient the lens). In addition, having two widely-spaced markings about 14 mm apart at the 3 and 9 o'clock positions, as opposed to one mark or a set of marks at the 6 o'clock position, makes it easier to quantify the angle of rotation. Many laboratories that opt for the 6 o'clock indication provide three lines on their lenses, each separated by the same known angle, thus also facilitating a determination of lens rotation. Unfortunately, there is no standardization with respect to the angles used by different manufacturers (Figure T.10).

Estimation is a straightforward and reasonable technique for assessing the degree of lens rotation, made simpler if the practitioner remembers that the difference between each hour on a clock face is 30°. Clinical experience has shown that this is a satisfactory method of assessing lens rotation, with errors more likely to occur when evaluating higher amounts of lens rotation. *See* stabilization of soft toric lenses; toric lens fitting, soft; toric lens, soft.

toric lens, soft

The use of soft toric lenses (in preference to soft spherical lenses) is indicated when there is ocular **astigmatism** present (whether corneal or non-corneal) that warrants correction. Unlike **rigid lenses**, **soft lenses** do not mask corneal astigmatism, but rather conform to the shape of the **cornea**. Consequently, correcting ocular astigmatism with soft lenses requires that cylinder be incorporated into the **back vertex power** (BVP) of the lens.

When deciding whether or not to prescribe a soft toric lens, the following factors need to be taken into account:

1. *The degree of astigmatism.* As a generalization, 1.00 D or more of astigmatism should be corrected, although there will be significant variability

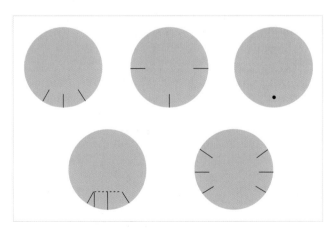

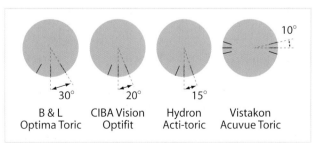

Figure T.9 Various markings used by different manufacturers to assist practitioners in determining the angle of rotation of soft toric lenses in the eye.

Figure T.10 Examples of the different angles between axis location marks adopted by some manufacturers of soft toric lenses.

between patients. About 45% of the population require a cylindrical correction of up to 0.75 D, and 25% of the population require a correction of 1.00 D or more.

2. *The cylinder axis.* An uncorrected cylinder with an oblique axis will cause greater degradation of the visual image compared with an equivalent amount of uncorrected with-the-rule or against-the-rule astigmatism.

3. *Ocular dominance.* Uncorrected astigmatism is far more likely to be accepted by the patient if it is in the non-dominant eye or in the eye with the poorer acuity.

4. *Viability of other alternatives.* The practitioner needs to consider whether soft toric lenses are the best option or if the patient would be better off with spectacles or rigid lenses. For example, a patient with high degrees (> 5.00 D) of both corneal and spectacle astigmatism would probably achieve better acuities with a rigid toric lens.

5. *Visual needs of the patient.* Usually, the less critical the visual task, the greater the amount of astigmatism that can be left uncorrected (and *vice versa*).

The two principal categories of surface optics of soft toric lenses are:

1. Toroidal back surface with a spherical front surface
2. Spherical back surface with toroidal front surface.

Regardless of which of these configurations is prescribed, the end result on the eye will be a bitoric lens form due to the wrapping of the front and back surface of the lens onto the cornea. The choice of design configuration is generally based more on considerations relating to manufacture. *See* stabilization of soft toric lenses; toric lens fitting, soft; toric lens rotation, soft.

toroidal back surface
See stabilization of rigid toric lenses; stabilization of soft toric lenses.

total diameter (TD)
The total diameter (TD) of a lens is measured from the very edge of the lens through the lens centre (Figure T.11; *see* also Figure B.1). The fact that the **water content** and therefore the dimensions of some **soft lens** materials vary with temperature makes it difficult to compare the labelled diameter of one lens to another. Most non-ionic soft lenses, particularly those containing n-vinyl pyrrolidone, shrink by approximately 0.5 mm when raised from room to eye temperature.

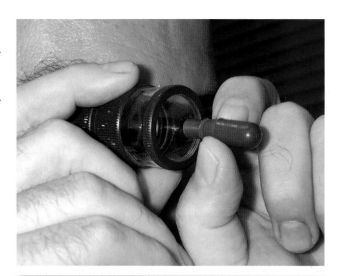

Figure T.11 Measuring the overall diameter of a rigid lens using a loupe with calibrated scale on clear base plate.

Ionic lenses are also temperature sensitive, although they shrink much less than non-ionic lenses. Some lenses are made larger in diameter to compensate for this. A further complicating factor is that the on-eye diameter is affected by the sagittal depth of the lens. Lenses of similar nominal diameter can vary in sagittal depth by as much as 1 mm and, since the periphery of a soft lens flattens to align with the bulbar **conjunctiva**, the sagittal depth can have a significant effect on lens diameter during lens wear.

training, patients
See patient education.

training, staff
See staff training in contact lens practice.

translating vision lenses
See alternating vision lenses for presbyopia.

trial fitting, soft lens
See fitting soft lenses.

trial lens set disinfection
The vast majority of patients who wear **soft lenses** are fitted using disposable, single-use trial lenses, which are often supplied free by the manufacturer for this purpose. However, certain complex soft lenses (e.g. high-powered lenticular lenses, special tints, custom-made bifocal designs) are best fitted from trial lens sets. Although excellent success rates in fitting **rigid lenses** empirically (i.e. the lens is ordered based on measures of refraction and ocular dimensions) have been demonstrated, certain ocular conditions can only be corrected by fitting

sophisticated designs from a trial lens set. An obvious case is **keratoconus**, and a practitioner who fits patients with this condition may have access to a number of trial fitting sets, each representing a different design concept. The issue arises as to how such trial fitting sets should be maintained so as to prevent cross-contamination of patients.

Proper application of the standard soft lens and rigid lens care protocols will be efficacious at killing most bacteria, viruses, fungi and protozoa, especially those known to cause infection in the eye. However, certain infectious agents that have more recently been identified are apparently resistant to current soft and rigid lens care regimens. Of particular concern at the present time is a proteinaceous vector known as a prion – a chameleon-like infectious agent that exists in different strains, has distinct biological properties, and can alter when the disease for which it is responsible crosses the species barrier. It has been suggested by health authorities in the UK that there is a remote theoretical risk of transmission of variant Creutzfeldt–Jacob disease (vCJD) between humans via transfer of bodily tissues and fluids such as tears. The prion is a vector for transmission of this disease.

An extension of the above argument leads to the conclusion that vCJD could theoretically be transmitted from an infected individual to another person via a trial contact lens contaminated with the offending prion. A solution containing 20 000 ppm of available chlorine of sodium hypochlorite is effective in reducing transmissible spongiform encephalopathy (vCJD) infectivity; such a solution can be employed for disinfecting reusable rigid trial lenses.

trichiasis
See eyelid pathology, therapeutic lenses for.

trigeminal neuralgia
See eyelid pathology, therapeutic lenses for.

truncation
See stabilization of rigid toric lenses; stabilization of soft toric lenses.

Tuohy, Kevin
See poly(methyl methacrylate) (PMMA) lenses.

two-step hydrogen peroxide disinfecting solution
See hydrogen peroxide disinfecting solution.

U

ultrasound disinfection, soft lens
This physical method of soft lens disinfection relies on sonic energy being imparted to micro-organisms to cause lethal cell changes. Such devices have a limited disinfection efficacy.

ultraviolet radiation disinfection, soft lens
Studies on the efficacy of ultraviolet radiation for contact lens disinfection have provided equivocal results. Using radiation of 253.7 nm at an energy of 44.3 $\mu W/cm^2$, **Acanthamoeba** cysts and trophozoites survive irradiation of 22 minutes in duration. Although the numbers of some micro-organisms are reduced by ultraviolet irradiation, the level of survivors is unacceptably high. However, adequate bacterial disinfection can be achieved at the same wavelength using an ultraviolet lamp with a higher energy output, 950 $\mu W/cm^2$; lens parameter changes with this level of radiation are not clinically important.

UltraVision Corporation
UltraVision Corporation was founded by two optometrists, Dr Vince Zuccaro and Dr Gary Edwards. The company was formed in 1993 to develop a carbosilfocon material for contact lens use, and was listed on the Alberta Stock Exchange in 1994. In 1999 it acquired UK-based IGEL and Australia-based Capricornia to increase product breadth and market depth. It has distribution and manufacturing facilities in North America, the United Kingdom, Australia and Singapore. The corporate headquarters are in St Hubert, Quebec, Canada. The company also operates rigid lens laboratories in some markets.
Website: www.ultravision. co.uk

unit-dose saline
See saline solutions.

USAN classification
See water content, hydrogel.

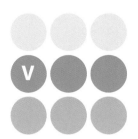

vacuoles

When the **cornea** is severely compromised, such as in the case of severe stromal **oedema** or an extensive **microcyst** response, the epithelium can also become oedematous; this manifests as the appearance of small fluid vacuoles in the epithelium. By observing the cornea using **indirect retro-illumination** on the **slit-lamp biomicroscope**, fluid vacuoles can be observed to display 'unreversed illumination'; that is, the distribution of light within the vacuole is the same as the light distribution of the background (Figure V.1). This indicates that the vacuole is acting as a diverging refractor, and therefore it must consist of material that is of a lower **refractive index** (fluid) than the surrounding epithelial tissue.

The aetiology of epithelial fluid vacuoles is two-fold. Epithelial oedema follows traumatic loss of surface epithelial cells. The fluid barrier (zonula occludens) that is normally found between surface epithelial cells is breached, resulting in the movement of fluid into the deeper layers of the epithelium. Since the cells are tightly fitted and attach snugly together, the oedema may not occur instantly, nor be widespread. Epithelial oedema can also form as a result of hypotonic ocular exposure, which can compromise the integrity of the fluid barrier. Epithelial oedema and the following thinning can co-exist during periods of **rigid lens** wear.

The flare observed with **fluorescein** in and around corneal abrasions is epithelial oedema. Histopatho-logical evaluation of corneas following hypotonic exposure demonstrates that the oedema is extracellular and is present throughout the full thickness of the epithelium. Reflex tears are of low tonicity and may also provoke epithelial oedema, such as during adaptation to rigid lenses.

Breakdown of the corneal fluid barrier, as indicated by the presence of fluid vacuoles, can lead to secondary problems. For example, contaminated low tonicity water – such as that which may be found in a jacuzzi or hot tub – has an association with contracting an **Acanthamoeba keratitis**. The amoeba may use the spaces created between cells by the oedematous state to gain entry to the cornea. This scenario is possible in both contact lens wearers and non-lens wearers. Fluid vacuoles can break through the anterior epithelial surface, leading to a very painful condition. Practitioners should therefore take action to eliminate fluid vacuoles from the epithelium by treating the underlying cause, which generally equates to the prescription of highly gas-permeable contact lenses that afford optimal corneal oxygenation.

variant Creutzfeldt–Jacob disease

See trial lens set disinfection.

vascularization

See neovascularization.

vascularized limbal keratitis

This condition is observed in patients wearing **rigid contact lenses** on an **extended wear** basis. It manifests as a limbal inflammation, typically at either the 3 or 9 o'clock positions, and an encroachment of limbal vessels (Figure V.2). The adjacent **conjunctiva** may be oedematous and hyperaemic, and the lesion may be surrounded by fine superficial punctate epithelial staining and mild corneal infiltration. The patient may only be mildly symptomatic, complaining of ocular **dryness**. The problem may be exacerbated if the lens surface is crazed or deposited.

This condition often occurs in regions of the limbus that have become desiccated due to poor wetting of the ocular surface. This problem is caused by bridging of the lids away from the globe, thus preventing the lids from distributing tears over the affected area. In this regard, vascularized limbal keratitis may be an advanced form of 3 and 9 o'clock

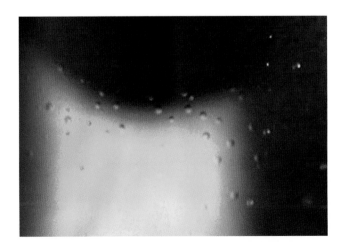

Figure V.1 Fluid vacuoles at the epithelial surface displaying unreversed illumination.

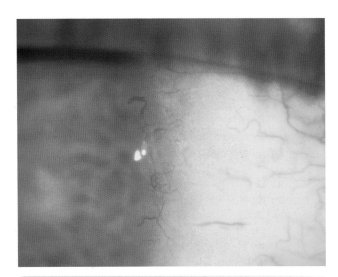

Figure V.2 Vascularized limbal keratitis.

staining. In late stages of this condition the lesion can become slightly raised, in the form of a thickened mass of epithelial tissue through which blood vessels traverse at various depths. This epithelial hypertrophy may be related to the fact that the limbus contains a high concentration of stem cells, creating a greater capacity for epithelial cell mitosis and movement. Also, the limbus hosts a vast array of immunologic mechanisms mediated via the mononuclear phagocyte system in limbal vessels.

Vascularized limbal keratitis is reversible, and cessation of lens wear for a few weeks will allow most of the pathology to resolve. Converting the patient from **extended-wear** to daily-wear lenses, and refitting with a smaller diameter rigid lens, may prevent the problem from recurring. Changing from rigid to **soft lenses** will certainly eliminate the problem.

vascular pannus
See pannus.

vat dye tinting
This process is used for creating translucent tints in **soft lenses**. The finished contact lens is soaked in a water-soluble dye for a fixed amount of time and at a specified temperature. The lens is then exposed to air, rendering the dye insoluble and trapped within the lens matrix. Because the dye only enters the lens surface to a depth of about 10 μm, the lens will appear to have a uniform tint across its entirety, the intensity of which will be independent of optical power. The dye is held in position by strong absorptive forces, resulting in a stable, permanent tint that can only be extracted by the use of powerful solvents. *See* tinted lenses.

vCJD
See trial lens set disinfection.

vertical analogue scale
This is a tool for quantifying subjective sensations (e.g. lens comfort). The patient is invited to mark the position on a vertical scale corresponding to the level of comfort (Figure V.3). The reason that the scale is oriented vertically is to avoid the potential bias, as a result of 'handedness', that may invalidate the use of a horizontal scale. The distance along the scale from the zero position is measured and taken as an index of the degree of sensation.

vertometer
See focimeter.

vessel ingrowth
See neovascularization.

V-gauge
The **total diameter** (TD) of a **rigid lens** can be measured using a V-gauge. This is a triangular channel cut into a plastic strip with markings and numerical diameter values arranged in descending order of magnitude towards the apex of the channel. The lens is placed at the wide end of the channel and pushed gently along towards the narrow end (or allowed to roll down within the channel as the V-gauge is tilted with the narrow end of the channel downwards) until it becomes lightly 'wedged' in the V-gauge channel (Figure V.4). Care must be taken to ensure that the V-gauge does not flex the lens, as this would underestimate lens diameter. The overall diameter is read off the pre-calibrated scale.

videokeratoscope for corneal measurement
See corneal topographic analysis.

videokeratoscope for lens measurement
Videokeratoscopes are ideal for checking aspheric front lens surfaces, with the lenses on or off the eye.

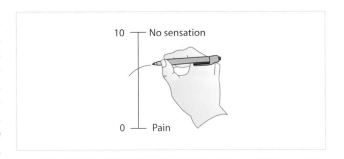

Figure V.3 Vertical analogue scale used to quantify subjective comfort, whereby a higher number indicates greater comfort.

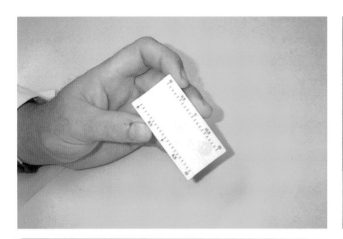

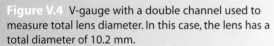

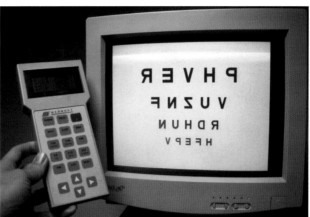

Figure V.4 V-gauge with a double channel used to measure total lens diameter. In this case, the lens has a total diameter of 10.2 mm.

Figure V.5 Computerized visual acuity chart. The letters on the screen are reversed for mirror display.

Also, videokeratoscopes can be used to monitor lens front surface shape in cases of suspected lens flexure or dimensional instability. Videokeratoscopes are not generally suited for lens back surface analysis because the inherent software packages are designed for analysing convex surfaces only.

visibility tints
See handling tints.

vision, measurement of
Vision should always be one of the first measurements in any contact lens examination. In this way, the vision measurement will be most indicative of the habitual vision of the patient and will be unaffected by the lights and ocular manipulations associated with later test procedures. It is equally important to establish a baseline measure of vision for medicolegal reasons.

The computer-presented visual acuity chart has advantages over other types of vision chart for contact lens practice (Figure V.5). Computer-generated optotypes can be randomized to prevent the contact lens patient from learning the letter sequences at successive visits. In addition, computerized vision charts can usually present letters down to 6/3 – a

level of vision that can be achieved by many younger contact lens wearers.

Vision should be measured with and without the habitual distance spectacles of the patient at both distance and near. The level of vision can be related to the clinical history and to the results of the refraction and the binocular vision examinations. The unaided vision is of interest because patients who are commonly or intermittently uncorrected will compare that to the level of acuity they achieve with contact lenses.

vision, poor
See poor vision, investigation of.

Vista Optics
This is a small company of about 20 employees that was established in 1979 by David Walker. It manufactures polymers for optical applications, including intra-ocular lenses and **soft and rigid contact lenses**. The company is also involved in specialist health-related areas, such as the surface coating of medical devices using polymeric grafting systems and prosthetic eyes. It distributes internationally, and its headquarters are in Stockport, UK. Website: www.vista-optics.com

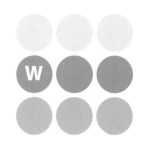

warpage

See corneal warpage; dimensional instability, rigid lens.

water content, soft lens

The function of the chemical groups in **hydrogels** is primarily to attract and bind water within the structure. The extent of this water-binding ability controls the equilibrium water content (EWC), which is the single most important property of a hydrogel. It is defined as:

$$EWC\ (\%) = \frac{\text{weight of water}}{\text{weight of hydrated gel}} \times 100\%$$

It is important to define the temperature at which the measurement was made and the nature of the hydrating medium (e.g. pure water or saline solution). The apparent equilibrium water content of a gel measured in water at 20°C in isotonic **saline** can be quite different from its value when maintained at 35°C in isotonic saline in a laboratory, or in the eye (at a presumed temperature of 35°C) (Figure W.1).

Poly-HEMA hydrogel has an equilibrium water content of approximately 38% (depending upon the degree of cross-linking and conditions of measurement). This can be reduced by co-polymerizing with a hydrophobic monomer such as methyl methacrylate, or increased by co-polymerizing with more hydrophilic monomers such as N-vinyl pyrrolidone (NVP) or methacrylic acid. By using a range of monomers in various combinations it is possible to purpose-design or tailor-make **polymers** for contact lens use. In order to achieve a particular water content, a mixture of monomers is chosen such that the balance of more hydrophilic and less hydrophilic monomers gives the required water content. A cross-linking agent (usually at around 1% of the total monomer mix) is added to produce a network that will give elastic stability.

A particular combination of monomers and cross-linking agent is classified in the USA in two ways. It is given a USAN (United States Adopted Name) identity (e.g. etafilcon-A), which is unique to that specific composition. It will also fall into one of the four groups of the **FDA** classification scheme, which offers a simple but effective subdivision of lens materials, on the basis of water content and ionic character, into four groups:

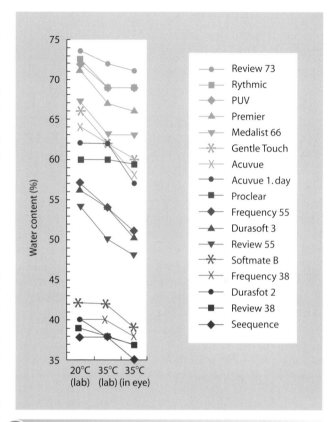

Figure W.1 Change in the water content of a wide range of hydrogel lenses when the environment is changed from (left) laboratory room temperature (20°C) to (centre) 35°C maintained in a temperature-controlled laboratory water bath to (right) lens wear (35°C).

1. Group I – low water content non-ionic
2. Group II – high water content non-ionic
3. Group III – low water content ionic
4. Group IV – high water content ionic.

The division between low and high water content is set at 50%, and an ionic hydrogel is defined as one containing more that 0.2% ionic material. Although the classification was designed many years ago to deal with differences in solution sensitivity, it remains a useful method for the broad segregation of materials, particularly those in Groups II and IV.

One or two types of classification anomaly do exist, however. The first arises in high water content polymers with levels of methacrylic acid only marginally above 0.2%, such as perfilcon. Although placed in Group IV, they do not behave like typical

Group IV materials such as etafilcon and vifilcon. The principal difference is found in the way that they interact with **tear** components. The second type of anomaly lies in the fact that, some years ago, the same USAN name appears to have been given to two or more different ratios of the same ingredients, and as a result the same USAN name is given to materials of different water content that appear in more than one FDA Group (e.g. bufilcon and phemfilcon). *See* refractometer, soft lens.

wearing schedule

In the past, all patients fitted with lenses for the first time were advised to adopt a wearing schedule, which means progressively increasing lens wearing time over the first few days or weeks of wear. Such advice was also given when lenses were worn following a period of prolonged cessation of lens wear. The said purpose of advising adherence to a wearing schedule was to allow patients to 'adapt' to lenses. Failure to adapt to early generation, low oxygen performance **PMMA** and thick **soft lenses** (by exceeding the adaptation wearing schedule) resulted in worsening discomfort and red and watery eyes towards the end of the wearing period. The physiological basis of this adaptation process remains unclear, but appears to be related to the effects of prolonged **hypoxia**. Guidelines relating to wearing schedules for soft and **rigid lenses** are as follows:

1. *Soft lenses.* Soft contact lens wearers used to be advised to wear their lenses for no more than 4 hours on the first day, and to increase the wearing time by no more than 2 hours each day over subsequent wearing days up to a maximum of 12 hours wear per day. New modalities and improvements in soft lens materials and design have now largely rendered this approach redundant. Some gradual adaptation may be advised if the patient is being prescribed lenses of relatively low oxygen performance (e.g. very high-powered lenses). Inevitably, the more frequently lenses are worn, the greater the level of adaptation. Patients should be warned not to over-wear daily-wear soft contact lenses in spite of how comfortable they may feel. The introduction of 1-day disposable soft lenses in the mid-1990s has meant that a number of patients wear their lenses on a part-time basis; however, adaptation is not required when wearing such lenses.

2. *Rigid lenses.* These lenses generally require some adaptation. Topical anaesthetics have been advocated by some practitioners, to alleviate **discomfort** during the fitting appointment and the dispensing visit. Nominally, patients are instructed to wear lenses on the first day for about 2 hours, building up by an extra 2 hours per day. Some practitioners accelerate this process by advising patients to wear lenses in the morning, followed by a break during the afternoon, and then to recommence wear in the evening. The adaptation process is patient-dependent, and the level of comfort can act as a guide. For a variety of reasons, it sometimes takes a few days for the surface of rigid lenses to attain an optimal level of wettability and comfort. First, some hydrophobic polishing compounds may not have been completely removed from the lens surface prior to delivery (although thorough lens cleaning prior to dispensing the lens to the patient can alleviate such problems). Secondly, until becoming coated with the natural constituents of the tears, rigid lenses may remain slightly hydrophobic on the first day of wear, especially if they have been delivered in a dry state. Storing 'dry-supplied' rigid lenses in solution for about 24 hours prior to dispensing will minimize this effect.

wetting solutions, rigid lens

In addition to their role in lens disinfection, most **rigid lens** 'storage' solutions also act to 'wet' or 'condition' the lens. This role is principally to act as a lubricant, affording a degree of protection to the **cornea** and lid margins when the lens is inserted. The cushioning effect minimizes **discomfort** at insertion. The secondary effects of successful lens wetting are that the lens surface is rendered hydrophilic to aid a stable pre-lens tear film, and is made more 'biocompatible', which might reduce protein deposition.

Various agents are incorporated into rigid lens solutions to aid surface conditioning. Polyvinyl alcohol is a positively charged polymer that is attracted to the negatively charged surface of lenses containing methacrylic acid to provide more wettable lenses. Another agent used to increase wettability is the viscosity agent hydroxyethylcellulose. In addition to preservatives and conditioning/wetting agents, rigid lens care solutions also contain buffering agents to maintain a stable pH, and chelating agents to increase antimicrobial action and assist in lens cleaning.

Wichterle, Otto

Initial attempts during the 1950s by Otto Wichterle (Figure W.2) to produce **soft lenses** from **hydroxyethyl methacrylate** (HEMA), and manufacture them using **cast moulding**, met with limited success. Unable to attract support from the Institute of

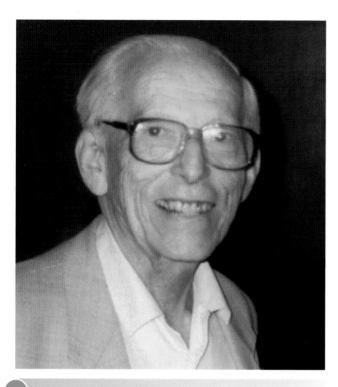

Figure W.2 Otto Wichterle.

Macromolecular Research in Czechoslovakia (now The Czech Republic), where he worked, and indeed discouraged by his superiors, Wichterle was forced to conduct further secret experiments in his own home. Working with his son's mechanical construction kit, Wichterle developed the **spin-casting** technique and eventually managed to persuade his peers to conduct further trials at the Institute. He claims to have produced 'the first suitable contact lenses' in late 1961, which presumably approximates to the first occasion when a soft lens was actually worn on a human eye. The patent to develop soft contact lenses commercially was subsequently acquired by **Bausch & Lomb** in the USA, who introduced soft lenses into the world market in 1972.

Wilhelmy plate measurement

This method of measuring contact lens **surface wettability** is also known as dynamic contact angle analysis (see Figure C.1). During the Wilhelmy plate technique, the sample is held in a microbalance and immersed into a liquid by means of a moveable platform. The angle that the meniscus of the immersion fluid makes with the test sample as it is lowered into the immersion fluid (the 'advancing angle'), and the angle that the meniscus of the immersion fluid makes with the test sample as it is removed from the immersion fluid (the 'receding angle'), is calculated from force measurements obtained during sequential immersion cycles. The difference between the advancing and receding angles is known as hysteresis, and this provides a measure of surface characterization.

wing cells of the epithelium
See corneal epithelium.

wrinkling
Corneal wrinkling is a rare but severe ocular complication of contact lens wear, characterized by the appearance of a series of deep parallel grooves, giving the impression of a 'wrinkled' **cornea**. In white light, the ridges of the wrinkles can be seen as bright reflexes (Figure W.3). These take the form of linear wave patterns of **fluorescein** pooling across the cornea and intersecting at different angles. Several discrete spots of fluorescence may be observed at the points of intersection of the two wave patterns.

This condition is observed in patients wearing **steeply fitted**, highly elastic, ultra-thin, middle **water content** lenses; such lenses are typically custom made and are not standard commercial products. Excessive elastic forces are thought to draw corneal tissue inwards from the limbus, causing the cornea essentially to 'collapse' in a concertina-like fashion, creating a wrinkled appearance. These forces could be derived from intrinsic elastic energy created when a relatively steep lens is compressed against the eye and then attempts to return to its original shape. Corneal wrinkling may also have an osmotic aetiology in view of the observation that complete evaporation of the **tear film** in normal

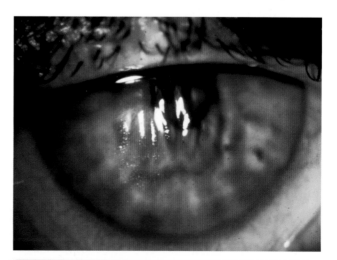

Figure W.3 Wrinkling of the corneal epithelium caused by an experimental soft lens of high elasticity (the lens is in the eye).

humans can cause an almost identical corneal wrinkling and vision loss to lens-induced wrinkling.

As would be expected with such a dramatic distortion of the corneal surface, vision drops to less than 6/60 within 5 minutes of lens insertion. The condition is also extremely painful. Clinical evaluation of corneal wrinkling is best achieved by **slit-lamp** examination under white light, and with fluorescein under cobalt blue light. Computerized **videokeratoscopy** can provide useful supplementary information by viewing both the unprocessed image of the reflected mires and the processed, colour-coded surface map.

Corneal wrinkling probably involves the epithelium and anterior stroma. This view is based upon observations of the extreme variance in intensity of fluorescence across the ridges of a wrinkled cornea, implying deep furrows, and the extreme distortion of photokeratometric mires. The intensity of the wrinkling pattern increases with time following a blink, indicating fluorescein pooling within deep troughs.

The treatment protocol for a patient experiencing corneal wrinkling is to cease lens wear immediately. Although the appearance of wrinkling will indeed have disappeared within 24 hours, the patient should not wear any lenses for 1 week as a precaution so as to allow possible sub-clinical compromise to resolve. The patient should then be refitted with a **soft lens** that is devoid of inherently high elastic forces. Alternatively, **rigid lenses** can be fitted because corneal wrinkling does not occur with such lenses. The time course of recovery of corneal wrinkling is directly related to the period of lens wear that induced the changes, whereby more intense wrinkling takes longer to recover.

Wolfring gland
See accessory lacrimal glands.

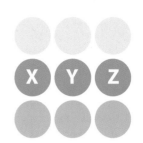

X-Chrom lens

A **rigid lens** with a red tint, designed to be worn in the non-dominant eye, with a clear lens in the contralateral eye. It has been claimed that wearing this lens combination improves colour perception in red–green colour-deficient patients. The lens transmits light above 570 nm. The true effect is probably the creation of inter-ocular colour rivalry, which serves to alter the colour world and shifts the axes of colour discrimination. *See* ChromaGen lenses.

Y

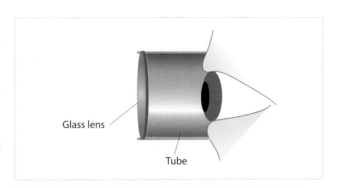

Glass lens

Tube

Figure Y.1 Eyecup design of Thomas Young.

young patients

See paediatric contact lens fitting.

Young, Thomas

As part of a series of experiments concerning the mechanisms of accommodation, in 1801 Thomas Young constructed a device that was essentially a fluid-filled eyecup that fitted snugly into the orbital rim (Figure Y.1). A microscope eyepiece was fitted into the base of the eyecup, thus forming a similar system to that used by **Descartes**. Young's invention was somewhat more practical in that it could be held in place with a headband and blinking was possible; however, he did not intend this device to be used for the correction of refractive errors.

Z

Zeis gland

See gland of Zeis.

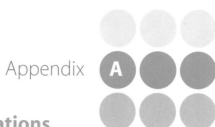

Efron grading scales for contact lens complications

The grading scales presented on the following two pages were devised by Professor Nathan Efron and painted by the ophthalmic artist, Terry R Tarrant.

These grading scales are designed to assist practitioners to quantify the level of severity of a variety of contact lens complications. The eight complications on the left hand page are those that are more likely to be encountered in contact lens practice. Many of these complications are graded routinely by some practitioners. The complications on the right-hand page are less commonly encountered in contact lens practice, and represent pathology that is rare or unusual.

The development of these grading scales was kindly sponsored by Biocompatibles–Hydron.

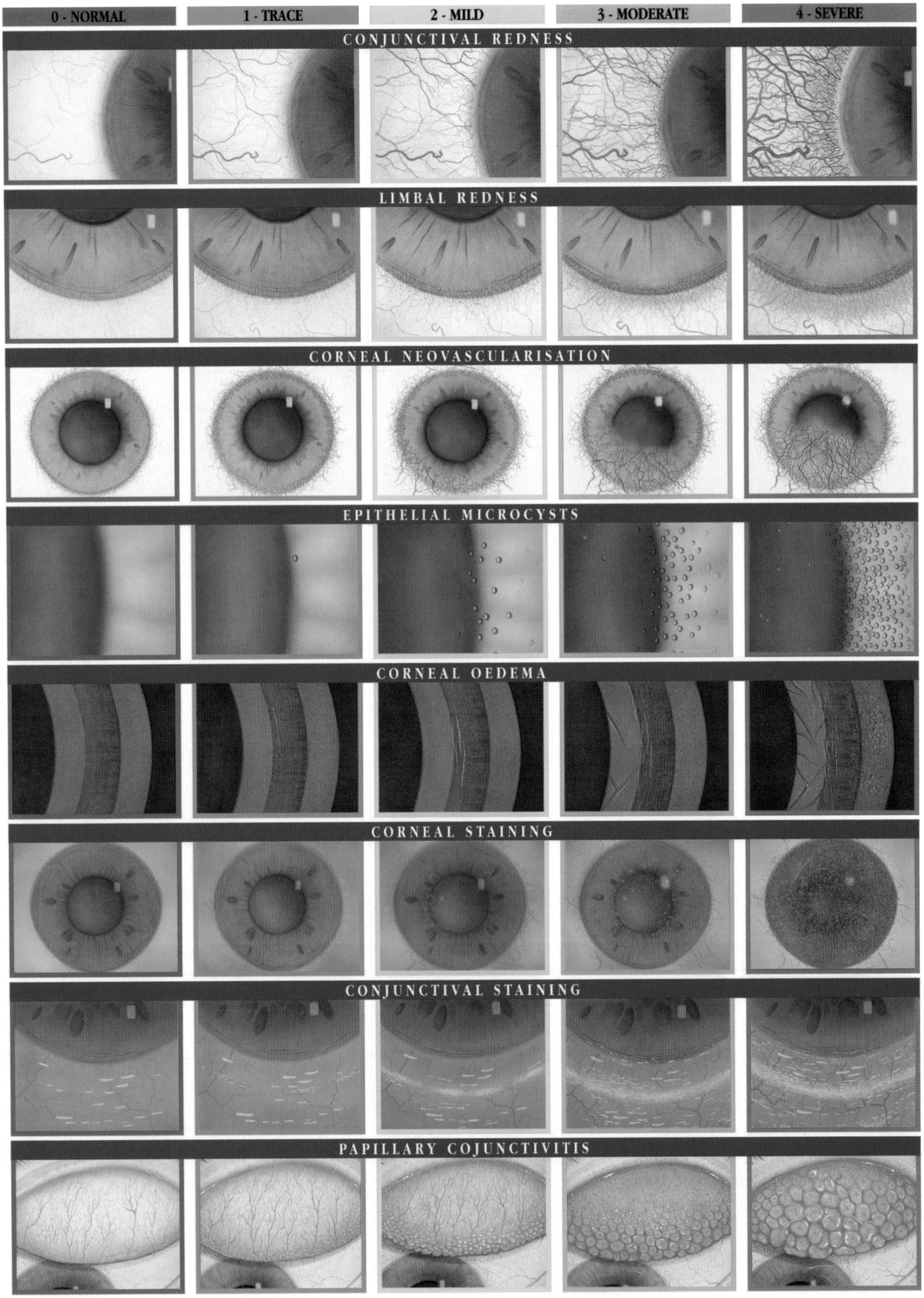

| | 0 - NORMAL | 1 - TRACE | 2 - MILD | 3 - MODERATE | 4 - SEVERE |

CONJUNCTIVAL REDNESS

LIMBAL REDNESS

CORNEAL NEOVASCULARISATION

EPITHELIAL MICROCYSTS

CORNEAL OEDEMA

CORNEAL STAINING

CONJUNCTIVAL STAINING

PAPILLARY COJUNCTIVITIS

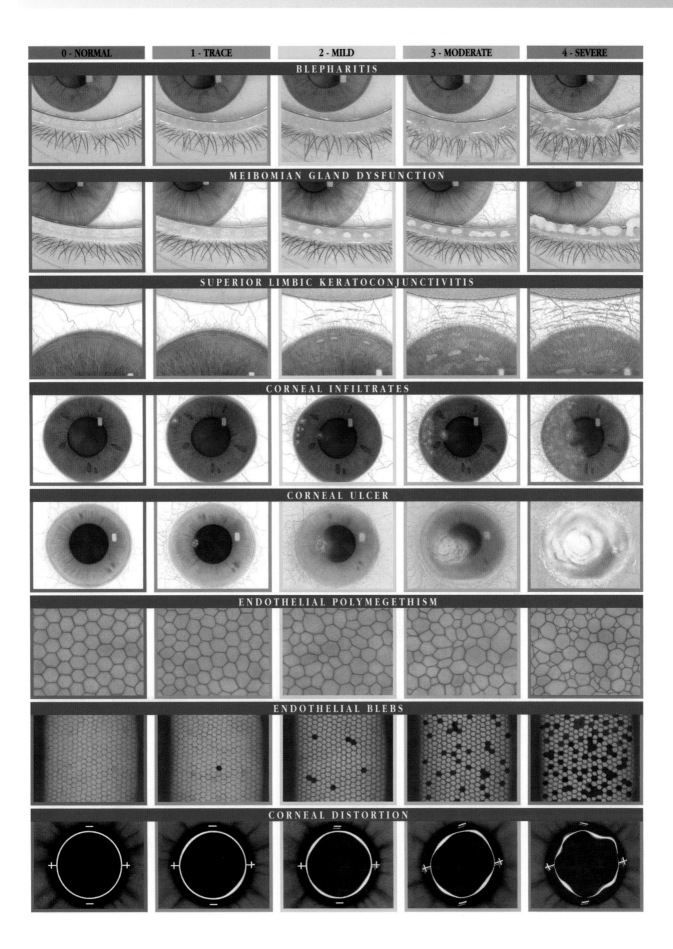

Vertex distance correction

Effective power (D) of plus- and minus-prescription spectacle lenses at the corneal plane for various vertex distances (mm)*. Courtesy of Adrian S. Bruce

Spec Rx (D)	Power (D) at Corneal Plane for Different Vertex Distances (mm)									
	8 mm		10 mm		12 mm		14 mm		16 mm	
	plus	minus	plus	minus	plus	minus	plus	minus	plus	minus
4.00	4.13	3.88	4.17	3.85	4.20	3.82	4.24	3.79	4.27	3.76
4.25	4.40	4.11	4.44	4.08	4.48	4.04	4.52	4.01	4.56	3.98
4.50	4.67	4.34	4.71	4.31	4.76	4.27	4.80	4.23	4.85	4.20
4.75	4.94	4.58	4.99	4.53	5.04	4.49	5.09	4.45	5.14	4.41
5.00	5.21	4.81	5.26	4.76	5.32	4.72	5.38	4.67	5.43	4.63
5.25	5.48	5.04	5.54	4.99	5.60	4.94	5.67	4.89	5.73	4.84
5.50	5.75	5.27	5.82	5.21	5.89	5.16	5.96	5.11	6.03	5.06
5.75	6.03	5.50	6.10	5.44	6.18	5.38	6.25	5.32	6.33	5.27
6.00	6.30	5.73	6.38	5.66	6.47	5.60	6.55	5.54	6.64	5.47
6.25	6.58	5.95	6.67	5.88	6.76	5.81	6.85	5.75	6.94	5.68
6.50	6.86	6.18	6.95	6.10	7.05	6.03	7.15	5.96	7.25	5.89
6.75	7.14	6.40	7.24	6.32	7.34	6.24	7.45	6.17	7.57	6.09
7.00	7.42	6.63	7.53	6.54	7.64	6.46	7.76	6.38	7.88	6.29
7.25	7.70	6.85	7.82	6.76	7.94	6.67	8.07	6.58	8.20	6.50
7.50	7.98	7.08	8.11	6.98	8.24	6.88	8.38	6.79	8.52	6.70
7.75	8.26	7.30	8.40	7.19	8.54	7.09	8.69	6.99	8.85	6.90
8.00	8.55	7.52	8.70	7.41	8.85	7.30	9.01	7.19	9.17	7.09
8.25	8.83	7.74	8.99	7.62	9.16	7.51	9.33	7.40	9.50	7.29
8.50	9.12	7.96	9.29	7.83	9.47	7.71	9.65	7.60	9.84	7.48
8.75	9.41	8.18	9.59	8.05	9.78	7.92	9.97	7.80	10.17	7.68
9.00	9.70	8.40	9.89	8.26	10.09	8.12	10.30	7.99	10.51	7.87
9.25	9.99	8.61	10.19	8.47	10.40	8.33	10.63	8.19	10.86	8.06
9.50	10.28	8.83	10.50	8.68	10.72	8.53	10.96	8.38	11.20	8.25
9.75	10.57	9.04	10.80	8.88	11.04	8.73	11.29	8.58	11.55	8.43
10.00	10.87	9.26	11.11	9.09	11.36	8.93	11.63	8.77	11.90	8.62
10.25	11.17	9.47	11.42	9.30	11.69	9.13	11.97	8.96	12.26	8.81
10.50	11.46	9.69	11.73	9.50	12.01	9.33	12.31	9.15	12.62	8.99
10.75	11.76	9.90	12.04	9.71	12.34	9.52	12.65	9.34	12.98	9.17
11.00	12.06	10.11	12.36	9.91	12.67	9.72	13.00	9.53	13.35	9.35
11.25	12.36	10.32	12.68	10.11	13.01	9.91	13.35	9.72	13.72	9.53
11.50	12.67	10.53	12.99	10.31	13.34	10.11	13.71	9.91	14.09	9.71
11.75	12.97	10.74	13.31	10.51	13.68	10.30	14.06	10.09	14.47	9.89
12.00	13.27	10.95	13.64	10.71	14.02	10.49	14.42	10.27	14.85	10.07

Effective power (D) of plus- and minus-prescription spectacle lenses at the corneal plane for various vertex distances (mm)*.
Courtesy of Adrian S Bruce – *continued*

Spec Rx (D)	Power (D) at Corneal Plane for Different Vertex Distances (mm)									
	8 mm		10 mm		12 mm		14 mm		16 mm	
	plus	minus	plus	minus	plus	minus	plus	minus	plus	minus
12.25	13.58	11.16	13.96	10.91	14.36	10.68	14.79	10.46	15.24	10.24
12.50	13.89	11.36	14.29	11.11	14.71	10.87	15.15	10.64	15.63	10.42
12.75	14.20	11.57	14.61	11.31	15.05	11.06	15.52	10.82	16.02	10.59
13.00	14.51	11.78	14.94	11.50	15.40	11.25	15.89	11.00	16.41	10.76
13.25	14.82	11.98	15.27	11.70	15.76	11.43	16.27	11.18	16.81	10.93
13.50	15.13	12.18	15.61	11.89	16.11	11.62	16.65	11.35	17.22	11.10
13.75	15.45	12.39	15.94	12.09	16.47	11.80	17.03	11.53	17.63	11.27
14.00	15.77	12.59	16.28	12.28	16.83	11.99	17.41	11.71	18.04	11.44
14.25	16.08	12.79	16.62	12.47	17.19	12.17	17.80	11.88	18.46	11.60
14.50	16.40	12.99	16.96	12.66	17.55	12.35	18.19	12.05	18.88	11.77
14.75	16.72	13.19	17.30	12.85	17.92	12.53	18.59	12.23	19.31	11.93
15.00	17.05	13.39	17.65	13.04	18.29	12.71	18.99	12.40	19.74	12.10
15.25	17.37	13.59	17.99	13.23	18.67	12.89	19.39	12.57	20.17	12.26
15.50	17.69	13.79	18.34	13.42	19.04	13.07	19.80	12.74	20.61	12.42
15.75	18.02	13.99	18.69	13.61	19.42	13.25	20.21	12.90	21.06	12.58
16.00	18.35	14.18	19.05	13.79	19.80	13.42	20.62	13.07	21.51	12.74
16.25	18.68	14.38	19.40	13.98	20.19	13.60	21.04	13.24	21.96	12.90
16.50	19.01	14.58	19.76	14.16	20.57	13.77	21.46	13.40	22.42	13.05
16.75	19.34	14.77	20.12	14.35	20.96	13.95	21.88	13.57	22.88	13.21
17.00	19.68	14.96	20.48	14.53	21.36	14.12	22.31	13.73	23.35	13.36
17.25	20.01	15.16	20.85	14.71	21.75	14.29	22.74	13.89	23.83	13.52
17.50	20.35	15.35	21.21	14.89	22.15	14.46	23.18	14.06	24.31	13.67
17.75	20.69	15.54	21.58	15.07	22.55	14.63	23.62	14.22	24.79	13.82
18.00	21.03	15.73	21.95	15.25	22.96	14.80	24.06	14.38	25.28	13.98
18.25	21.37	15.92	22.32	15.43	23.37	14.97	24.51	14.54	25.78	14.13
18.50	21.71	16.11	22.70	15.61	23.78	15.14	24.97	14.69	26.28	14.27
18.75	22.06	16.30	23.08	15.79	24.19	15.31	25.42	14.85	26.79	14.42
19.00	22.41	16.49	23.46	15.97	24.61	15.47	25.89	15.01	27.30	14.57
19.25	22.75	16.68	23.84	16.14	25.03	15.64	26.35	15.16	27.82	14.72
19.50	23.10	16.87	24.22	16.32	25.46	15.80	26.82	15.32	28.34	14.86
19.75	23.46	17.06	24.61	16.49	25.88	15.97	27.30	15.47	28.87	15.01
20.00	23.81	17.24	25.00	16.67	26.32	16.13	27.78	15.63	29.41	15.15

* Based on the equation: $OR = SR/(1 - [d \times SR])$, where

   OR = ocular refraction

   SR = spectacle refraction

   d = vertex distance (m)

● The lens powers enclosed within the heavy border relate to the standard vertex distance of 12 mm that will apply in most cases.

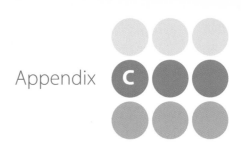

Extended keratometer range conversion

Conversion of keratometer reading (D) to its extended value (D) when a +1.25 D lens (for steep corneas) or a −1.00 D lens (for flat corneas) is held in front of the keratometer*. Courtesy of Adrian S. Bruce.

Steep Corneas (using a +1.25 D lens)[a]					
Keratometer Reading (D)	Extended Value (D)	Keratometer Reading (D)	Extended Value (D)	Keratometer Reading (D)	Extended Value (D)
43.00	50.13	46.13	53.78	49.25	57.42
43.13	50.28	46.25	53.92	49.38	57.57
43.25	50.42	46.38	54.07	49.50	57.71
43.38	50.57	46.50	54.21	49.63	57.86
43.50	50.72	46.63	54.36	49.75	58.00
43.63	50.86	46.75	54.51	49.88	58.15
43.75	51.01	46.88	54.65	50.00	58.30
43.88	51.15	47.00	54.80	50.13	58.44
44.00	51.30	47.13	54.94	50.25	58.59
44.13	51.44	47.25	55.09	50.38	58.73
44.25	51.59	47.38	55.23	50.50	58.88
44.38	51.74	47.50	55.38	50.63	59.02
44.50	51.88	47.63	55.53	50.75	59.17
44.63	52.03	47.75	55.67	50.88	59.32
44.75	52.17	47.88	55.82	51.00	59.46
44.88	52.32	48.00	55.96	51.13	59.61
45.00	52.47	48.13	56.11	51.25	59.75
45.13	52.61	48.25	56.25	51.38	59.90
45.25	52.76	48.38	56.40	51.50	60.04
45.38	52.90	48.50	56.55	51.63	60.19
45.50	53.05	48.63	56.69	51.75	60.34
45.63	53.19	48.75	56.84	51.88	60.48
45.75	53.34	48.88	56.98	52.00	60.63
45.88	53.49	49.00	57.13		
46.00	53.63	49.13	57.27		

[a] Based on the equation: Extended = (1.166 × Keratometer) − 0.005

Flat Corneas (using a –1.00 D lens)[b]

Keratometer Reading (D)	Extended Value (D)	Keratometer Reading (D)	Extended Value (D)	Keratometer Reading (D)	Extended Value (D)
36.00	30.87	38.12	32.70	40.25	34.52
36.12	30.98	38.25	32.80	40.37	34.63
36.25	31.09	38.37	32.91	40.50	34.73
36.37	31.19	38.50	33.02	40.62	34.84
36.50	31.30	38.62	33.12	40.75	34.95
36.62	31.41	38.75	33.23	40.87	35.06
36.75	31.52	38.87	33.34	41.00	35.16
36.87	31.62	39.00	33.45	41.12	35.27
37.00	31.73	39.12	33.55	41.25	35.38
37.12	31.84	39.25	33.66	41.37	35.48
37.25	31.94	39.37	33.77	41.50	35.59
37.37	32.05	39.50	33.88	41.62	35.70
37.50	32.16	39.62	33.98	41.75	35.81
37.62	32.27	39.75	34.09	41.87	35.91
37.75	32.37	39.87	34.20	42.00	36.02
37.87	32.48	40.00	34.30		
38.00	32.59	40.12	34.41		

[b] Based on the equation: Extended = (1.858 × Keratometer) −0.014

* Derived from data in: Mandell, R.B. (1988) Dioptral and mm curves for extended keratometer range. Appendix 7. In *Contact Lens Practice* 4th ed. pp. 998–999. Charles C. Thomas.

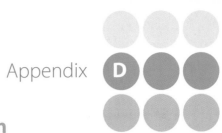

Appendix **D**

Corneal curvature – corneal power conversion

Conversion between corneal front surface radius of curvature (r; mm) and corneal power (K; D)*. Courtesy of Adrian S. Bruce

r (mm)	K (D)	r (mm)	K (D)	r (mm)	K (D)	r (mm)	K (D)	r (mm)	K (D)
6.30	53.57	6.99	48.28	7.63	44.23	8.27	40.81	8.91	37.88
6.36	53.07	7.00	48.21	7.64	44.18	8.28	40.76	8.92	37.84
6.37	52.98	7.01	48.15	7.65	44.12	8.29	40.71	8.93	37.79
6.38	52.90	7.02	48.08	7.66	44.06	8.30	40.66	8.94	37.75
6.39	52.82	7.03	48.01	7.67	44.00	8.31	40.61	8.95	37.71
6.40	52.73	7.04	47.94	7.68	43.95	8.32	40.56	8.96	37.67
6.41	52.65	7.05	47.87	7.69	43.89	8.33	40.52	8.97	37.63
6.42	52.57	7.06	47.80	7.70	43.83	8.34	40.47	8.98	37.58
6.43	52.49	7.07	47.74	7.71	43.77	8.35	40.42	8.99	37.54
6.44	52.41	7.08	47.67	7.72	43.72	8.36	40.37	9.00	37.50
6.45	52.33	7.09	47.60	7.73	43.66	8.37	40.32	9.01	37.46
6.46	52.24	7.10	47.54	7.74	43.60	8.38	40.27	9.02	37.42
6.47	52.16	7.11	47.47	7.75	43.55	8.39	40.23	9.03	37.38
6.48	52.08	7.12	47.40	7.76	43.49	8.40	40.18	9.04	37.33
6.49	52.00	7.13	47.34	7.77	43.44	8.41	40.13	9.05	37.29
6.50	51.92	7.14	47.27	7.78	43.38	8.42	40.08	9.06	37.25
6.51	51.84	7.15	47.20	7.79	43.32	8.43	40.04	9.07	37.21
6.52	51.76	7.16	47.14	7.80	43.27	8.44	39.99	9.08	37.17
6.53	51.68	7.17	47.07	7.81	43.21	8.45	39.94	9.09	37.13
6.54	51.61	7.18	47.01	7.82	43.16	8.46	39.89	9.10	37.09
6.55	51.53	7.19	46.94	7.83	43.10	8.47	39.85	9.11	37.05
6.56	51.45	7.20	46.88	7.84	43.05	8.48	39.80	9.12	37.01
6.57	51.37	7.21	46.81	7.85	42.99	8.49	39.75	9.13	36.97
6.58	51.29	7.22	46.75	7.86	42.94	8.50	39.71	9.14	36.93
6.59	51.21	7.23	46.68	7.87	42.88	8.51	39.66	9.15	36.89
6.60	51.14	7.24	46.62	7.88	42.83	8.52	39.61	9.16	36.84
6.61	51.06	7.25	46.55	7.89	42.78	8.53	39.57	9.17	36.80
6.62	50.98	7.26	46.49	7.90	42.72	8.54	39.52	9.18	36.76
6.63	50.90	7.27	46.42	7.91	42.67	8.55	39.47	9.19	36.72
6.64	50.83	7.28	46.36	7.92	42.61	8.56	39.43	9.20	36.68
6.65	50.75	7.29	46.30	7.93	42.56	8.57	39.38	9.21	36.64
6.66	50.68	7.30	46.23	7.94	42.51	8.58	39.34	9.22	36.61
6.67	50.60	7.31	46.17	7.95	42.45	8.59	39.29	9.23	36.57
6.68	50.52	7.32	46.11	7.96	42.40	8.60	39.24	9.24	36.53
6.69	50.45	7.33	46.04	7.97	42.35	8.61	39.20	9.25	36.49
6.70	50.37	7.34	45.98	7.98	42.29	8.62	39.15	9.26	36.45

Conversion between corneal front surface radius of curvature (r; mm) and corneal power (K; D)*. Courtesy of Adrian S. Bruce – *continued*

r (mm)	K (D)	r (mm)	K (D)	r (mm)	K (D)	r (mm)	K (D)	r (mm)	K (D)
6.71	50.30	7.35	45.92	7.99	42.24	8.63	39.11	9.27	36.41
6.72	50.22	7.36	45.86	8.00	42.19	8.64	39.06	9.28	36.37
6.73	50.15	7.37	45.79	8.01	42.13	8.65	39.02	9.29	36.33
6.74	50.07	7.38	45.73	8.02	42.08	8.66	38.97	9.30	36.29
6.75	50.00	7.39	45.67	8.03	42.03	8.67	38.93	9.31	36.25
6.76	49.93	7.40	45.61	8.04	41.98	8.68	38.88	9.32	36.21
6.77	49.85	7.41	45.55	8.05	41.93	8.69	38.84	9.33	36.17
6.78	49.78	7.42	45.49	8.06	41.87	8.70	38.79	9.34	36.13
6.79	49.71	7.43	45.42	8.07	41.82	8.71	38.75	9.35	36.10
6.80	49.63	7.44	45.36	8.08	41.77	8.72	38.70	9.36	36.06
6.81	49.56	7.45	45.30	8.09	41.72	8.73	38.66	9.37	36.02
6.82	49.49	7.46	45.24	8.10	41.67	8.74	38.62	9.38	35.98
6.83	49.41	7.47	45.18	8.11	41.62	8.75	38.57	9.39	35.94
6.84	49.34	7.48	45.12	8.12	41.56	8.76	38.53	9.40	35.90
6.85	49.27	7.49	45.06	8.13	41.51	8.77	38.48	9.41	35.87
6.86	49.20	7.50	45.00	8.14	41.46	8.78	38.44	9.42	35.83
6.87	49.13	7.51	44.94	8.15	41.41	8.79	38.40	9.43	35.79
6.88	49.06	7.52	44.88	8.16	41.36	8.80	38.35	9.44	35.75
6.89	48.98	7.53	44.82	8.17	41.31	8.81	38.31	9.45	35.71
6.90	48.91	7.54	44.76	8.18	41.26	8.82	38.27	9.46	35.68
6.91	48.84	7.55	44.70	8.19	41.21	8.83	38.22	9.47	35.64
6.92	48.77	7.56	44.64	8.20	41.16	8.84	38.18	9.48	35.60
6.93	48.70	7.57	44.58	8.21	41.11	8.85	38.14	9.49	35.56
6.94	48.63	7.58	44.53	8.22	41.06	8.86	38.09	9.50	35.53
6.95	48.56	7.59	44.47	8.23	41.01	8.87	38.05	9.51	35.49
6.96	48.49	7.60	44.41	8.24	40.96	8.88	38.01	9.52	35.45
6.97	48.42	7.61	44.35	8.25	40.91	8.89	37.96	9.53	35.41
6.98	48.35	7.62	44.29	8.26	40.86	8.90	37.92	9.54	35.38

* Based on the equation: Surface power (D) = (1.3375 − 1.0)/radius (m)

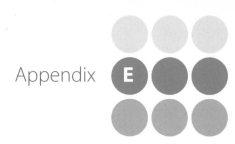
Contact lens manufacturing tolerances

Table A Dimensional tolerances for soft, PMMA and rigid lenses (all units in mm)

Dimension	Soft Lenses	PMMA Lenses	Rigid Lenses
Back optic zone radius	±0.20	±0.025	±0.05
Back optic zone radii of toroidal surfaces where the difference in radii is:			
<0.20		±0.25	±0.05
0.2–0.4		±0.35	±0.06
0.4–0.6		±0.55	±0.07
>0.6		±0.75	±0.09
Sagitta at specified diameter	±0.05		
Back optic zone diameter	±0.20	±0.025	±0.05
Back peripheral radius		±0.10	±0.10
Front peripheral radius		±0.10	±0.10
Back peripheral diameter		±0.20	±0.20
Total diameter	±0.20	±0.10	±0.10
Front optic zone diameter	±0.20	±0.20	±0.20
Bifocal segment height		−0.10 to +0.20	−0.10 to +0.20
Centre thickness		±0.02	±0.02
Centre thickness, where the nominal value is:			
≤0.10	±0.010 + 10%		
>0.10	±0.015 + 5%		

Table B Optical tolerances for soft, PMMA and rigid lenses

Dimension	Soft Lenses	PMMA Lenses	Rigid Lenses
Back vertex power			
≤5D		±0.12D	±0.12D
≤10D	±0.25D	±0.18D	±0.18D
≤15D		±0.25D	±0.25D
≤20D	±0.50D	±0.37D	±0.37D
>20D	±1.00D	±0.50D	±0.50D
Cylinder power			
≤2D	±0.25D	±0.25D	±0.25D
2–4D	±0.37D	±0.37D	±0.37D
>4D	±0.50D	±0.50D	±0.50D
Cylinder axis	±5°	±5°	±5°
Prismatic error			
(measured at the geometric			
centre of the optic zone)			
Back vertex power ≤6D		±0.25cm/m	±0.25cm/m
Back vertex power >6D		±0.50cm/m	±0.50cm/m
Prescribed prism		±0.25cm/m	±0.25cm/m

Table C Material property tolerances for soft lenses

Material Property	Tolerance
Refractive index	±0.005
Water content	±2%
Oxygen permeability	±20%

- The tolerances outlined in this appendix were obtained from the following standards:
  ISO 8321–1:1991 Optics and optical instruments – Contact Lenses – Part 1: Specification for rigid corneal and scleral contact lenses.
  BS EN ISO 8321–2: 2000 (BS 7208–24:2000) Ophthalmic optics – Specifications for material, optical and dimensional properties of contact lenses – Part 2: Single-vision hydrogel contact lenses.
- PMMA tolerances are given here because trial lens fitting sets are often fabricated from this material due to its resilience.
- See also: Hough, T. (2000) *A Guide to Contact Lens Standards*. British Contact Lens Association.

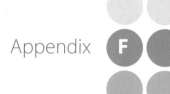

Terms, symbols and abbreviations

Terms, symbols and abbreviations used to describe contact lenses

Term	Symbol	Abbreviation
Back optic zone radius	r_0	BOZR
Back peripheral radius	$r_1, r_2, \ldots$	BPR1, BPR2, …
Front optic zone radius	r_{a0}	FOZR
Front peripheral radius	$r_{a1}, r_{a2}, \ldots$	FPR1, FPR2, …
Back optic zone diameter	$\varnothing_0$	BOZD
Back peripheral zone diameters	$\varnothing_1, \varnothing_2, \ldots$	BPZD1, BPZD2, …
Total diameter	$\varnothing_T$	TD
Front optic zone diameter	$\varnothing_{a0}$	FOZD
Front peripheral zone diameters	$\varnothing_{a1}, \varnothing_{a2}, \ldots$	FPZD1, FPZD2, …
Geometric centre thickness	t_c	tc
Carrier junction thickness	t_{a0}	tj
Peripheral junction thickness	$t_{a1}, t_{a2}, \ldots$	ta1, ta2, …
Radial edge thickness	t_e	RET
Axial edge thickness	t_{ak}	AET
Radial edge lift	l_r	REL
Axial edge lift	l_a	AEL
Front vertex power	F_v	FVP
Back vertex power	F'_v	BVP
Oxygen flux	j	j
Oxygen permeability	Dk	Dk
Oxygen transmissibility	Dk/t	Dk/t

- The terms and symbols outlined above were obtained from the following standard:
  ISO8320–1986 Optics and optical instruments – Contact Lenses – Vocabulary and symbols.
- The abbreviations given above were modified from those suggested by:
  Hough, T. (2000) *A Guide to Contact Lens Standards*. British Contact Lens Association.